MEDICAL
INTELLIGENCE
UNIT

LOCAL
IMMUNOSUPPRESSION
OF ORGAN TRANSPLANTS

Scott A. Gruber, M.D., Ph.D.

Albany Medical College
Albany, New York, U.S.A.

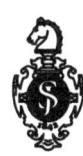

Springer-Verlag
Berlin Heidelberg GmbH

R.G. LANDES COMPANY
AUSTIN

MEDICAL INTELLIGENCE UNIT
LOCAL IMMUNOSUPPRESSION OF ORGAN TRANSPLANTS

R.G. LANDES COMPANY
Austin, Texas, U.S.A.

International Copyright © 1996 Springer-Verlag Berlin Heidelberg
Originally published by Springer-Verlag Heidelberg, Germany in 1996
Softcover reprint of the hardcover 1st edition 1996

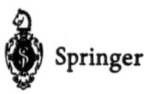 Springer

International ISBN 978-3-662-22107-5

While the authors, editors and publisher believe that drug selection and dosage and the specifications and usage of equipment and devices, as set forth in this book, are in accord with current recommendations and practice at the time of publication, they make no warranty, expressed or implied, with respect to material described in this book. In view of the ongoing research, equipment development, changes in governmental regulations and the rapid accumulation of information relating to the biomedical sciences, the reader is urged to carefully review and evaluate the information provided herein.

Library of Congress Cataloging-in-Publication Data

Gruber, Scott A., 1957-
Local immunosuppression of organ transplants / Scott A. Gruber.
p. cm. -- (Medical intelligence unit)
Includes bibliographical references and index.
ISBN 978-3-662-22107-5   ISBN 978-3-662-22105-1 (eBook)
DOI 10.1007/978-3-662-22105-1
1. Transplantation immunology. I. Title. II. Series.
[DNLM: 1. Organ Transplantation. 2. Immunosuppression. WO 680
G885L 1996]
QR188.8.G78   1996
617.9'5--dc20
DNLM/DLC   96-17732
for Library of Congress   CIP

Publisher's Note

R.G. Landes Company publishes six book series: *Medical Intelligence Unit, Molecular Biology Intelligence Unit, Neuroscience Intelligence Unit, Tissue Engineering Intelligence Unit, Biotechnology Intelligence Unit* and *Environmental Intelligence Unit.* The authors of our books are acknowledged leaders in their fields and the topics are unique. Almost without exception, no other similar books exist on these topics.

Our goal is to publish books in important and rapidly changing areas of bioscience and environment for sophisticated researchers and clinicians. To achieve this goal, we have accelerated our publishing program to conform to the fast pace in which information grows in bioscience. Most of our books are published within 90 to 120 days of receipt of the manuscript. We would like to thank our readers for their continuing interest and welcome any comments or suggestions they may have for future books.

Deborah Muir Molsberry
Publications Director
R.G. Landes Company

CONTENTS

EDITOR

Scott A. Gruber, M.D., Ph.D.
Albany Medical College
Albany, New York, U.S.A.
Chapters 1, 2, 3, 9

CONTRIBUTORS

Edward J. Alfrey, M.D.
Stanford University Medical Center
Stanford, California, U.S.A.
Chapter 8

Nancy L. Ascher, M.D., Ph.D.
University of California
San Francisco Medical Center
San Francisco, California, U.S.A.
Chapter 11

Kirby S. Black, Ph.D.
CryoLife, Inc.
Marietta, Georgia, U.S.A.
Chapter 14

Steven F. Bolling, M.D.
The University of Michigan
Ann Arbor, Michigan, U.S.A.
Chapter 16

Jonathan S. Bromberg, M.D., Ph.D.
University of Michigan
Ann Arbor, Michigan, U.S.A.
Chapter 17

Gilbert J. Burckart, Pharm.D.
University of Pittsburgh
   Medical Center
Pittsburgh, Pennsylvania, U.S.A.
Chapter 13

A. Alfred Chahine, M.D.
The Children's Hospital of Philadelphia
University of Pennsylvania School
   of Medicine
Philadelphia, Pennsylvania, U.S.A.
Chapter 18

Donald C. Dafoe, M.D.
Stanford University Medical Center
Stanford, California, U.S.A.
Chapter 8

Ali R. Djalilian, M.D.
University of Minnesota
Minneapolis, Minnesota, U.S.A.
Chapter 15

M. Wayne Flye, M.D., Ph.D.
Washington University School
   of Medicine
St. Louis, Missouri, U.S.A.
Chapter 6

Chris E. Freise, M.D.
University of California
San Francisco Medical Center
San Francisco, California, U.S.A.
Chapter 11

Bartley P. Griffith, M.D.
University of Pittsburgh Medical Center
Pittsburgh, Pennsylvania, U.S.A.
Chapter 13

Charles W. Hewitt, Ph.D.
Robert Wood Johnson Medical School
Camden, New Jersey, U.S.A
Chapter 14

Edward J. Holland, M.D.
University of Minnesota
Minneapolis, Minnesota, U.S.A.
Chapter 15

Stephen E. Hughes, Ph.D.
Albany Medical College
Albany, New York, U.S.A.
Chapters 1-3, 9

Aldo T. Iacono, M.D.
University of Pittsburgh
   Medical Center
Pittsburgh, Pennsylvania, U.S.A.
Chapter 13

Barry D. Kahan, Ph.D., M.D.
University of Texas Medical School
Houston, Texas, U.S.A.
Chapter 5

Robert Keenan, M.D.
University of Pittsburgh Medical Center
Pittsburgh, Pennsylvania, U.S.A.
Chapter 13

Saiho Ko, M.D.
Nara Medical University
Nara, Japan
Chapters 10, 12

Vinod Labhasetwar, Ph.D.
University of Michigan
Ann Arbor, Michigan, U.S.A.
Chapter 16

Henry T. Lau, M.D.
The Children's Hospital of Philadelphia
University of Pennsylvania School
   of Medicine
Philadelphia, Pennsylvania, U.S.A.
Chapter 18

Chol Joo Lee, M.D., Ph.D.
Kyoto First Red Cross Hospital
Kyoto City, Japan
Chapter 7

Robert J. Levy, M.D.
The University of Michigan
Ann Arbor, Michigan, U.S.A.
Chapter 16

Yoshiyuki Nakajima, M.D.
Nara Medical University
Nara, Japan
Chapters 10, 12

Hiroshige Nakano, M.D.
Nara Medical University
Nara, Japan
Chapters 10, 12

Takahiro Oka, M.D., Ph.D.
Kyoto Prefectural University
  of Medicine
Kyoto City, Japan
Chapter 7

Sardha Perera, M.D.
Albany Medical College
Albany, New York, U.S.A.
Chapters 2, 3

LiHui Qin, M.D., Ph.D.
University of Michigan
Ann Arbor, Michigan, U.S.A.
Chapter 17

John P. Roberts, M.D.
University of California
San Francisco Medical Center
San Francisco, California, U.S.A.
Chapter 11

T. J. M. Ruers, M.D., Ph.D.
University Hospital Maastricht
The Netherlands
Chapter 4

Helena P. Selawry, M.D., Ph.D.
University of Tennesee College
  of Medicine
Memphis, Tennesee, U.S.A.
Chapter 19

Stanislaw M. Stepkowski, Ph.D.
The University of Texas Medical School
Houston, Texas, U.S.A.
Chapter 5

Christian Stoeckert, Ph.D.
The Children's Hospital of Philadelphia
University of Pennsylvania School
  of Medicine
Philadelphia, Pennsylvania, U.S.A.
Chapter 18

Mou-er Wang, M.D.
The University of Texas Medical School
Houston, Texas, U.S.A.
Chapter 5

Shengguang Xiao, M.D.
Albany Medical College
Albany, New York, U.S.A.
Chapters 1, 9

Norio Yoshimura, M.D., Ph.D.
Kyoto Prefectural University of Medicine
Kyoto City, Japan
Chapter 7

Samuel Yu
Washington University School
  of Medicine
St. Louis, Missouri, U.S.A.
Chapter 6

Ming Yu, M.D.
The Children's Hospital of Philadelphia
University of Pennsylvania School
  of Medicine
Philadelphia, Pennsylvania, U.S.A.
Chapter 18

PREFACE

Although the results of organ transplantation have improved dramatically over the past decade, several long-term problems continue to exist with systemically-administered immunosuppressive agents, including late opportunistic infections, spontaneous neoplasms, metabolic alterations, and drug toxicities. One approach toward reducing the drug-specific and general adverse consequences of systemic immunosuppression in allograft recipients, and thereby improving the quality and duration of life following transplantation, is the utilization of local drug administration systems to establish a more selective presence of currently available immunosuppressive agents in the transplanted organ through the spatial and temporal control of drug delivery, with a concomitant reduction in systemic drug exposure.

This book brings together for first time in a single volume a complete review of the research done over the past 30 years by leading investigators around the world in targeting immunosuppressants to both solid-organ and cellular transplants. In the first section of the book, a background discussion of the local regulation of allograft rejection and the pharmacokinetic advantage of regional drug delivery, as well as a review of studies of local immunosuppression performed prior to 1984, are provided. The rest of the volume is devoted to research performed over the past decade, with the second section consisting of studies conducted in rat allograft models using osmotic minipumps for delivery of a variety of immunosuppressants.

My laboratory was the first to both validate the principles governing the pharmacokinetics of target-aimed drug delivery and to demonstrate the efficacy of local immunosuppressive therapy in a large-animal model, and these canine renal allograft studies using a programmable, implantable pump/catheter system are discussed in the third section of the book. The final section consists of a potpourri of studies utilizing a variety of drug-targeting systems for achieving local immunosuppression, including liposomes, aerosol inhalation, topical application, controlled-release drug matrices, gene transfer, and cellular cotransplantation.

SECTION A: BACKGROUND

CHAPTER 1

LOCAL REGULATION OF ALLOGRAFT REJECTION

Scott A. Gruber, Shengguang Xiao and Stephen E. Hughes

The rationale behind local immunosuppression is based on the following two hypotheses: first, that rejection can be effectively suppressed by controlling only those immunologic events occurring at the graft site and second, that by administering appropriately chosen immunosuppressive agents directly into the allograft, one can simultaneously prevent rejection and diminish or eliminate the drug-specific and general adverse consequences of systemic immunosuppression. The second hypothesis is addressed by the studies contained within the remaining sections of the book, which employ a variety of drug-targeting systems for achieving local immunosuppression. This chapter will review the available data in support of the first hypothesis by detailing the evidence for and the mechanisms of local regulation of allograft rejection.

When this subject was last discussed in detail as part of two overviews of local immunosuppressive therapy,[1,2] the immunobiology of the rejection response was arbitrarily divided into continuous, overlapping phases for the purpose of analysis, with an attempt to compartmentalize the response into 'peripheral' events occurring within the transplanted tissue and 'central' events occurring within the lymph nodes, blood and spleen. In this way, the potential role for local therapy could be assessed throughout both the afferent and efferent arcs of allograft immunity. New information obtained from intense research conducted over the past 5 years, particularly regarding dendritic cell (DC) function and migration, adhesion molecule expression and distribution, leukocyte-endothelial cell and leukocyte-extracellular matrix (ECM) interactions, chemoattractants, T helper cell 1 (Th1)/Th2 responses, graft cytokine expression and nitric oxide (NO) production, has further emphasized the role played by the local environment of the graft in setting the course for the inflammatory response of acute allograft rejection. The discussion which follows highlights the new data available for each phase of the rejection process against

Local Immunosuppression of Organ Transplants, edited by Scott A. Gruber.
© 1996 R.G. Landes Company.

a summarized background of previously-reviewed material, and the reader is referred to the above-mentioned overviews for further details and references.[1,2]

SENSITIZATION/ IMMUNOSTIMULATION

The results of early studies regarding the route of allograft sensitization gave rise to the notion that sensitization to skin grafts occurred 'centrally' in the regional lymph nodes,[3,4] while sensitization to immediately-vascularized grafts occurred 'peripherally' within the graft itself.[5-7] This notion was supported by the subsequent studies of von Willebrand, Häyry and colleagues,[8-10] in which the Helsinki group isolated and identified the infiltrating inflammatory cells from rejecting rat renal transplants by enzymatic dispersion and noted that the lymphocyte proliferative and blast responses occurred earlier and with greater magnitude in the graft than in the central lymphatic system of the host (lymph nodes, blood and spleen). Furthermore, specific killer cells were first demonstrated in the renal parenchyma, and peak cytotoxic activity in the spleen was seen only after activity in the transplant had declined.

In contrast, more recent studies by Larsen and colleagues[11-13] examining the migration patterns of murine DC suggest that sensitization of both neovascularized and immediately-vascularized allografts occurs 'centrally' via the migration of donor-derived DC from the graft to peripheral lymph nodes and spleen. Along these lines, Kripke et al[14] have shown that cells isolated from the draining lymph nodes of skin allografts painted with the contact sensitizer FITC were able to transfer major histocompatibility complex (MHC)-restricted FITC hypersensitivity, implying that the antigen presenting cells (APCs) within the nodes were of donor origin. Moreover, Codner et al[15] demonstrated migration of donor-derived MHC class I-positive leukocytes with DC morphology from rat hindlimb allografts into the T cell rich areas of local (but not distant) lymph nodes and spleen within the first 3 days posttransplant.

Although this work supports the 'centralization' concept of sensitization, the Oxford group has also demonstrated that the ability of DCs to undergo in situ functional maturation and attainment of full immunostimulatory and migrational capabilities is dependent upon the local production of cytokines within the iso- or allograft during the nonspecific inflammatory response to surgical implantation. More specifically, their work suggests that in nonlymphoid, solid organs such as heart and kidney, functionally immature Ia+ leukocytes are present which, following transplantation, locally develop into mature DC.[16,17] Granulocyte/macrophage colony-stimulating factor, and to a lesser extent, interferon-gamma (IFN-γ), appear to be important regulators of this maturation via up-regulation of the CTLA4 counter-receptor (increased levels of B7-1 and B7-2), and tumor necrosis factor-alpha (TNF-α) and interleukin-1 alpha (IL-1α) may promote DC migration from nonlymphoid tissues to central lymphoid depots.[18-20] These cytokines may be derived from cells of the donor tissue (fibroblasts, endothelial cells) and perhaps also from early graft-infiltrating lymphocytes and macrophages. Therefore, intragraft events appear to be important even in initiating proposed 'central' sensitization mechanisms, and could theoretically serve as a target for local immunosuppressive treatment. Indeed, Freise et al[21] demonstrated that instillation of methylprednisolone directly into the allogeneic sponge of mice receiving both allogeneic and syngeneic sponge matrix grafts prevented the animals from becoming systemically sensitized to the presented donor alloantigen, so that the animal rejected a subsequent donor-type or third-party skin graft with first set kinetics.

GRAFT ANTIGEN PRESENTATION/RECOGNITION

Sensitized, allospecific CD4+ and CD8+ T lymphoblasts that are released from the host lymphoid tissues require restimulation with antigen for further growth and release of lymphokines and cytolysins, respectively.[22] These cells are among those randomly arriving at the graft as a result of nonspecific inflammatory stimuli, and may adhere to and be restimulated by activated graft endothelium, which is capable of presenting antigen to T lymphocytes and is clearly an important initial target for the antiallograft immune response (see below). Recent work by Tullius et al[23] suggests that the first interaction between host cells and graft is guided by the immunogenicity of the foreign tissue itself via up-regulation of adhesion molecules rather than the state of allosensitization of infiltrating lymphocytes. The Boston group examined the in vitro binding patterns of specifically-sensitized, nonsensitized and third-party lymphocyte populations to renal allografts, isografts and kidneys from naive animals, as well as patterns of intercellular adhesion molecule-1 (ICAM-1) and lymphocyte function-associated antigen-1 (LFA-1) expression, in a rodent model of acute kidney allograft rejection. Lymphocyte source (peripheral blood versus lymph node) or state of sensitization (naive versus allosensitized) did not affect the binding process regardless of stage of acute rejection; adherence was dependent only upon whether the transplant was an allo- or isograft. However, the time course and magnitude of lymphocyte adherence to various allograft compartments (first vascular endothelium, then tubules) correlated well with that of the immunohistological expression of ICAM-1, and lymphocyte binding could be diminished by 40% in the presence of anti-ICAM-1 and anti-LFA-1 monoclonal antibodies (mAbs).

ATTACHMENT OF LEUKOCYTES TO GRAFT VASCULAR ENDOTHELIUM AND TRANSMIGRATION THROUGH THE VESSEL WALL

Adhesion to the vascular endothelium is a necessary prelude to leukocyte migration into the allograft. As part of the antigen-independent inflammatory response to organ transplantation resulting from harvest, storage, engraftment and ischemia/reperfusion injury, the expression of E (endothelial)- and P (platelet)-selectins on the surface of graft endothelial cells and L (leukocyte)-selectin on the surface of locally-circulating leukocytes is up-regulated. This permits intravascular leukocyte rolling via temporary, weak, reversible adhesions mediated by lectin/carbohydrate interactions, and selectively reduces the flow of leukocytes within the graft circulation. The probability that the host cells will recognize further inflammatory stimuli emanating from the graft parenchymal cells, such as the chemoattractants interleukin-8 (IL-8), macrophage inflammatory protein-1α (MIP-1α), MIP-1β and RANTES, is thereby increased.[24] These chemokines, as well as the cytokines IL-1, IL-6 and TNF-α derived from donor cells or nonspecifically recruited monocyte/macrophages, stimulate the enhanced expression and activation of T lymphocyte integrins and their counter-receptors on the endothelium (LFA-1/ICAM-1; very late antigen-4 (VLA-4)/vascular cell adhesion molecule-1 (VCAM-1); CD2/LFA-3), resulting in strong adhesion. This late phase of definitive or strong adhesion enables additional signaling to take place which may lead to full cytokine stimulation and graft endothelial antigen presentation to host T cells (CD8/MHC class I; CD4/MHC class II), with the integrins providing a costimulatory signal that is essential for T cell receptor (TCR)-mediated T cell activation. Finally, release of IFN-γ by antigen-stimulated T cells activates macrophages and may further increase lymphocyte LFA-1 and endothelial ICAM-1, VCAM-1 and class II expression, perpetuating the inflammatory response within the allograft to a level beyond that seen in isografts.

The variable infiltration of leukocyte populations during early ischemic injury as opposed to later phases of graft rejection appears to relate to the degree and time course of selected endothelial cell adhesion molecules expressed. For example, Pelletier, Morgan and colleagues[25,26] found that increased expression of IL-1, IL-6, TNF-α, TNF-β and transforming growth factor β were found together with increased endothelial ICAM-1 expression and MECA-32 mAb reactivity in both murine cardiac isografts and allografts on day 1, but only the allografts expressed IL-2, IFN-γ and VCAM-1 on day 3. Antagonists to TNF-α and IL-4 abrogated the endothelial expression of VCAM-1 and reduced interstitial leukocytic infiltration, but surprisingly did not alter the tempo of the rejection process.[27]

Following attachment to the endothelial lining, the invading lymphocytes must breach the basement membrane before reaching the tissue, and IL-1 and TNF-α, as well as IFN-γ, appear to alter protease/antiprotease balances, resulting in basement membrane protein degradation by endothelial cells.[28] In addition, direct endothelial injury by lymphocytes,[29] with retraction of cells from the basement membrane, may also permit cells to transmigrate into the perivascular interstitial tissue. Along these lines, Simon et al[30] demonstrated that activated mouse CD8+ T cells release the enzyme serine proteinase 1, which selectively degrades basement membrane type IV collagen and may facilitate transmigration of the endothelium. Finally, VLA-4 binding may mediate changes in the shape of and cleavage of basement membrane proteins by host leukocytes as they begin to insinuate themselves between endothelial cells, moving along gradients of chemoattractants into the ECM.[31]

MIGRATION AND SELECTIVE RETENTION OF CELLS WITHIN THE GRAFT

Interstitial migration of leukocytes within the allograft is made possible by the increased and generalized expression of VLA-4 and the de novo expression of additional β1 integrin receptors (VLA-1, VLA-5 and VLA-6) to the ECM components: collagen, fibronectin (FN) and laminin (LN). It has become increasingly clear that ECM components, by virtue of their binding to the very late antigens, are active participants in the processes of allogeneic T cell activation, tissue localization and function, and that the role played by VLA-4 in mediating both cell-ECM (FN) and cell-cell (VCAM-1) adhesion is an important one.[32] Initial studies by Kupiec-Weglinski and De Sousa[33] noted a decreased accumulation of adoptively transferred labeled peripheral lymph node cells in cardiac allografts and lymph nodes of T cell deficient B rat recipients following treatment with anti-LN antibody. More recently, Coito et al[34,35] demonstrated that markedly increased intragraft production of both LN and FN in the early phase after transplantation precedes cellular infiltration, and that treatment of rats with a neutralizing anti-TNF-α antibody significantly prolongs cardiac allograft survival and down-regulates local production of FN at both mRNA and protein levels. Finally, the VLA-5 receptor on human CD4+ T cells has been shown to regulate expression of the IL-2 gene and to play a costimulatory role in CD3-TCR-mediated signal transduction by interacting with its FN ligand.[36] These studies provide an important link between the antiallograft response and the local environment of the graft, and support a key role for ECM components as in vivo adhesive factors for activated lymphocytes to home to the transplanted organ.

IN SITU MATURATION/PROLIFERATION

Ascher et al[37,38] utilized the sponge matrix allograft model to demonstrate that local expansion of donor-specific T cells may mediate graft rejection after the fifth posttransplant day without any contribution from the circulating pool of lymphocytes. Cytotoxic infiltration of the sponge appeared by day 8, rapidly proceeded to a day 14 peak, but was never preceded by the development of cytotoxic T lymphocytes (CTLs) within local lymph nodes or spleen. These findings support the hypothesis that precytotoxic specifically-sensitized T lymphocytes are recruited from the central lymphoid depots, where initial allo-sensitization occurs, to the graft site, where they locally expand and mature to effect rejection. The finding of host-independence at a certain stage of rejection coincides with the results of migration studies by Nemlander et al[39] who found that the size of the white cell traffic to and from the untreated rat renal allograft was approximately equal in both directions and exponentially increased up to day 4 posttransplant, with little exchange between the graft and host thereafter.

As part of a series of studies examining the in vivo mechanisms of alloreactivity in murine sponge grafts,[40-42] Orosz et al[43] developed a limiting dilution analysis technique that permits discrimination between graft-reactive naive cytotoxic T cell precursors (pCTL) and CTL that have been activated by specific alloantigen contact in vivo (allograft-conditioned CTL or cCTL). These investigators found that (1) cCTL comprise the vast majority of donor-reactive CTL at the graft site, a low percentage of donor-reactive CTL in the regional lymph nodes (the majority being pCTL), and virtually none of the donor-reactive CTL in the peripheral blood (all being pCTL); (2) all the antigenically-irrelevant CTL accumulating at the graft site are present as pCTL; (3) accumulation of cCTL in sponge implants is dependent upon the deposition of specific alloantigen therein; and (4) direct subsponge, but not intramuscular, cyclosporine A (CsA) injection markedly reduced the accumulation of donor-reactive CTL. These data suggest that there is rapid and efficient acquisition of cCTL by the graft site via local activation/maturation of pCTL following exposure to alloantigen or via recruitment from the periphery that can be inhibited by maintaining high intra-graft concentrations of immunosuppressive agents.

Ford et al[44] determined the time course of cytokine levels within rejecting sponge matrix allografts and found measurable concentrations of the macrophage products TNF, IL-1 and colony stimulating factor (M-CSF). Peak TNF levels preceded maxi-mal M-CSF and IL-1 levels, which coincided with the initial appearance of allospecific CTL. The fact that maximal CTL activity was seen after M-CSF and IL-1 levels had already begun to fall suggests that these monokines, together with IL-6,[45,46] may influence the local maturation or recruitment of precytotoxic T lymphocytes.

Ruers et al[47] have investigated the degree of cellular proliferation occurring within rat heterotopic cardiac allografts and the influence of local steroid therapy on this proliferation. Utilizing a bromodeoxy-uridine-labeling technique, these authors found that both T cytotoxic/suppressor and Th cell phenotypes showed significant in situ proliferative activity in untreated recipients, and that this pattern did not change in the budesonide-treated rats despite the absence of signs of graft destruction. These data demonstrate that inhibition of cellular proliferation may not be required for effective local immunosuppression. Finally, it is now clear that allograft rejection is associated with a sizable in situ proliferative response involving B cells[48,49] and macrophages[50] as well as T cells.

EFFECTOR/INFLAMMATORY AND REGULATORY MECHANISMS

The identification of two functional subsets of Th cells (Th1 and Th2) developing from precursor Th0 cells has brought with it new information and hypotheses regarding both effector and regulatory mechanisms of allograft rejection. Th1 cells produce IL-2, IFN-γ and TNF-β, while Th2 cells produce IL-4, IL-5, IL-6 and IL-10. It has become clear that the secreted products of each subset have the potential to down-regulate clonal expansion and/or functional activities of the reciprocal T cell subpopulation, and that the ultimate phenotype of the immune response generated in any given instance will reflect the relative frequency and activation status of both Th1 and Th2 cells in the local millieu.

IL-12 derived from macrophages, B cells and NK cells is thought to promote development of proinflammatory Th1 cells,[51] which, via IL-2 and IFN-γ, mediate delayed-type hypersensitivity and antibody-dependent cellular cytotoxicity responses and promote CTL development. Both of these cytokines are prominently expressed in the human renal allograft prior to or during rejection, and both Dallman et al[52] and Orosz and co-workers[25] have reported that the IL-2 gene product appears at a very early stage of mouse heart allograft rejection, but not in syngeneic grafts. On the other hand, IL-2 is required for IL-4 and IL-5 production by naive T cells in vitro and for Th2-predominant responses in vivo,[53,54] and IFN-γ, while serving to promote macrophage activation, also induces macrophage expression of IL-4 receptors[55] and release of IL-10.[56]

IL-4 and IL-10 released by activated Th2 cells up-regulate B cell antibody production but have the potential to inhibit or down-regulate the following:[57] (1) local generation of Th1 cells from precursors; (2) activation of existing mature Th1 cells via down-regulation of macrophage B7 expression and IL-12 production; (3) ICAM-1 and E-selectin expression; (4) CTL effector function; (5) monocyte FcγR membrane expression and FcγR-mediated cytotoxic activity and (6) release of IL-1, IL-6 and TNF-α by cells of the monocyte-macrophage lineage. Using molecular and/or immunohistochemical techniques, several laboratories have documented that the expression of Th1 cytokines is dramatically suppressed but that of Th2 cytokines persists in heart grafts recovered from tolerant recipients (in various different models), suggesting that Th2 cells may exert immunosuppressive or tolerogenic effects. Along these lines, intragraft infusion of IL-4 significantly prolonged rat heart allograft survival in donor-specific transfusion/CsA-treated animals.[58]

Soluble factors present within the allograft may affect the predominant Th1/Th2 phenotype of the response. For example, prostaglandin E_2 (PGE$_2$) and PGI$_2$ block proliferation and cytokine release by Th1, but not Th2, cells[59] (see chapter 6). Recent work in the sponge matrix allograft model

has demonstrated that IFN-γ and IL-2 produced by alloactivated Th1 cells induce macrophage NO synthesis, and that the resulting NO production inhibits lymphocyte proliferation and the development of donor-specific cytolytic activity, but not macrophage APC function nor cytokine synthesis.[60-62] Furthermore, more evidence is accumulating that, depending on the local microenvironment, Th2 responses may not be tolerogenic and may promote the recruitment of alternate effector mechanisms (e.g., eosinophil infiltration and increased IgG1 alloantibody) for allograft rejection.[63] It therefore appears that the balance of antagonistic factors released by Th1 and Th2 cells within the millieu of the graft will ultimately determine its fate.

SUMMARY

Intragraft events appear to be important in initiating hypothesized 'central' mechanisms of allosensitization. Following the random migration of sensitized T cells back to the graft and their reactivation by alloantigen, the inflammatory response in the allograft diverges from that in the isograft, and further lymphocyte recruitment, graft infiltration, lymphocyte maturation and proliferation and effector mechanisms are all regulated by chemokines, cytokines and adhesion molecules present in situ. It is certainly conceivable that the appropriately-timed local administration of agents which block several of these phases, including currently available immunosuppressants, as well as specific antibodies to cytokines, cytokine receptors, matrix/basement membrane components and adhesion, MHC, and other cell-surface molecules, could effectively arrest the rejection response.

REFERENCES

1. Gruber SA. The case for local immunosuppression. Transplantation 1992; 54:1.

2. Gruber SA. Locoregional immunosuppression of organ transplants. Immunol Rev 1992; 129:5.

3. Barker CF, Billingham RE. The role of afferent lymphatics in the rejection of skin homografts. J Exp Med 1968; 128:197.

4. Tilney NL, Gowans JL. The sensitization of rats by allografts transplanted to alymphatic pedicles of skin. J Exp Med 1970; 133:951.

5. Hume DM, Egdahl RH. Progressive destruction of renal homografts isolated from the regional lymphatics of the host. Surgery 1955; 38:194.

6. Strober S, Gowans JL. The role of lymphocytes in the sensitization of rats to renal homografts. J Exp Med 1965; 122:347.

7. Pedersen NC, Morris B. The role of the lymphatic system in the rejection of homografts: a study of lymph from renal transplants. J Exp Med 1970; 131:936.

8. Häyry P, von Willebrand E., Soots A. In situ effector mechanisms in rat kidney allograft rejection. III. Kinetics of the inflammatory response and generation of donor-directed killer cells. Scand J Immunol 1979; 10:95.

9. von Willebrand E, Soots A, Häyry P. In situ effector mechanisms in rat kidney allograft rejection. I. Characterization of the host cellular infiltrate in rejecting allograft parenchyma. Cell Immunol 1979; 46:309.

10. von Willebrand E, Soots A, Häyry P. In situ effector mechanisms in rat kidney allograft rejection. II. Heterogeneity of the effector cells in the inflammatory infiltrate vs that in the spleen of the recipient rat. Cell Immunol 1979; 46:327.

11. Larsen CP, Barker H, Morris PJ et al. Failure of mature dendritic cells of the host to migrate from the blood into cardiac or skin allografts. Transplantation 1990; 50:294.

12. Larsen CP, Morris PJ, Austyn JM. Migration of dendritic leukocytes from cardiac allografts into host spleens: a novel pathway for initiation of rejection. J Exp Med 1990; 171:307.

13. Larsen CP, Steinman RM, Witmer-Pack M et al. Migration and maturation of Langerhans cells in skin transplants and explants. J Exp Med 1990; 172:1483.

14. Kripke ML, Munn CG, Jeevan A et al. Evidence that cutaneous antigen-presenting cells migrate to regional lymph nodes during contact sensitization. J Immunol 1990; 145:2833.

15. Codner MA, Shuster BA, Steinman RM et al. Migration of donor leukocytes from limb allografts into host lymphoid tissues. Ann Plastic Surg 1990; 25:353.

16. Austyn JM, Hankins DF, Larsen CP et al. Isolation and characterization of dendritic cells from mouse heart and kidney. J Immunol 1994; 152:2401.

17. Rao AS, Roake JA, Larsen CP et al. Isolation of dendritic leukocytes from non-lymphoid organs. Adv Exp Med Biol 1993; 329:507.

18. Larsen CP, Ritchie SC, Hendrix R et al. Regulation of immunostimulatory function and costimulatory molecule (B7-1 and B7-2) expression on murine dendritic cells. J Immunol 1994; 152:5208.

19. Larsen CP, Ritchie SC, Pearson TC et al. Functional expression of the costimulatory molecule, B7/BB1, on murine dendritic cell populations. J Exp Med 1992; 176:1215.

20. Roake JA, Rao AS, Morris PJ et al. Dendritic cell loss from nonlymphoid tissues after systemic administration of lipopolysaccharide, tumor necrosis factor, and interleukin 1. J Exp Med 1995; 181:2237.

21. Freise CE, Clemmings S, Clemens LE et al. Demonstration of local immunosuppression with methylprednisolone in the sponge matrix allograft model. Transplantation 1991; 52:318.

22. Inaba K, Steinman RM. Resting and sensitized T lymphocytes exhibit distinct stimulatory (antigen-presenting cell) requirements for growth and lymphokine release. J Exp Med 1984; 160:1717.

23. Tullius SG, Heemann UW, Zeilinger K et al. Binding of lymphocytes to acutely rejecting rat kidney allografts in vitro is guided by events in the graft itself rather than by sensitization of host lymphocytes. Transplant Immunol 1995; 3:91.

24. Taub DD, Conlon K, Lloyd AR et al. Preferential migration of activated CD4+ and CD8+ T cells in response to MIP-1α and MIP-1β. Science 1993; 260:355.

25. Pelletier RP, Morgan CJ, Sedmak DD et al. Analysis of inflammatory endothelial changes, including VCAM-1 expression, in murine cardiac grafts. Transplantation 1993; 55:315.

26. Morgan CJ, Pelletier RP, Hernandez CJ et al. Alloantigen-dependent endothelial phe-

notype and lymphokine mRNA expression in rejecting murine cardiac allografts. Transplantation 1993; 55:919.

27. Bergese SD, Huang EH, Pelletier RP et al. Regulation of endothelial VCAM-1 expression in murine cardiac grafts. Expression of allograft endothelial VCAM-1 can be manipulated with antagonist of IFN-alpha or IL-4 and is not required for allograft rejection. Am J Pathol 1995; 147:166.

28. Stolpen AH, Guinan EC, Fiers W et al. Recombinant tumor necrosis factor and immune interferon act singly and in combination to reorganize human vascular endothelial cell monolayers. Am J Pathol 1986; 123:16.

29. Pober JS, Cotran RS. The role of endothelial cells in inflammation. Transplantation 1990; 50:537.

30. Simon MM, Kramer MD, Prester M et al. Mouse T-cell associated serine proteinase 1 degrades collagen type IV: a structural basis for migration of lymphocytes through vascular basement membranes. Immunology 1991; 73:117.

31. Schrader B, Steinhoff G. Models of inflammatory cascade reactions by adhesion molecules. In: Steinhoff G, ed. Cell adhesion molecules in human organ transplants. Austin: RG Landes Co., 1993.

32. Kupiec-Weglinski JW, Coito AJ, Gorski A et al. Lymphocyte migration and tissue positioning in allograft recipients: the role played by extracellular matrix proteins. Transplant Rev 1995; 9:29.

33. Kupiec-Weglinski JW, De Sousa M. Lymphocyte traffic is modified in vivo by anti-laminin antibody. Immunology 1991; 72:312.

34. Coito AJ, Binder J, de Sousa M et al. The expression of extracellular matrix proteins during accelerated rejection of cardiac allografts in sensitized rats. Transplantation 1994; 57:599.

35. Coito AJ, Binder J, Van de Water L et al. Anti-TNF-a antibody treatment down-regulates the expression of fibronectin and decreases cellular infiltration of cardiac allografts in rats. J Immunol 1995; 154:2949.

36. Yamada A, Nikaido T, Nojima Y et al. Activation of human CD4 T lymphocytes.

Interaction of fibronectin with VLA-5 receptor on CD4 cells induces AP-1 transcription factor. J Immunol 1991; 146:53.

37. Ascher NL, Chen S, Hoffman R et al. Maturation of cytotoxic effector cells at the site of allograft rejection. Transplant Proc 1981; 13:1105.

38. Ascher NL, Chen S, Hoffman R et al. Maturation of cytotoxic T cells within sponge matrix allografts. J Immunol 1983; 131:617.

39. Nemlander A, Soots A, von Willebrand E et al. Redistribution of renal allograft responding leukocytes during rejection: II. Kinetics and specificity. J Exp Med 1982; 156:1987.

40. Orosz CG, Zinn NE, Sirinek LP et al. In vivo mechanisms of alloreactivity—IV. Cyclosporine differentially impairs accumulation of donor-reactive CTL but not donor-reactive alloantibody in murine sponge matrix allografts. Int J Immunopharmacol 1988; 10:305.

41. Orosz CG, Horstemeyer B, Zinn NE et al. In vivo mechanisms of alloreactivity—V. Influence of graft implantation on the activation and redistribution of graft-reactive CTL. Transplantation 1989; 48:519.

42. Orosz CG, Bishop DK, Ferguson RM. In vivo mechanisms of alloreactivity—VI. Evidence that alloantigen deposition initiates both local and systemic mechanisms that influence CTL accumulation at a graft site. Transplantation 1989; 48:818.

43. Orosz CG, Horstemeyer B, Zinn NE et al. Development and evaluation of a limiting dilution analysis technique that can discriminate in vivo alloactivated cytotoxic T lymphocytes from their naive cell precursors. Transplantation 1989; 47:189.

44. Ford HR, Hoffman RA, Wing EJ et al. Tumor necrosis factor, macrophage colony-stimulating factor, and interleukin 1 production within sponge matrix allografts. Transplantation 1990; 50:460.

45. Ford HR, Hoffman RA, McIntyre LA et al. Interleukin-6 production within the rejecting allograft coincides with cytotoxic T lymphocyte development. Surg Forum 1989; 40:360.

46. Vandenbroecke C, Caillat-Zucman S,

Legendre C et al. Differential in situ expression of cytokines in renal allograft rejection. Transplantation 1991; 51:602.

47. Ruers TJM, Schutte B, van der Linden CJ et al. Cellular proliferation at the site of organ allografts and the influence of immunosuppressive therapy. Transplantation 1990; 50:568.

48. Garovoy MR, Reddish MA, Busch GJ et al. Immunoglobulin-secreting cells recovered from rejected human renal allografts. Transplantation 1982; 33:109.

49. Renkonen R, Soots A, von Willebrand E et al. Lymphoid cell subclasses in rejecting renal allograft in the rat. Cell Immunol 1983; 77:187.

50. Kerr PG, Nikolic-Paterson DJ, Lan HY et al. Deoxyspergualin suppresses local macrophage proliferation in rat renal allograft rejection. Transplantation 1994; 58:596.

51. Hsieh CS, Macatonia SE, Tripp CS et al. Development of Th1 CD4+ T cells through IL-12 produced by Listeria-induced macrophages. Science 1993; 260:547.

52. Dallman MJ, Larsen CP, Morris PJ. Cytokine gene transcription in vascularised organ grafts—analysis using semiquantitative polymerase chain reaction. J Exp Med 1991; 174:493.

53. Ben-Sasson SZ, Le-Gros G, Conrad DH et al. IL-4 production by T cells from naive donors: IL-2 is required for IL-4 production. J Immunol 1990; 145:1127.

54. Steel C, Nutman TB. Regulation of IL-5 in Onchocerciasis. A critical role of IL-2. J Immunol 1993; 150:5511.

55. Feldman GM, Finbloom DS. Induction and regulation of IL-4 receptor expression on murine macrophage cell lines and bone marrow-derived macrophages by IFN-gamma. J Immunol 1990; 145:854.

56. de Waal Malefyt R, Abrams J, Bennett B et al. Interleukin 10 (IL-10) inhibits cytokine synthesis by human monocytes: An autoregulatory role of IL-10 produced by monocytes. J Exp Med 1991; 174:1209.

57. Lowry RP, Takeguchi T. The TH1, TH2 paradigm and transplantation tolerance. Austin: RG Landes Co., 1994.

58. Levy AE, Alexander JW. Administration of intragraft interleukin-4 prolongs cardiac allograft survival in rats treated with donor-specific transfusion/cyclosporine. Transplantation 1995; 60:405.

59. Betz M, Fox BS. Prostaglandin E2 inhibits production of Th1 lymphokines but not of Th2 lymphokines. J Immunol 1991; 146:108.

60. Langrehr JM, Hoffman RA, Billiar TR et al. Nitric oxide synthesis in the in vivo allograft response: A possible regulatory mechanism. Surgery 1991; 110:335.

61. Langrehr JM, Dull KE, Ochoa JB et al. Evidence that nitric oxide production by in vivo allosensitized cells inhibits the development of allospecific CTL. Transplantation 1992; 53:632.

62. Hoffman RA, Langrehr JM, Dull KE et al. Macrophage synthesis of nitric oxide in the mouse mixed leucocyte reaction. Transpl Immunol 1994; 2:313.

63. Chan SY, DeBruyne LA, Goodman RE et al. In vivo depletion of CD8+ T cells results in Th2 cytokine production and alternate mechanisms of allograft rejection. Transplantation 1995; 59:1155.

CHAPTER 2

PHARMACOKINETIC ADVANTAGE OF REGIONAL DRUG DELIVERY

Stephen E. Hughes, Sardha Perera and Scott A. Gruber

The pharmacokinetic advantage of intraarterial (i.a.) drug administration was initially articulated by Eckman et al[1] and has been subsequently reviewed in several reports.[2-6] The theory states that arterial infusion may provide increased drug delivery to the target organ and decreased drug delivery to the systemic circulation when compared with same-dose intravenous (i.v.) administration, and is based on two assumptions: (1) the kinetics of drug distribution in the body can be represented by linear compartmental analysis and (2) the rate coefficients remain constant over the entire range of drug concentrations and for the time periods involved.[1]

There are two kinds of pharmacokinetic advantage of i.a. over i.v. drug administration. The regional advantage reflects the degree to which target organ drug concentration can be increased when drug is infused locally rather than systemically. This advantage increases as the clearance of drug outside the target organ increases or as blood flow to the target organ decreases. The regional advantage is established during the first passage of drug through the target organ, since the drug then returns to the systemic circulation and is distributed as though injected intravenously.[1,3] The systemic advantage reflects the degree to which drug delivery to the systemic circulation can be reduced by local infusion via the first-pass elimination or metabolism of drug by the target organ. The systemic advantage increases as the extraction ratio of drug by the target organ increases.

The most commonly used mathematical approach to analyze pharmacokinetic data involves the use of open compartment models. The body may be described as a set of compartments, representing tissues and organs, each possessing unique kinetic parameters.[4] When considering the pharmacokinetics of regional drug delivery, the body can be portrayed using a two-compartment model: a regional compartment representing the target organ, and a peripheral, or systemic, compartment representing the rest of the body. By analyzing the time course of drug concentrations in the plasma in the two compartments, it is possible to determine the elimination half-life, total body clearance and steady-state level of the drug.

CALCULATION OF THE SYSTEMIC ADVANTAGE

When a drug is delivered locally to an organ that eliminates it from the body or metabolizes it, there is a first-pass effect. In this case, i.a. administration will produce lower systemic concentrations than will i.v. delivery of the same dose. Therefore, the systemic advantage ($R_{systemic}$) of i.a. drug administration to a target organ is given by the following equation:[3]

$$R_{systemic} = C_{systemic}(i.a.)/C_{systemic}(i.v.) = 1 - E$$
$$(Eq. 1)$$

where $C_{systemic}(i.a.)$ is the steady-state systemic drug concentration during i.a. infusion, $C_{systemic}(i.v.)$ is the steady-state systemic drug concentration during i.v. infusion, and E is the extraction ratio of drug by the target organ. Clearly, the greatest reduction in systemic drug delivery will occur when there is a large extraction of drug by the target organ.

If it is possible to sample both the arterial blood supplying the target organ and the venous blood returning from the target organ, E may be calculated more directly as the ratio of the rate of drug delivery to the rate of drug extraction. The rate of delivery of drug to a target organ is the product of organ blood flow (Q_T) and the arterial concentration of the drug (C_a):

$$Rate\ of\ delivery = Q_T \bullet C_a$$

The rate at which drug leaves the target organ in the venous effluent is similarly defined as $Q_T \bullet C_v$, where C_v is the venous concentration of the drug. The rate of extraction is the difference between these rates:

$$Rate\ of\ extraction = Q_T \bullet (C_a - C_v)$$

These two terms can be combined to yield the extraction ratio, E:[4]

$$E = rate\ of\ extraction/rate\ of\ delivery =$$
$$Q_T \bullet (C_a - C_v)/\ Q_T \bullet C_a = (C_a - C_v)/C_a =$$
$$1 - C_v/C_a$$

CALCULATION OF THE REGIONAL ADVANTAGE

The regional advantage (R_{target}) is determined from the following ratio:[3]

$$R_{target} = C_{target}(i.a.)/C_{target}(i.v.) = 1 + Cl_s/Q_T$$
$$(Eq. 2)$$

where $C_{target}(i.a.)$ is the steady-state drug concentration in the target organ during i.a. infusion, $C_{target}(i.v.)$ is the steady-state drug concentration in the target organ during i.v. infusion and Cl_s is the systemic clearance of drug outside the target organ calculated during i.v. administration. The numerator, $C_{target}(i.a.)$, represents the steady-state drug concentration in the target organ during i.a. infusion, and is given by the sum of two components: the concentration of drug directly infused into the target organ + the concentration of drug present in the blood returning to the target at steady state. Therefore,

$$C_{target}(i.a.) = inf/Q_T + C_{systemic}(i.a.)$$
$$(Eq. 3)$$

where inf is the constant infusion rate of drug. The denominator in Eq.2, $C_{target}(i.v.)$, is equivalent to $C_{systemic}(i.v.)$ since steady-state target organ and systemic drug concentrations would be expected to be equal during a continuous i.v. infusion.

CALCULATION OF SELECTIVITY

Equations 1 and 2 for regional and systemic pharmacokinetic advantage are valid at steady state during constant-rate infusion or when considering the total amount of drug (concentration integrated over time) delivered to the target organ and systemic circulation following i.a. and i.v. bolus injection.[1,2] The overall pharmacokinetic advantage of local drug delivery, or selectivity (R_d), has been defined as the ratio of the regional and systemic advantages:[3]

$$R_d = R_{target}/R_{systemic} = 1 + Cl_s/[Q_T \cdot (1 - E)]$$
(Eq. 4)

ADDITIONAL CONSIDERATIONS

Thus, local drug administration achieves an advantage over systemic administration when the infused drug is extracted efficiently by the target organ or when the drug has a high systemic clearance relative to target organ blood flow.[4,5] As Equation 4 indicates, if the drug clearance outside the target is small with respect to organ blood flow, then R_d approaches one, indicating no regional advantage. It is also important to note that, even in cases where the target organ is the sole source of elimination of the drug ($Cl_s = 0$), higher concentrations are delivered to the target by i.a. than i.v. infusion as long as steady state has not yet been reached. This situation may result in reduced systemic toxicity but not in an improvement in therapeutic response.[3] Moreover, nonlinearity in pharmacokinetics as a result of saturation of plasma and/or tissue protein binding, carrier transport systems and elimination mechanisms may alter the expected gain from target-directed drug delivery.[5]

In an overview of the pharmacokinetic problems and pitfalls of arterial drug infusion published in 1988, Dedrick[6] emphasized that data rigorously supporting the above principles governing the advantages of i.a. infusions are rare, and that determination of simultaneous drug concentrations in both regional and systemic compartments is very difficult since relatively few organs provide access to the venous blood that drains the entire territory served by the infused artery. At this time, three research groups were examining the pharmacokinetic advantage of i.a. infusions in experimental models. Daeman[4] performed a detailed evaluation of the advantage of re-

gional over systemic drug administration to the rat kidney, liver, testis and transplanted heart utilizing a variety of different drugs and infusion techniques. Ruers et al[7,8] discussed the regional and systemic advantage obtainable from intrarenal prednisolone and intracardiac budesonide infusion, respectively, in rodent transplant models (see chapter 4). Finally, our laboratory was the first to validate the theoretical considerations concerning regional drug delivery in a large-animal (canine renal allograft) model using completely implantable devices for arterial cannulation and drug administration which can be directly applied to man[9] (see chapter 9).

However, extrapolation from animal studies into the clinical setting may not be a routine matter. When comparisons are made across species, the physiological property of interest is considered proportional to some power of the body weight according to the allometric equation. With regard to Equation 4, blood flow (Q_T), or tissue perfusion, tends to be similar across species, while large differences can occur in total body clearance (Cl_s).[6,10] If the differences in Cl_s can be determined, then an allometric basis for interspecies scaling of pharmacokinetic advantage can be established.

Different organs differ in their suitability for regional drug delivery depending on their blood flow, their capacity for drug elimination and the pharmacokinetics of the agent chosen for administration.[4] For example, although the kidney may be an excellent target organ for achieving systemic advantage of locally-infused immunosuppressants which are excreted unchanged in the urine, it is really unsuited for achieving regional advantage because it is a high-flow organ. Under most circumstances, extrarenal clearance will be less than renal blood flow, and only a minimal regional advantage will be attainable. Possibilities for overcoming this pharmacokinetic obstacle are as follows: (1) Use of immunosuppressive agents with vasoconstrictor properties or supplementary use of vasoconstrictors to decrease renal blood flow;[4] (2) Supplementary use of agents which enhance extrarenal drug clearance (e.g., phenobarbital to enhance liver metabolism);[4] (3) Design of intermittent, short-lasting (relative to the elimination half-life of the drug) infusions which avoid steady-state conditions and maintain a persistent differential in the time integrals of arterial drug levels obtained by i.a. and i.v. infusion.[5] Systemic advantage may be further enhanced by concomitantly administering drugs which alter urinary pH to increase elimination of weak acids and bases. Finally, when designing immunosuppressive regimens for chronic intrarenal administration, one must be cognizant of the fact that transplant blood flow and first-pass drug extraction may increase gradually with time as a result of hypertrophy of the single kidney or may decrease acutely during rejection episodes.

Finally, calculation of the pharmacokinetic advantage depends on total regional blood flow and assumes that drug is equally distributed throughout the target organ. For this assumption to be valid, complete mixing of drug in the bloodstream must occur prior to the first bifurcation of the distal arterial tree. However, drug streaming from the tip of an indwelling arterial catheter may produce inhomogeneous drug distribution within the target organ, leading to a localized saturation of elimination mechanisms and a decreased first-pass extraction.[4,6,10,11] As a consequence of this, portions of the target region may receive a suboptimal dose of drug, while other areas could receive toxic levels.[11,12] Thus, pharmacokinetic and therapeutic studies involving i.a. infusion should be evaluated in light of the unknown effects of streaming on drug distribution.

REFERENCES

1. Eckman WW, Patlak CS, Fenstermacher JD. A critical evaluation of the principles governing the advantages of intraarterial infusions. J Pharmacokinet Biopharmacol 1974; 2:257.
2. Øie S, Huang JD. Influence of administration route on drug delivery to target organ. J Pharm Sci 1981; 70:1344.
3. Collins JM. Pharmacologic rationale for regional drug delivery. J Clin Oncol 1984; 2:498.
4. Daeman M. Local drug administration. An experimental study on its possibilities and limitations. Doctoral dissertation: University of Limburg, Maastricht, The Netherlands 1987.
5. Smits JF, Thijssen HH. Spatial control of drug action: theoretical considerations on the pharmacokinetics of target-aimed drug delivery. In: Struyker-Boudier HAJ, ed. Rate controlled drug administration and action. Boca Raton: CRC Press, 1987.
6. Dedrick RL. Arterial drug infusion: pharmacokinetic problems and pitfalls. J Natl Cancer Inst 1988; 80:84.
7. Ruers TJM, Buurman WA, Smits JFM et al. Local treatment of renal allografts, a promising way to reduce the dosage of immunosuppressive drugs. Transplantation 1986; 41:156.
8. Ruers TJM, Daeman MJAP, Thijssen HHW et al. Sensitivity of graft rejection in rats to local immunosuppressive therapy. Transplantation 1988; 46:820.
9. Gruber SA, Canafax DM, Erdmann GR et al. The pharmacokinetic advantage of local 6-mercaptopurine infusion in a canine renal transplant model. Transplantation 1989; 48:928.
10. Dedrick RL. Interspecies scaling of regional drug delivery. J Pharm Sci 1986; 75:1047.
11. Blacklock JB, Wright DC, Dedrick RL et al. Drug streaming during intraarterial chemotherapy. J Neurosurg 1986; 64:2841.
12. Lutz RJ, Dedrick RL, Boretos JW et al. Mixing studies during intracarotid artery infusions in an in vitro model. J Neurosurg 1986; 64:277.

CHAPTER 3

EARLY STUDIES OF LOCAL IMMUNOSUPPRESSION (1964-1984)

Stephen E. Hughes, Sardha Perera and Scott A. Gruber

REGIONAL DRUG DELIVERY

The possibility that regional administration of a drug might prolong the survival of transplanted tissue arose during the early 1950s, when Billingham et al[1] treated rabbit skin allografts with 5 mg of cortisone acetate suspended in 0.2 ml of saline with 1.5% benzyl alcohol. This suspension was applied directly to the grafted skin every third day, beginning immediately before the grafts were placed on the prepared site. The topical application of cortisone more than doubled the survival time of the allografts, while systemic administration of the same quantity of cortisone on the same schedule was completely ineffective in delaying rejection. Although the potential clinical advantage of applying cortisone locally in quantities that would inhibit the rejection response and simultaneously avoid deleterious systemic side effects was apparent to these investigators, the idea languished until the next decade.

The development of small, portable infusion pumps opened up the possibility of continuously delivering drug to unrestrained experimental animals for sufficient periods of time to study the effects of intraarterial (i.a.) drug administration on the rejection of solid-organ transplants. Investigation of the efficacy of locoregional treatment of renal allografts began when Miura et al[2] utilized such a pump to deliver methotrexate into the arterial blood supply of the transplanted dog kidney. In their model, a teflon catheter was inserted into the aorta some distance upstream from the take-off of, rather than directly into, the iliac artery feeding the allograft. Because of this design, methotrexate was delivered not only to the kidney, where it could be cleared from the body, but

Local Immunosuppression of Organ Transplants, edited by Scott A. Gruber.
© 1996 R.G. Landes Company.

also to the systemic circulation. In addition, some animals were supplemented with daily intramuscular methotrexate injections. All kidneys ceased functioning due to rejection within 4 days. Eight of 13 dogs receiving high-dose methotrexate (up to 0.5 mg/kg/day) and 5 of 13 animals receiving low-dose methotrexate (0.02 mg/kg/day) died with concomitant systemic drug toxicity.

Two years later, Retik et al[3] reported results from a canine model in which a polyvinyl catheter was implanted in the common iliac artery proximal to its end-to-end anastomosis with the donor renal artery, a design which restricted drug delivery through the catheter to the transplanted kidney. Unlike the previously-discussed model, drugs were administered through the catheter by slow bolus injection, not constant infusion. These investigators showed that intrarenal injection of actinomycin C reversed 16 of 18 rejection episodes in animals receiving a background of systemic azathioprine and azaserine. Intermittent i.a. azathioprine alone, in maintenance doses as low as 0.5-1.0 mg/kg/day and in antirejection doses as high as 10-12 mg/kg/day, moderately improved survival compared with that previously reported in the literature for oral or intravenous (i.v.) administration. In addition, autografts receiving i.a. azathioprine, azaserine and intermittent actinomycin C in doses similar to those used in the allografts suffered no alterations in renal function, and overall, the indwelling arterial catheter was relatively free of complications. However, while the doses of immunosuppressive agents delivered via the catheter were generally less than those typically used by other investigators,[4] systemic drug toxicity was still a major cause of death, and several animals required i.a. doses similar to oral or i.v. doses to control rejection. The authors concluded that, in general, intermittent local infusion of immunosuppressive drugs suffered from a poor therapeutic index and was not warranted.

These negative findings were corroborated 3 years later in a report by Terz et

al[5] who delivered various antimetabolites into canine renal allografts via continuous i.a. infusion. Specifically, the authors utilized a polyvinyl catheter placed in the suprapubic branch of the left external iliac artery connected to a microflow syringe pump to locally administer 6-mercaptopurine to 7 dogs and methotrexate to 16 dogs beginning on the day of transplantation. In the 6-mercaptopurine group, one animal receiving 5 mg/kg/day died in 8 days with gross and histologic evidence of rejection. Of six dogs receiving 7.5 mg/kg/day, two animals died in four days from leukopenia, while the remaining four animals died between days 4 and 18 with renal failure and histologic evidence of rejection. The methotrexate group was divided into two subgroups. Ten dogs were infused with either 0.1 or 0.2 mg/kg/day and received daily injections of citrovorum factor. Mean survival times were 18.5 days for the low-dose dogs (n = 4) and 9.9 days for the high-dose animals (n = 6), with all animals dying from rejection. The other six dogs received either 0.05 or 0.1 mg/kg/day methotrexate with no citrovorum rescue. All of these animals died from systemic toxicity. The authors concluded that regional infusion of these immunosuppressive agents provided no significant benefit over what was achievable with systemic therapy.

Investigation of the efficacy of local steroid treatment of renal allografts began in the mid-1960s when it was demonstrated that continuous i.a. infusion of cortisone (8.5-12.5 mg/kg/day),[6] hydrocortisone (12.5-16.5 mg/kg/day),[7] prednisolone (2.5-3.0 mg/kg/day)[7] or high-dose prednisone (200 mg/day)[5] into canine renal transplants using external syringe pumps or i.v. infusion sets produced no significant differences in survival time or time to rejection when compared with untreated controls. Ackerman and Barnard[6] did notice less graft size increase, interstitial round cell infiltrate and vascular endothelial reaction in the cortisone-treated kidneys than in the controls, but three of the seven animals died from systemic drug toxicity, with massive gastrointestinal hemorrhage and typical ulceration at postmortem.

At the same time, Kountz and Cohn[8] reported that in dogs receiving two grafts from the same donor and a background of oral azathioprine, the kidney treated directly with a solution containing methylprednisolone, heparin and actinomycin D for the first 24-72 h posttransplant showed less histologic rejection after 2 weeks than its mate. This same solution was then administered intrarenally to 61 living-related donor renal allograft recipients from 1 to 3 days posttransplant, and was capable of reversing all but 1 of 18 rejection crises occurring in the first 3 months if administered intrarenally (within 3 weeks posttransplant) or systemically (3 weeks to 3 months posttransplant).[9] Finally, Laupacis et al[10] reported successful treatment of 26 out of 54 severe, refractory rejection episodes occurring within 2 months posttransplant with i.a. methylprednisolone and heparin infusion in 46 kidney transplant patients. However, some of these patients received other antirejection modalities (antilymphocyte globulin, leukopheresis, plasmapheresis or cyclophosphamide) simultaneously, and there were nine significant catheter-related complications.

In 1984, Campbell et al[11] utilized an implantable Infusaid pump to deliver a constant infusion of PGE_1 directly into the renal transplant artery. In this nonphysiologic, four-kidney canine model, the recipient's native kidneys were not removed and renal transplantation was performed to the iliac vessels bilaterally (both allografts coming from the same donor), with continuous infusion of PGE_1 to one kidney. Although the type of cellular infiltrate in the two kidneys differed, allograft failure, as assessed by decreasing renal blood flow, occurred similarly in both treated and untreated kidneys.

LOCAL GRAFT IRRADIATION

In an early study, local irradiation of canine renal allografts with daily doses of 100 rads begun on the day of transplantation did not prolong graft survival nor alter the histologic response within the kidney.[12] Kauffman et al[13] corroborated this initial finding, but further demonstrated that a higher dose of 150 rads delivered every other day up to a total of 900 rads was sufficient to significantly prolong graft survival, with no leukopenia or generalized immunosuppression. Increasing the dose beyond 150 rads did not provide an additional antirejection effect. The greatest enhancement of survival occurred if the first dose of radiation was administered on the day of transplantation. Delaying the first dose until day 2, 3 or 4 posttransplant prolonged graft survival in some animals, but when considered as groups, no significant prolongation of renal function beyond that in the control group was seen. The dog that was first irradiated on day 4 was already showing signs of rejection at the time, indicated by worsening azotemia. Following radiation treatment, however, the blood urea nitrogen in this animal dropped to 55% of its peak level, suggesting that at least a partial reversal of the rejection process had occurred.[13]

The same local irradiation protocol was followed by Wolf et al[14] in their study of canine renal allografts, with the exception that irradiation commenced 1 day after transplantation and was performed every other day from that point to a total of 900 rads. The mean functional survival time of the nonirradiated control kidneys was 5.7 days, while that of the irradiated kidneys was 12.1 days. During the course of irradiation, biopsies showed reduced lymphocytic infiltration compared with that in the untreated controls. However, following cessation of radiation treatment, rejection supervened in the normal fashion. At the time of rejection, the irradiated kidneys were indistinguishable from the control kidneys.

Local graft irradiation was also shown to be effective in prolonging the function of heterotopic cardiac allografts in rats[15] and dogs.[16] In 15 rats, irradiation was initiated on the day of transplantation, and a total dose of 900 rads was administered as a series of 150 rad doses given on alternate days. Although the treated allografts survived significantly longer (14.7 ± 3.1 days) than those in a group of 15 untreated rats (9.9 ± 1.5 days), all hearts functioned at a subnormal level (decreased pulse rate) beginning on days 5-9. The authors postulated that this might be due to interstitial infiltration by lymphocytes, which is reduced but not eliminated by local irradiation.[15] In contrast to other investigators, Gergely and Coles[16] utilized a higher total dose of radiation (2400 rads, administered in six biweekly doses of 400 rads), and found that treated canine heart transplants maintained viability for up to 10 weeks, while the nonirradiated controls were rejected after 12 days. Biospies revealed a reduced lymphocytic infiltrate as well as alterations in the vasculature within the irradiated grafts, both of which may have contributed to the prolonged survival observed. Finally, Ascher et al[17] used the sponge matrix allograft to correlate the effects of early local irradiation with cellular events associated with graft rejection, and demonstrated decreased cytotoxic cell infiltration in irradiated sponges.

Development of severe infections often requires reduction of immunosuppressive drug doses in transplant patients, which in turn increases the risk of acute rejection. When acute rejection occurs in such situations, local irradiation has proven to be of therapeutic value. In a report of four renal allograft recipients suffering rejection episodes following discontinuation of drug therapy due to infection, local irradiation of the allografts with 150 rads per treatment, for a total of 300 to 900 rads, resulted in complete reversal of rejection and return to normal renal function.[18]

More recent clinical studies have examined the role of local irradiation in the prophylaxis and treatment of acute renal allograft rejection. Halperin et al[19] found that irradiation with 600 rads, delivered in four daily doses of 150 rads, was of limited benefit to some patients with refractory rejection, particularly those suffering from tubulointerstitial, as opposed to vascular, rejection. In a 3-year, randomized study, the efficacy of local irradiation in combination with high-dose i.v. methylprednisolone therapy was compared with

that of steroid treatment alone.[20] Radiation was delivered as 175 rads every other day for a total of 525 rads. Rejection was reversed in 84.5% of the control group, but in only 75% in the irradiated group. The irradiated patients also suffered more frequent recurrent rejections, and overall graft survival was significantly lower than that in the control group.

CONCLUSION

This chapter has summarized the conflicting reports regarding the effectiveness of local pharmacologic and radiologic treatment of experimental and human allografts appearing prior to 1985. In 1986, Ruers et al[21] demonstrated that continuous i.a. infusion of prednisolone in rat renal allograft recipients produced a significant increase in graft survival when compared with same-dose systemic administration, and ushered in the 'modern era' of local immunosuppressive therapy. In light of the recent development of more specific and potent immunosuppressive agents, the technological advances in design of local drug-delivery systems, the elucidation of the pharmacokinetics of target-aimed drug delivery, and the advances made in understanding the cellular mechanisms of allograft rejection, it is clear that the concept of local immunosuppression deserves reexploration.

REFERENCES

1. Billingham RE, Krohn PL, Medawar PB. Effect of locally applied cortisone acetate on survival of skin homografts in rabbits. Br Med J 1951; 1:1049.
2. Miura T, Shah S, Khazei AM. Continuous chronometric infusion of immunosuppressive drugs into the arterial blood supply of a transplanted kidney. Lahey Clin Bull 1964; 13:136.
3. Retik AB, Dubernard J-M, Hester WJ et al. A study of the effects of intraarterial immunosuppressive drug therapy on canine renal allografts. Surgery 1966; 60:1242.
4. Calne RY, Alexandre GPJ, Murray JE. A study of the effects of drugs in prolonging survival of homologous renal transplants in dogs. Ann NY Acad Sci 1962; 99:743.

5. Terz JJ, Crampton R, Miller D et al. Regional infusion chemotherapy for prolongation of kidney allografts. J Surg Res 1969; 9:13.

6. Ackerman RW, Barnard CN. The effect of direct infusions of cortisone into the renal artery of a transplanted kidney. S A Med J 1966; 40:83.

7. Dougherty JC, Nehlsen SL, Minick R et al. Failure of regional immunosuppressive therapy to modify renal allograft rejection. Transplantation 1968; 6:554.

8. Kountz SL, Cohn RB. Successful intrarenal treatment of the allograft reaction. Surg Forum 1967; 18:251.

9. Kountz SL, Cohn RB. Initial treatment of renal allografts with large intrarenal doses of immunosuppressive drugs. Lancet 1969; 1:338.

10. Laupacis A, Keown PA, Rankin RN et al. Intraarterial methylprednisolone and heparin (IAT) for the treatment of refractory renal transplant rejection episodes. Transplant Proc 1982; 14:693.

11. Campbell D, Wiggins R, Kunkel S et al. Constant intrarenal infusion of PGE_1 into a canine renal transplant using a totally implantable pump. Transplantation 1984; 38:209.

12. Banks DE, Auburn RP, Hubay CA et al. Effects of intermittent irradiation in situ on renal homotransplantation. J Urol 1961; 86:181.

13. Kauffman Jr HM, Cleveland RJ, Dwyer JJ et al. Prolongation of renal homograft function by local graft radiation. Surg Gynecol Obstet 1965; 120:49.

14. Wolf JS, McGavic JD, Hume DM. Inhibition of the effector mechanism of transplant immunity by local graft irradiation. Surg Gynecol Obstet 1969; 128:584.

15. Ono K, Lindsey ES, Creech O Jr. Transplanted rat heart: local graft irradiation. Transplantation 1969; 7:176.

16. Gergely NF, Coles JC. Prolongation of heterotopic cardiac allografts in dogs by topical radiation. Transplantation 1970; 9:193.

17. Ascher NL, Hoffman RA, Simmons RL. Local graft irradiation: effect on cytotoxic cell infiltration. Surg Forum 1984; 16:272.

18. Fidler JP, Alexander JW, Smith EJ et al. Radiation reversal of acute rejection in patients with life-threatening infections. Arch Surg 1973; 107:256.

19. Halperin EC, Delmonico FL, Nelson PW et al. The use of local allograft irradiation following renal transplantation. J Rad Oncol Biol Phys 1984; 10:987.

20. Pilepich MV, Sicard GA, Breaux SR et al. Renal graft irradiation in acute rejection. Transplantation 1983; 35:208.

21. Ruers TJM, Buurman WA, van der Linden CJ et al. Renal pro-drugs offer new perspectives in immunosuppressive therapy. Transplant Proc 1986; 18:907.

SECTION B:
PUMP-BASED LOCAL INFUSION IN RAT ALLOGRAFT MODELS

CHAPTER 4

SELECTIVE IMMUNOSUPPRESSION BY LOCAL TREATMENT OF THE ALLOGRAFT:
STUDIES ON INTRARENAL PREDNISOLONE AND INTRACARDIAC BUDESONIDE DELIVERY IN THE RAT

T. J. M. Ruers

So far immunosuppressive therapy after organ transplantation consists of systemic inhibition of the immune response. Recently however, controversy has increased concerning the role of systemic versus local regulatory mechanisms in the cellular immune response.[1,2] Immune stimulation by major histocompatibility complex (MHC) antigen expression has been seen as a local as well as a systemic process in both allograft rejection and autoimmune disease.[3-9] The same controversy holds true for the effector mechanisms during cellular immune responses.[1,2,10-13] If however, local regulatory mechanisms within the graft are of major importance during the rejection response, the allograft would be a favorable subject for local immunosuppressive therapy. In this way, allograft survival could be induced by local immunosuppression within the graft, while systemic side effects of immunosuppressive therapy are avoided. We have investigated this approach by local drug delivery to rat renal and cardiac allografts and were able to demonstrate that local treatment of allograft rejection is indeed an effective approach to induce selective immunosuppression.

IMMUNOLOGICAL ASPECTS OF LOCAL TREATMENT

Initially, it was studied whether local treatment of the allograft resulted in effective immunosuppression and hence prolongation of graft

Local Immunosuppression of Organ Transplants, edited by Scott A. Gruber.
© 1996 R.G. Landes Company.

survival.[14] Next, investigations were directed to the mechanisms by which local immunosuppression interfered with the rejection response.[15]

Kidneys were transplanted from Brown Norway (BN) rats to Lewis rats. Both recipient native kidneys were removed and graft survival was assessed by animal survival. Local immunosuppression was provided by delivery of prednisolone into the renal artery of the transplanted kidney.[4] For this purpose, a polyethylene catheter was introduced in the suprarenal or testicular artery of the transplanted kidney (Fig. 4.1). The catheter was secured to the vessel, preventing the tip of the cannula from protruding into the arterial lumen. The cath-eter was connected to an osmotic mini-pump implanted in the abdominal cavity. The osmotic minipump delivered the drug in a continuous fashion for 13 days. For systemic intravenous (i.v.) drug delivery, a catheter was introduced into the jugular vein, guided to the abdominal cavity, and connected to the osmotic minipump. The technique of intrarenal drug delivery itself proved to have no detrimental or enhancing effects on renal allograft survival (Table 4.1). To study the effect of local immunosuppression on renal allograft survival, various prednisolone treatments were tested. The drug was administered by continuous infusion (intrarenal, i.v. or intraperitoneal [i.p.]) or by i.p. bolus injection,

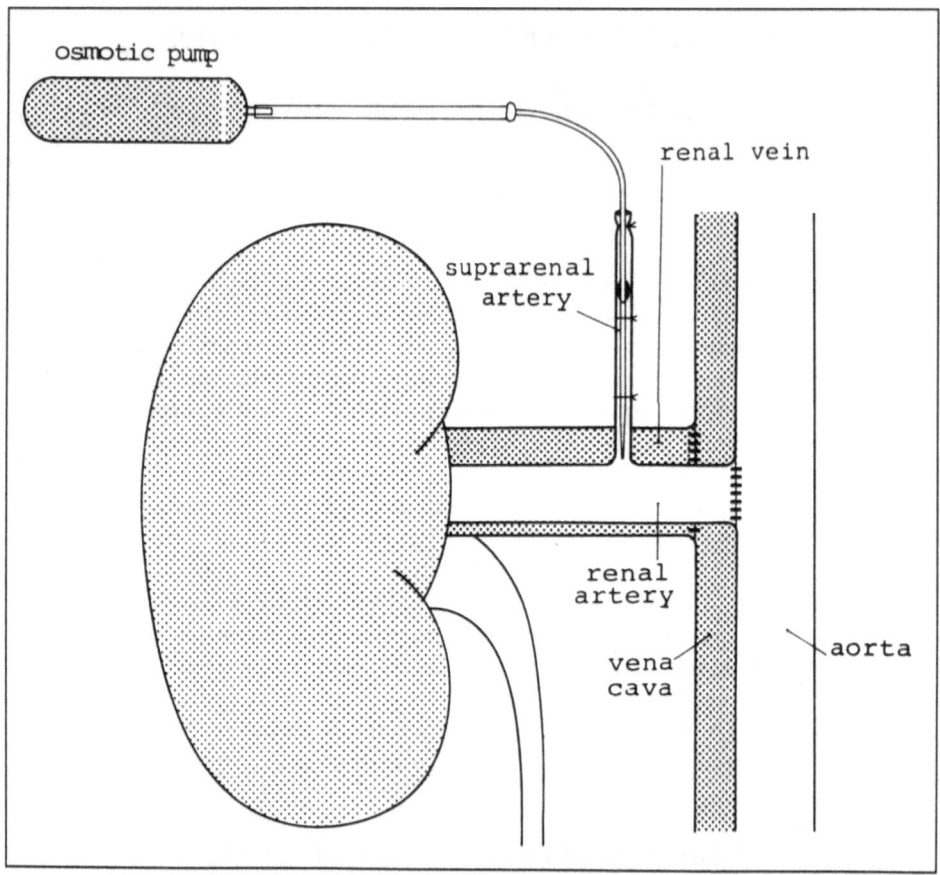

Fig. 4.1. Schematic outline of the experimental model used for drug infusion into the renal artery of a transplanted kidney. A catheter is introduced into the suprarenal (or testicular) artery of the transplanted kidney and connected to an osmotic minipump implanted in the abdominal cavity. The osmotic minipump delivers the drug in a continuous fashion from day 0 until day 13. Reproduced with permission from Ruers TJM et al, Local treatment of renal allografts, a promising way to reduce the dosage of immunosuppressive drugs. Transplantation 1986; 41:156.

and dose response studies were performed (Table 4.2). Intrarenal administration of prednisolone appeared to be superior to any other way of drug administration. A low dose of 4 mg/kg/day, given by continuous intrarenal infusion, resulted in significant prolongation of graft survival, whereas continuous systemic administration of this dose was not effective. In order to induce prolongation of graft survival with systemic administration, the dose had to be at least doubled. Intrarenal prednisolone delivery (4 mg/kg/day) produced kidney prednisolone levels twice as high as those during same-dose systemic i.p. administration of the drug,[15] whereas systemic drug levels during both intrarenal and i.p. administration were comparable (Table 4.3). These systemic drug levels were by themselves not sufficiently immunosuppressive to induce graft survival since systemic prednisolone infusion at a dose of 4 mg/kg/day did not result in significant prolongation of graft survival. These findings

Table 4.1. Effect of the intrarenal infusion technique upon the survival and the serum urea levels of Lewis rats receiving BN renal allografts

Treatment	Survival (days)	MST[a]	Day 3 urea (mg/100ml)[b]
–	7.7.8.8 8.9.9	8	111 ± 50
Saline Intrarenal	6.7.7.7.7 7.8.12	7	127 ± 47

a. MST = median survival time
b. Mean serum urea levels ± SD
Reproduced with permission from Ruers TJM et al, Local treatment of renal allografts, a promising way to reduce the dosage of immunosuppressive drugs. Transplantation 1986; 41:156.

Table 4.2. Effect of various prednisolone treatments upon the survival of Lewis rats receiving BN renal allografts

Daily i.p. Injection			Continuous Infusion					
Prednisolone (mg/kg/day)	Survival (days)	MST[a]	Intraperitoneal Survival (days)	MST	Intravenous Survival (days)	MST	Intrarenal Survival (days)	MST
4	7.7.7.7.7 8.8.10.11	7	9.9.9.9 9.10.10	9	7.7.7.8 9.15.18 11	8.5	17.17.18 26.26>50 >50	26[b]
8	7.7.7.8.8 8.8.32	8	9.9.10.14 18.20.41 >50	16[c]				
12	7.7.7.8 8.10.10	8						

a MST = Median survival time (days).
b Wilcoxon rank test for difference between animals treated with continuous intrarenal infusion of prednisolone (4 mg/kg body wt/day) and animals treated with this dose by continuous i.v. infusion (P < 0.05), continuous i.p. infusion (P < 0.01), or i.p. bolus injections (P < 0.01).
c Wilcoxon rank test for difference between animals treated with continuous i.p. infusion (8 mg/kg body wt/day) and animals treated with this dose by i.p. bolus injections (P < 0.01).
Reproduced with permission from Ruers TJM et al, Local treatment of renal allografts, a promising way to reduce the dosage of immunosuppressive drugs. Transplantation 1986; 41:156.

Table 4.3. Graft survival and mean prednisolone levels in plasma and renal allografts during continuous delivery of prednisolone intrarenally or intraperitoneally

Therapy	Mean ($\pm$ SD) Prednisolone Level on Day 3		MST* (days)	n
	Plasma (ng/ml)	Renal Allograft (ng/kidney)		
4 mg/kg continuously intraperitoneally	$46 \pm 8^+$	$126 \pm 21^§$	9**	9
4 mg/kg continuously intrarenally	$53 \pm 14^+$	$213 \pm 80^§$	28**	9

* MST = median graft survival time as determined in graft survival studies. MST in untreated controls is 8 days.

\+ Wilcoxon rank test for difference between plasma prednisolone levels in animals treated i.p. and intrarenally is not significant.

§ Wilcoxon rank test for difference between prednisolone levels in renal allografts of animals treated i.p. and intrarenally ($P < 0.05$).

** Wilcoxon rank test for difference between MST in animals treated i.p. and intrarenally with prednisolone ($P < 0.01$).

Reproduced from The Journal of Experimental Medicine 1987; 166:1205 by copyright permission of The Rockefeller University Press.

indicate that local drug levels within the graft were responsible for the immunosuppressive effect obtained during local graft treatment.

Next we investigated local regulatory mechanisms in graft rejection and their response to local immunosuppressive therapy.[15] For this purpose, local immunosuppression was provided by intrarenal prednisolone infusion at a dose of 4 mg/kg/day, and control animals were either untreated or received prednisolone 4 mg/kg/day i.p. Animals were sacrificed on days 3, 7 and 12 after transplantation, and immunohistological studies were performed. Untreated animals showed intense infiltration of host MHC class II positive cells throughout the kidney together with marked destruction of renal tissue (Table 4.4). In animals treated with prednisolone i.p. (median survival time [MST] 9 days), cellular infiltration was somewhat postponed compared with the untreated animals; however, eventually dense infiltration of MHC class II cells was observed together with marked destruction of the graft.

The histological picture of animals treated intrarenally was completely different from that in untreated and i.p.-treated animals. Intrarenally treated grafts also showed distinct cellular infiltration with host MHC class II positive cells, but in contrast, extensive tissue damage and necrosis of the graft was absent (Table 4.4). The phenotypic composition of the cellular infiltrate in the renal allografts after various treatments was comparable, except for the fact that intrarenally-treated grafts showed less infiltration with macrophages than the untreated and i.p.-treated animals (Table 4.5). Apparently, the cellular infiltrate that was present in the intrarenally-treated grafts was not able to induce graft destruction. To study this observation in further detail, grafts were stained for IL-2 receptor expression, the presence of interferon-gamma (IFN-γ), and the expression of MHC class II antigens on renal tissue (Table 4.4). Untreated rats and rats treated with prednisolone i.p. showed cells positive for IL-2 receptor and IFN-γ within the graft, as well as distinct staining of MHC class II antigens on renal tissue. Completely different results were obtained in animals treated intrarenally. Grafts from these animals showed almost no staining for IL-2 receptor expression and IFN-γ, despite the presence of cellular infiltrates. Moreover, these animals failed to show MHC class II expression on renal tissue, except for some weak staining on day 7. From these observations, it may be concluded that local prednisolone levels within the graft do not primarily interfere with cellular infiltration

Table 4.4. Immunohistological observations in rat renal allografts after various prednisolone treatments

Therapy	Area Infiltrated by MHC Class II Positive Host Cells (His19+)*	IL–2 Receptor on Infiltrating cells (ART18+)	Presence of IFN–γ (DB1⁺)	MHC Class II Expression on Tubules (OX6+)	Graft Destruction, Edema, Hemorrhage, Necrosis**
BN → BN Untreated Day 7***	6 ± 1	–	–	–	–
BN →Lewis Untreated					
Day 3	15 ± 4	+/–	+/–	+	–
Day 7	30 ± 7	+	+	+++	+++
BN→Lewis 4 mg/kg i.p.					
Day 3	6 ± 1	–	–	–	–
Day 7	33 ± 7	+	+	++	++/+++
BN→Lewis 4 mg/kg intrarenally					
Day 3	5 ± 1	–	–	–	–
Day 7	27 ± 6	+/–	+/–	+	–
Day 12	20 ± 5	–	–	–	–

Data represent consistent observations made in all rats of the experimental group (n = 4 or 5).

* In the BN (Rtⁿ) → Lewis (Rtˡ) strain combination, MHC class II antigens on host cells were identified with the monoclonal antibody His19, which reacts with MHC class II antigens of rat strains of haplotype L, but not with class II antigens of rat strains of haplotype N. In the BN → BN strain combination, class II antigens on infiltrating cells were identified with OX6, which recognizes rat class II antigens of the rat strains of haplotype L and N. Results are expressed as the percentage area of the tissue section infiltrated by class II positive cells. Data given are mean values ± SD.

** Examined on routine H and E staining.

*** Day after grafting

Reproduced from The Journal of Experimental Medicine 1987; 166:1205 by copyright permission of The Rockefeller University Press.

within the graft but interfere with IL-2 receptor expression, IFN-γ production and MHC class II induction on grafted tissue.

In conclusion, these data demonstrate that local prednisolone levels within the graft can result in effective immunosuppression. Moreover, the data indicate the presence of local regulatory mechanisms in graft rejection. To further strengthen the evidence for the efficacy of local graft treatment, a special heart transplantation model was developed.[16] In this model, systemic blood levels of the immunosuppressive drug could be minimized by transplanting cardiac allografts in such way that venous blood flow from the graft directly entered the liver of the recipient via an anastomo-sis between the graft and the portal vein. These heterotopic cardiac transplants were performed from BN to Lewis strain rats, while the native heart of the recipient animal remained functionally in situ. Donor hearts were anastomosed to the recipient using an end-to-side anastomosis between donor descending aorta and recipient abdominal aorta. Venous outflow was created by end-to-side anastomosis of donor pulmonary artery to recipient portal vein (Fig. 4.2). In this heart transplantation model, blood flow is reversed in the thoracic aorta. The aortic valves are automatically closed and blood runs via the coronary arteries, myocardium and coronary veins into the right atrium and ventricle.

Table 4.5. Phenotypic composition of the cellular infiltrate in rat renal allografts after various prednisolone treatments*

Therapy	Percentage Area Infiltrated by Positive Cells**				
	OX19 T cells	W3/25 Th	OX8 Tc/s	W3/25 + OX8*** Th, Tc/s	ED2 Macro-phages
BN → Lewis untreated	24 ± 6	28 ± 5	29 ± 7	37 ± 6	38 ± 11
BN → Lewis 4 mg/kg i.p.	21 ± 5	25 ± 6	27 ± 7	37 ± 9	31 ± 8
BN → Lewis 4 mg/kg intrarenally	20 ± 4	23 ± 4	26 ± 6	32 ± 8	18± 6

*   Immunohistological studies were performed on grafts removed on day 7 after transplantation.
** Data given are mean values ± SD. n = 5 per group.
*** Stained simultaneously with W3/25 and OX8.
Reproduced from The Journal of Experimental Medicine 1987; 166:1205 by copyright permission of The Rockefeller University Press.

Venous blood passes via the pulmonary artery into the portal vein and enters the liver. Heartbeat can be checked daily by palpation through the abdominal wall, and rejection is taken to be the complete absence of ventricular contraction (MST of untreated animals is 7 days). Local immunosuppression was provided by infusion of the steroid budesonide directly into the transplanted aorta for 13 days. For this purpose, a catheter was introduced into the left carotid artery of the transplant and connected to an osmotic minipump implanted into the abdominal cavity. The steroid budesonide is rapidly cleared by the liver and cardiac tissue binding of the drug is high, which means that the pharmacological properties of the drug in combination with the characteristics of the transplantation model made it possible to accurately measure the effect of local immunosuppressive therapy.[16] Hence, local budesonide administration,120 µg/kg/day, produced high drug levels within the graft (29.6 ng/mg) and low systemic drug levels (0.34 ng/ml) (Table 4.6), whereas budesonide 120 µg/kg/day administered directly into the jugular vein produced comparable drug levels within the graft (31.0 ng/mg) but significantly higher drug levels systemically (1.65 ng/ml). To analyze whether the low systemic plasma levels during local budesonide administration had any systemic biological effects, normal nontransplanted Lewis rats were treated with budesonide 120 µg/kg/day for 10 days delivered directly into the portal vein. At that time, body weight, spleen weight, thymus weight, adrenal weight and leukocyte count were determined. For comparison, another group of normal animals was treated with budesonide 120 µg/kg/day administered systemically into the jugular vein.

As shown in Table 4.7, budesonide delivered directly into the portal vein, which mimics the situation during local graft treatment, did not induce systemic toxicity. All data obtained in this group were similar to the data of control animals, which received only the solvent (propandiol 66%) administered directly into the portal vein. In contrast, however, budesonide administered i.v. showed strong systemic toxicity. Body weight, spleen weight, thymus weight, and adrenal weight of the systemically-treated animals were significantly lower than of those of the control animals

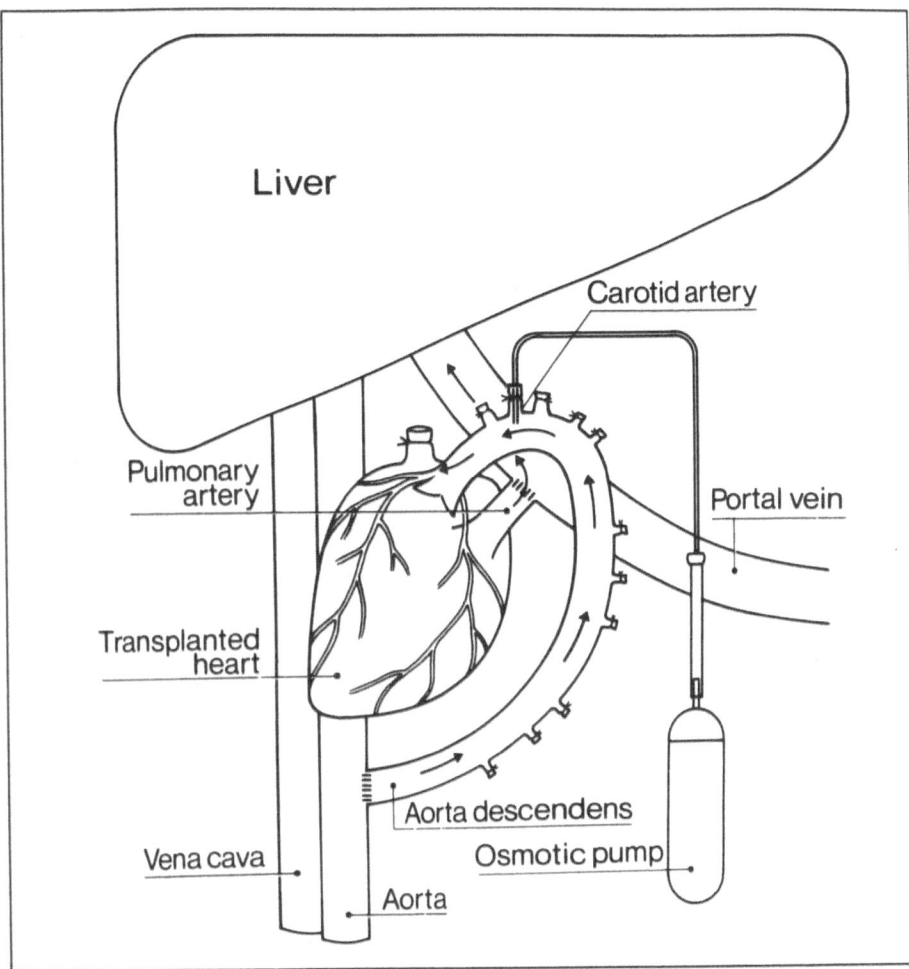

Fig. 4.2. Schematic outline of the experimental model used. Cardiac transplants were performed with end-to-side anastomosis between donor descending aorta and recipient abdominal aorta. Venous outflow was created by end-to-side anastomosis between donor pulmonary artery and recipient portal vein. In the transplantation model, blood flow is reversed as indicated. For local drug administration, a catheter was introduced into the left carotid artery of the transplanted aorta and connected to an osmotic minipump. Reproduced with permission from Ruers TJM et al, Sensitivity of grafy rejection in rats to local immunosuppresive therapy. Transplantation 1988; 46:820.

and the animals treated with budesonide administered directly into the portal vein. Both local and systemic administration of budesonide, 120 µg/kg/day for 13 days, resulted in significant prolongation of graft survival (Table 4.8); MST was 19.5 days and 20 days, respectively, compared with 7 days in controls. These data demonstrate that allograft rejection can be treated locally without significant systemic immunosuppression and confirmed our earlier results using prednisolone in the rat kidney transplantation model.

The data obtained in the studies mentioned above clearly demonstrate that local treatment of the graft is an effective way to induce selective immunosuppression. Our findings are in agreement with those studies advocating a central role of local regulatory mechanisms during allograft rejection.[4,5,9-13] For example, it was demonstrated that cytotoxic T-lymphocytes (Tc cells) could mature in sponge matrix allografts independent of the host systemic immune response from day 5 after transplantation.[11] This observation stimulated us

Table 4.6. Plasma and tissue levels of budesonide[a]

	Continuous Locally	Continuous i.v.
Infusion rate	25 ng/min	25 ng/min
Blood flow through graft	7.2 ± 0.5 ml/min	7.2 ± 0.5 ml/min
Systemic plasma (blood) concentration (Cs)	0.34 ± 0.1 ng/ml[b]	1.65 ± 0.6 ng/ml[b]
Concentration in graft[c]	29.6 ± 10.1 ng/mg	31.0 ± 11.0 ng/mg
Plasma (blood) clearance	15.2 ml/min	15.2 ml/min
Cs loc./Cs syst.	0.2	

a After transplantation, animals were treated for 5 days with budesonide 120 µg/kg body weight/day given by continuous local infusion or continuous i.v. infusion. At day 5, pharmacokinetic studies were performed. ^{3}H-budesonide and cold, unlabeled budesonide were infused together for 5 hr, while the total budesonide dose remained 120 µg/kg body weight/day. At t = 300 min, plasma levels and tissue levels of unchanged ^{3}H-budesonide were determined by HPLC. Budesonide concentrations are given as the total amount of unchanged budesonide calculated from the amount of unchanged ^{3}H-budesonide measured by HPLC. Animals weighed 300 ± 10 g, n = 6 per group. All data given are mean values ± SD.

b Wilcoxon rank test for difference between plasma levels in animals treated locally and intravenously, $P < 0.01$.

c Expressed in ng per mg tissue.

Reproduced with permission from Ruers TJM et al, Sensitivity of graft rejection in rats to local immunosuppressive therapy. Transplantation 1988; 46:820.

Table 4.7. Systemic biological effects of budesonide with different methods of administration[a]

	Propandiol 66%	Budesonide 120 µg/kg/day	
	Continuous Into Portal Vein	Continuous Into Portal Vein	Continuous Into Jugular Vein
Initial body weight (grams) day 0	313 ± 25	319 ± 24	322 ± 26
Data at day 10			
Body weight (grams)	297 ± 20	296 ± 12[b]	249 ± 20[d]
Leukocyte count x 10^6 cells/ml	18.5 ± 4.7	15.7 ± 3.0	14.8 ± 4.8
Spleen weight (mg)	768 ± 121	797 ± 150[c]	591 ± 137[e]
Thymus weight (mg)	293 ± 48	263 ± 22[b]	123 ± 67[d]
Adrenal weight (mg)	39.6 ± 4.4	37.5 ± 2.2[b]	25.5 ± 6.8[d]
n =	7	7	6

a   Normal Lewis rats received budesonide by continuous infusion into the jugular vein or by continuous infusion into the portal vein. Control animals received propandiol 66% by continuous infusion into the portal vein. All data given are mean values ± SD.

b,c Wilcoxon rank test for difference between animals treated with budesonide administered into the portal vein and animals treated with budesonide administered into the jugular vein: $^b P < 0.01$, $^c P < 0.05$. Differences between control animals and animals treated with budesonide administered into the portal vein were not significant.

d,e Wilcoxon rank test for difference between animals treated with budesonide administered into the jugular vein and control animals: $^d P < 0.01$, $^e P < 0.05$.

Reproduced with permission from Ruers TJM et al, Sensitivity of graft rejection in rats to local immunosuppressive therapy. Transplantation 1988; 46:820.

Table 4.8. The effect of various budesonide treatments upon heart allograft survival

| Budesonide µg/kg body weight/day | Continuous Locally | | Continuous i.v. | |
	Graft survival (days)	MST[a]	Graft Survival (days)	MST[a]
40	11,12,13,13, 14,15,16,20	13.5 ± 2.9[b]	8,9,12,13, 14,14,22	13 ± 4.6[b]
90	15,16,16, 18,18	16 ± 1.5[b]	13,16,16 16,18,19,22	16 ± 3.1[b]
120	15,17,18,19 20,20,21,21	19.5 ± 2.2[b]	17,17,18,19 21,22,22,23	20 ± 2.4[b]

a MST = median graft survival time ± SD.
b Wilcoxon rank test for difference between animals treated with budesonide and animals treated with the solvent ($P < 0.01$).
- Control animals were untreated or received continuous local infusion of the solvent.
   In both groups, MST was 7 days. Graft survival times (in days) in the untreated group were 6,6,6,7,7,8,8,9; graft survival times (in days) in the group treated locally with the solvent were 6,7,7,7,7,8,10,12.
- Rejection was taken as the complete absence of ventricular contraction and was confirmed by histopathological examination.
Reproduced with permission from Ruers TJM et al, Sensibility of graft rejection in rats to local immunosuppressive therapy. Transplantation 1988; 46:820.

to study in more detail to what extent infiltrating cells proliferate at the site of the allograft and whether proliferative behavior is changed during immunosuppressive therapy.

For this purpose, a 5'bromodeoxyuridine (BrdU) labeling technique was introduced[17,18] which allows the accurate detection of both proliferative activity and phenotypic characterization of cellular infiltrates within the allograft.[17] Heterotopic cardiac transplantation from BN to Lewis rats was performed as described earlier. To detect proliferative activity within the cardiac allografts, animals received BrdU, 50 mg/kg, by i.p. bolus injection. One hour after BrdU was administered, animals were killed and allografts excised. BrdU is incorporated into DNA during the S phase of the cell cycle and hence detection of BrdU is indicative of proliferative activity. Control tissues were removed together with the cardiac allografts. For immunosuppression, the steroid budesonide was administered by continuous infusion into the jugular vein for 13 days at a dose of 120 µg/kg/day, which produced a MST of 20 days versus 7 days in controls.

BrdU positive cells could clearly be identified among the infiltrating cells within the graft (Table 4.9). In the untreated recipients, T-cytotoxic/suppressor (Tc/s) cells as well as T helper (Th) cells showed proliferative activity at the site of the graft (Table 4.10). The percentage of OX8 positive cells within the grafts that showed proliferation ranged from 15% to 37%. The percentage of W3/25 positive cells within the grafts that showed proliferation ranged from 25% to 30%. In contrast, macrophages (ED2 positive cells) hardly demonstrated any proliferative activity within the graft, with only 1-4% of these cells staining positive for BrdU. In addition to the sponge matrix experiments performed by others, which showed proliferation of Tc cells within the graft,[11] we were able to detect proliferation of Th cells within the graft, which supports the link between delayed-type hypersensitivity and allograft rejection as suggested by others.[1,19-21] During systemic treatment with budesonide, a remarkable number of proliferative cells was still observed within the grafts, although signs of graft destruction were absent during treatment (Table 4.9).

Table 4.9. Histopathological observations and proliferative activity in untreated and budesonide-treated cardiac allografts

	Cellular Infiltrate	BrdU Positive Cells	Graft Destruction, Edema, Hemorrhage, Necrosis
Day 3 untreated[a]	+	+	-
Day 5 untreated	+++	+++	++
Day 3 budesonide [b]	+	+	-
Day 5 budesonide	++	++	-
Day 15 budesonide	+++	+++	++

a Cardiac transplantation was performed from BN to Lewis rats. On days 3 and 5 after transplantation, BrdU labeling was performed and grafts were subsequently excised. Grafts were analyzed for the presence of cellular infiltrate, BrdU positive cells and signs of graft destruction. Data represent consistent observations made in all rats of the experimental group (n = 4).

b Lewis recipients were treated with budesonide, 120 μg/kg/day, for 13 days. After BrdU labelling, grafts were excised on days 3, 5 and 15 after transplantation. Grafts were analyzed for the presence of cellular infiltrate, BrdU positive cells, and signs of graft destruction. Data represent consistent observations made in all rats of the experimental group (n = 4).

Reproduced with permission from Ruers TJM, et al. Cellular proliferation of the site of organ allografts and the influence of immunosuppressive therapy. Transplantation 1990; 50:568.

In the treated grafts, overall cellular infiltration was lower when compared with that in the untreated grafts; however, the percentage of Th cells and Tc/s cells that showed proliferation was comparable (Table 4.10). Cellular infiltration during effective immunosuppressive therapy has also been observed by others.[9,22-24] The fact, however, that infiltrating cells showed proliferative activity during treatment, while signs of graft destruction were absent, is striking. This finding questions the importance of the antiproliferative effect of steroids described extensively in vitro.[25-27] In contrast, it suggests the importance of other immunosuppressive effects of the drug, such as blocking the production of lymphokines and cytokines,[25,28-34] which may both play an essential role in mediating tissue destruction.[1,35] The observation that in budesonide-treated animals signs of graft destruction are absent despite the presence of proliferative cells within the graft is in concordance with our earlier findings that showed cellular infiltrates without graft destruction in kidney allografts in animals treated with prednisolone.

From the studies described above,[14-17] it can be concluded that inhibition of the immune response within the graft by local immunosuppressive treatment is an effective way to induce selective immunosuppression and represents a potentially important way to manipulate the immune response in organ transplantation. More recently our findings have been confirmed by Gruber et al[36-39] who demonstrated the efficacy of local immunosuppressive therapy in a canine renal transplant model (chapter 9).

PHARMACOLOGICAL AND THERAPEUTIC ASPECTS OF LOCAL TREATMENT

So far, it has been demonstrated that allograft rejection can be treated locally. Moreover, it was shown that local immunosuppression can reduce systemic side effects while treatment of the target organ, the allograft, still remains optimal. Generally, the advantage of local over systemic drug delivery is related to the ratio of drug concentrations produced (locally and systemically) during local and systemic drug administration[40,41] (see chapter 2). Accordingly, the pharmacokinetic advantage of local drug delivery can be classified as regional or systemic. Regional advantage is defined as the gain in drug concentration at the target organ (e.g., the graft) during

Table 4.10. *Phenotypic composition of the cellular infiltrate and relation to proliferative activity in cardiac allografts on day 5 after transplantation in untreated and budesonide-treated animals*

	Percentage Area Infiltrated by Positive Cells				Percentage of Cells Positive for Relevant Phenotype Positively Staining for BrdU*		
	OX8 Tc, Ts	W3/25 Th	ED2 mφ		OX8 Tc, Ts	W3/25 Th	ED2 mφ
Untreated Animals							
510	18	8	17		37	27	3
511	20	11	20		18	30	4
512	26	10	26		15	25	1
513	19	9	21		30	26	3
Budesonide Animals							
540	9	3	13		22	31	2
541	6	3	6		35	34	9
542	11	4	8		20	32	5
543	11	5	12		30	26	3

mφ = macrophage
Cardiac transplantation was performed from BN to Lewis rats. After BrdU labeling, allografts were excised on day 5 after transplantation and immunohistological studies were performed.

$$* = \frac{\text{cells positive for relevant phenotype as well as positive for BrdU staining}}{\text{cells positive for relevant phenotype}} \times 100\%$$

Reproduced with permission from Ruers TJM, et al. Cellular proliferation of the site of organ allografts and the influence of immunosuppressive therapy. Transplantation 1990; 50:568.

local over systemic drug administration, and was obtained in the kidney transplantation model. During intrarenal prednisolone infusion, drug levels within the graft were twice as high as those obtained during systemic drug delivery, while systemic drug levels were comparable. The regional advantage achieved by local administration could be used to lower the dose of prednisolone during local delivery, when compared with systemic delivery, without losing immunosuppressive effect. A reduction in systemic drug concentration, or systemic advantage, is obtained during local drug administration if the drug is rapidly cleared by the target organ to which it is delivered or shortly thereafter. Systemic advantage was obtained in the heart transplantation model in which budesonide was rapidly cleared by the liver shortly after it was infused into the target organ, the transplanted heart. Compared with systemic budesonide administration, this approach resulted in lower systemic drug levels.

Regarding local immunosuppressive therapy, several options exist by which an immunosuppressive drug, suitable for local application, can be delivered to the graft (target tissue). In our studies, local immunosuppression was produced by continuous infusion of the drug into the artery supplying the graft. In this model, the advantage of local immunosuppressive therapy can be realized when the immunosuppressant is cleared by the graft or shortly thereafter. This approach, mainly leading to systemic advantage, is applicable to kidney and liver transplants, since both organs possess clearing capacities. When the immunosuppressive drug infused into the artery supplying the graft is not cleared by the graft, local drug delivery can still be of advantage (regional) when the systemic clearance of the drug is high and the blood flow through the target organ (graft) is low.[40,41] Since blood flow through rejecting allografts decreases significantly, this approach would be applicable to antirejection therapy. In 1969, Kountz and Cohn,[42] and later Laupacis et al[43] demonstrated excellent graft survival rates in renal transplant patients treated with intrarenal delivery of methylprednisolone over a short period of time immediately after transplantation or during rejection episodes (chapter 3). However, at that time, intra-arterial infusion of the drug into the graft had serious drawbacks, such as infection and thrombosis, both of which limited clinical application. Nowadays, intraarterial drug delivery to the graft may become clinically applicable by means of biocompatible catheters and programmable, implantable infusion pumps. Depending, however, on the site of the graft and the pharmacokinetic properties of the drug, other routes of administration may be used for local treatment. For example, oral administration and aerosols may be used in liver and lung transplant recipients, respectively.

Besides the possibilities mentioned above, several drug targeting systems are under investigation at the moment. For organ transplants, site-specific drug delivery via prodrugs may be an attractive approach to local immunosuppression.[41,44,45] Pro drugs are agents which must undergo biotransformation prior to exerting their pharmacological effects. Taking advantage of unique characteristics of cells or tissues, it is possible to design prodrugs which are cell- or tissue-specific.[44] According to these principles, drugs can be developed which are by themselves inactive, but within the specific organ, e.g., kidney or liver, they undergo change into the active drug by local enzymatic reactions highly specific for the organ. When the active compound fulfils the above pharmacokinetic criteria, such as high clearance by the target organ or shortly thereafter, this approach can result in high local drug levels and low systemic drug levels. According to the results of our experiments described herein as well as the findings of others,[36-39] the development of prodrugs which permit localized immunosuppression of certain defined grafts would open new perspectives in immunosuppressive therapy.

References

1. Ascher NL, Hoffman R, Hanto DW et al. Intragraft rejection mechanisms. Immunol Rev 1984; 77:217.
2. Häyry P. Intragraft events in allograft destruction. Transplantation 1984; 38:1.
3. Hanafusa T, Pujol-Borell R, Chiovato L et al. Aberrant expression of HLA-DR antigen on thymocytes in Grave's disease: relevance for auto-immunity. Lancet 1983; 2:1111.
4. De Waal RMV, Bogman MJJ, Maass CN et al. Variable expression of Ia antigens on vascular endothelium of mouse skin grafts. Nature 1983; 303:426.
5. Hall BM, Bishop GA, Duggin GG et al. Increased expression of HLA-DR antigens on renal tubular cells in renal transplants: relevance to the rejection response. Lancet 1984; 2:247.
6. Sobel RA, Blanchette BW, Bahn AK et al. The immunopathology of experimental allergic encephalomyelitis. II. Endothelial cell Ia increases prior to inflammatory cell infiltration. J Immunol 1984; 132:2402.
7. Wadgymar A, Urmson J, Baumal R et al. Changes in Ia expression in mouse kidney during acute graft versus host disease. J Immunol 1984; 132:1826.
8. Clarke Forbes RD, Parfrey NA, Gomersall M et al. Dendritic cell-lymphoid cell aggregation and major histocompatibility antigen expression during rat cardiac allograft rejection. J Exp Med 1986; 164:1239.
9. Häyry P, von Willebrand E. The influence of the pattern of inflammation and admin-

istration of steroid on class II MHC antigen expression in renal transplants. Transplantation 1986; 42:358.

10. Nemlander A, Soots A, von Willebrand E et al. Redistribution of renal allograft-responding leucocytes during rejection. II. Kinetics and specificity. J Exp Med 1982; 156:1087.

11. Ascher NL, Chen S, Hoffman RA et al. Maturation of cytotoxic T cells within sponge matrix allografts. J Immunol 1983; 131:617.

12. Orosz CG, Zinn NE, Sirinek L et al. In vivo mechanisms of alloreactivity. I. Frequency of donor-reactive cytotoxic T lymphocytes in sponge matrix allografts. Transplantation 1986; 41:75.

13. Orosz CG, Zinn NE, Sirinek L et al. In vivo mechanisms of alloreactivity. II. Allospecificity of cytotoxic T lymphocytes in sponge matrix allografts as determined by limiting dilution analysis. Transplantation 1986; 41:84.

14. Ruers TJM, Buurman WA, Smits JFM et al. Local treatment of renal allografts, a promising way to reduce the dosage of immunosuppressive drugs. Transplantation 1986; 41:156.

15. Ruers TJM, Buurman WA, van Boxtel CJ et al. Immunohistological observations in rat kidney allografts after local steroid administration. J Exp Med 1987; 166:1205.

16. Ruers TJM, Daemen MJAP, Thijssen HHW et al. Sensitivity of graft rejection in rats to local immunosuppressive therapy. Transplantation 1988; 46:820.

17. Ruers TJM, Schutte B, van der Linden CJ et al. Cellular proliferation at the site of organ allografts and the influence of immunosuppressive therapy. Transplantation 1990; 50:568.

18. Schutte B, Reynders MMJ, Bosman FT et al. Studies with anti-bromodeoxyuridine antibodies. II Simultaneous immunocytochemical detection of antigen expression and DNA synthesis by in vivo labeling of mouse intestinal mucosa. J Histochem Cytochem 1987; 35:371.

19. Loveland BE, Hogarth PM, Ceredig RH et al. Cells mediating graft rejection in mouse. I. Lyt-1 cells mediate skin graft rejection. J Exp Med 1981; 153:1044.

20. Lowry RP, Gurley KE, Clarke Forbes RD. Immune mechanisms in organ allograft rejection. I. Delayed-type hypersensitivity and lymphocytotoxicity in heart graft rejection. Transplantation 1983; 36:391.

21. Lowry RP, Margehesco DM, Blackburn JH. Immune mechanisms in organ allograft rejection. VI. Delayed-type hypersensitivity and lymphotoxin in experimental renal allograft rejection. Transplantation 1985; 40:183.

22. Homan WP, Fabre JW, Wiliams KA et al. Studies on the immunosuppressive properties of cyclosporin A in rats receiving renal allografts. Transplantation 1980; 29:361.

23. Homan WP, Fabre JW, Millard PR et al. Effect of cyclosporin A upon second set rejection of rat renal allografts. Transplantation 1980; 30:354.

24. Mason DW, Morris PJ. Inhibition of the accumulation in rat kidney allografts of specific but not non-specific-cytotoxic cells by cyclosporine. Transplantation 1984; 37:46.

25. Cupps TR, Fauci AS. Corticosteroid-mediated immunoregulation in man. Immunol Rev 1982; 65:133.

26. Roath S, Cuppari G. The effects of steroids on cultured lymphocytes. Clin Res 1965; 13:542.

27. Rosenberg JC, Lysz K. Suppression of the immune response by steroids. Transplantation 1980; 29:425.

28. Dupont E, Wybran J, Toussaint C. Glucocorticosteroid and organ transplantation. Transplantation 1984; 37:331.

29. Dupont E, Huygen K, Schandené L et al. Influence of in vivo immunosuppressive drugs on production of lymphokines. Transplantation 1985; 39:143.

30. Arya SK, Wong-Staal F, Gallo RC. Dexamethasone-mediated inhibition of human T cell growth factor and gamma-interferon mRNA. J Immunol 1984; 133:273.

31. Snyder DS, Unanue ER. Corticosteroids inhibit murine macrophage Ia expression and interleukin 1 production. J Immunol 1982; 129:1803.

32. Larsson EL. Cyclosporin A and dexamethasone suppress T cell responses by selectively acting at distinct sites of the triggering process. J Immunol 1980; 124:2828.

33. Gillis S, Crabtree GR, Smith KA. Glucocorticoid induced inhibition of T cell growth factor production. I. The effect on mitogen induced lymphocyte proliferation. J Immunol 1979; 123:16.

34. Waage A, Bakke O. Glucocorticosteroids suppress the production of tumor necrosis factor by lipopolysaccharide stimulated human monocytes. Immunology 1988; 63:299.

35. Lowry RP, Blais D, Marghesco D et al. Immune effector mechanisms in organ allograft rejection. VIII: Inflammatory mediators and cytotoxins in rejecting rat cardiac allografts. Transplants Proc 1987; 19:426.

36. Gruber SA, Canafax DM, Erdmann GR et al. The pharmacokinetic advantage of local 6-mercaptopurine infusion in a canine renal transplant model. Transplantation 1989; 48:928.

37. Gruber SA. The case for local immunosuppression. Transplantion 1992; 54:1.

38. Gruber SA, Erdmann GR, Burke BA et al. Mizoribine pharmacokinetics and pharmacodynamics in a canine renal allograft model of local immunosuppression. Transplantation 1992; 53:12.

39. Gruber SA, Hrushesky WJM, Cipolle RJ et al. Local immunosuppression with reduced systemic toxicity in a canine renal allograft model. Transplantation 1989; 48:936.

40. Daemen M. Local drug administration: an experimental study on its possibilities and limitations. Thesis, M. Daemen, 1987, University of Limburg, The Netherlands.

41. Smits JFM, Thijssen HHW. Spatial control of drug action: theoretical considerations on the pharmacokinetics of target-aimed drug delivery. In: HAJ Struyker-Boudier, ed. Rate controlled drug administration and action. CRC Press, 1986.

42. Kountz SL, Cohn R. Initial treatment of renal allografts with large intrarenal doses of immunosuppressive drugs. Lancet 1969; 1:338.

43. Laupacis A, Keown PA, Rankin RN et al. Intraarterial methylprednisolone and heparin for the treatment of refractory renal transplant rejection episodes. Tranplant Proc 1982; 14:693.

44. Bundgaard H. Design of pro-drugs. Amsterdam: Elsevier Science Publisher B.V., 1985.

45. Orlowski M, Mizoguchi H, Wilk S. N-acyl-γ-glutamyl derivatives of sulfamethoxazole as models of kidney selective prodrugs. J Pharmacol Exp Ther 1980; 212:167.

LOCAL IMMUNOSUPPRESSION OF RAT CARDIAC, LIVER, AND SMALL BOWEL ALLOGRAFTS

Mou-er Wang, Stanislaw M. Stepkowski and Barry D. Kahan

INTRODUCTION

Allotransplantation plays a critical role in the treatment of patients with end-stage renal, cardiac, hepatic and pulmonary diseases. Although systemic administration of immunosuppressive agents prevents graft rejection, toxic side effects cause the dysfunction of vital organs including kidney, liver and bone marrow.[1-3] In addition, current immunosuppression is associated with an increased incidence of infection, diabetes, hypertension and malignancy in transplant recipients. To overcome these problems, different approaches are under consideration: (1) improvement of immunosuppressive protocols by development of new nontoxic drugs;[4] (2) application of synergistic drug combinations to reduce individual drug doses, hence to decrease toxic side effects;[5] (3) donor or graft pretreatment to reduce graft-versus-host immune response for small bowel transplantation[6] and (4) local delivery of immunosuppressive agents to directly block intragraft events with reduction of systemic drug concentrations.[7]

INTRAGRAFT IMMUNE RESPONSE

The rationale for local immunosuppression is based upon the fact that the majority of immunological events during rejection occur at the graft site. Alloantigens are recognized either directly as intact molecules present on cell membranes (direct recognition) or indirectly as allopeptides following antigen processing and presentation by antigen presenting cells (APC; indirect recognition).[8] T cells recognize allodeterminants through the T cell receptor (TCR); activation of T cells requires a second signal

Local Immunosuppression of Organ Transplants, edited by Scott A. Gruber.
© 1996 R.G. Landes Company.

that is delivered by the interaction of B7 and CD28 molecules.[2] In similar fashion, B cells recognize allodeterminants through the B cell receptor (BCR); activation of B cells also requires a second signal that is delivered via CD40/CD40-ligand molecules.[10] Adhesion molecules facilitate the interaction of T cells, B cells and other leukocytes, and control attachment of host cells to the endothelium of and extravasation of cells into the allograft.[11] The local immune events are regulated by cytokines that are produced by different cells. T helper 1 (Th1) and Th2 cells have distinct profiles of cytokine production, and these cytokines activate leukocytes by binding to specific dimer receptors, each consisting of one private and one public chain.[12] Activated effector cells mediate graft destruction. Thus, interference with the immune events directly at the graft site may be the most effective way to block allograft rejection.

The cell surface structures recognized by T cells include major histocompatibility complex (MHC) antigens. The class I and II MHC genes exhibit extreme polymorphism.[13] The class I MHC molecule is expressed as a membrane-bound glycoprotein heavy chain (65 kD), that is nonconvalently associated with a β_2-microglobulin (β_2m; 12 kD) light chain. The heavy chain consists of polymorphic $\alpha1$ and $\alpha2$ and nonpolymorphic $\alpha3$ extracellular [90 amino acid (a.a.) residues], transmembrane (25 a.a.) and intracellular (12 a.a.) domains.[14] The class II MHC consists of two extracellular domains of α ($\alpha1$ and $\alpha2$) and β ($\beta1$ and β_2) chains.[15] Class I MHC molecules are expressed on the surface of almost all nucleated cells, whereas class II MHC molecules are expressed on lymphoid tissue including dendritic cells and B cells, both of which are involved in antigen presentation.

The direct recognition of alloantigens at the graft site induces a strong immune response, because the frequencies of host alloantigen-specific T cell precursors are 10- to 100-fold higher in comparison to those against other nominal antigens.[9] Acute allograft rejection is primarily mediated following direct recognition of allogeneic MHC molecules. Alloantigens shed from the graft migrate to the lymph nodes and spleen to be processed and presented as allopeptides by APC.[16-24] Selection of allopeptides for presentation depends upon peptide concentration, the efficiency of peptide transport through the endoplasmic reticulum, and most importantly, upon the presence of motif-residues (anchors) on peptides. Allopeptides of 8-10 residues in length bind to class I MHC and peptides of 12-24 residues in length bind to class II MHC. Activated T effector cells migrate from lymph nodes and spleen through the blood stream to the allograft where they mediate graft destruction.[19-21]

A TCR consists of covalently linked α and β chains;[25] both chains have variable (v) and constant regions, and the diversity in v regions allows for the selection of T cells with different specificities. The activation of T cells results from the complex signals delivered by the TCR, and the CD28/B7 molecules.[26] In addition, T cell activation may be facilitated by coreceptors (CD4/class II MHC, CD8/class I MHC) and molecules that increase avidity β_2 integrins/ immunoglobulin (Ig)-related cell adhesion molecules (Ig-CAM)]. Activated CD4$^+$ Th1 cells produce interleukin-2 (IL-2), interferon-γ (IFN-γ), and tumor necrosis factor (TNF), and Th2 cells produce IL-4, IL-5, IL-6, IL-10, and IL-13. Furthermore, CD4$^+$ T cells may differentiate into T delayed-type hypersensitivity (T$_{DTH}$) cells and CD8$^+$ T cells into T cytotoxic (T$_c$) effector cells that mediate allograft destruction.

Resting B cells bind antigen by Ig that serves as the BCR.[10] The diversity of BCRs is generated by the v regions of light and heavy chains, but in contrast to T cells, the B cell response is not MHC-restricted.[10] The activation of B cells and Ig class switching depends upon signals delivered by the BCR and CD40/CD40 ligand interaction.[27] In the mouse system, IL-4 and IL-13 control Bμ (IgM) class switching to Bγ1(IgG1) and Bϵ(IgE), transforming growth factor-β (TGF-β) regulates Bμ

switching to Bγ2a(IgG2a); and IFN-γ regulates Bμ switching to Bγ2b(IgG2b). Antibodies may mediate hyperacute, acute or chronic allograft rejection.

LOCAL IMMUNOSUPPRESSION OF HEART ALLOGRAFTS

The effectiveness of local versus systemic low-dose cyclosporine (CsA; 2.0 mg/kg/day) treatment delivered by a 14 day osmotic pump was examined in a rat heterotopic cardiac allograft model.[28] Systemic intravenous (i.v.) continuous infusion of CsA (2.0 mg/kg/day) to Wistar Furth (WF; RT1^u) recipients slightly prolonged the mean survival time (MST ± SD) of Buffalo (BUF; RT1^b) heart allografts from 6.8 ± 1.2 days in untreated controls to 13.6 ± 1.3 days (Table 5.1). In contrast, intragraft delivery of CsA (2.0 mg/kg/day) significantly extended graft survival (40.4 ± 2.0 days; P < 0.001). Furthermore, local CsA infusion achieved high drug levels within the graft (11.08 ± 5.44 ng/mg), in contradistinction to drug concentrations at the graft site after systemic drug delivery (1.3 ± 0.3 ng/mg). Interestingly, local and systemic CsA therapy produced similar drug levels in whole blood, 558 ± 13.1 ng/ml and 518 ± 7.0 ng/ml, respectively. In vitro analysis of T cells from recipients treated with local CsA immunosuppression documented development of cellular suppressor elements and reduction in the frequency of T$_c$. Thus, local intraarterial (i.a.) delivery of a subtherapeutic CsA dose protects heart allografts from rejection and allows the induction of specific systemic unresponsiveness.

Prostaglandins are among the lipid inflammatory mediators which regulate the immune response.[29] Prostaglandins of the E series (PGE) and prostacyclin (PGI$_2$) inhibit T cell proliferation, IL-2 synthesis, and generation of T$_c$ cells. Administration of the PGE$_1$ analog, 15(S)-15-methyl PGE$_1$, prolongs the survival of heart and kidney allografts in rats.[30] In addition, subtherapeutic doses of the prostaglandin analog enisoprost combined with low-dose CsA significantly extend heart allograft survival in rats.[31] Defibrotide (DF), a single-stranded polydeoxyribonucleotide extracted from bovine pulmonary tissue, has antithrombotic and profibrinolytic activities without affecting blood coagulation parameters.[32] Furthermore, DF induces the synthesis of PGE$_2$, which inhibits T and B cell responses as well as neutrophil activation. The effect of local or systemic infusion of DF alone or in combination with CsA was examined on rat cardiac allograft rejection.[33] Daily intraperitoneal injections of DF (150 mg/kg) failed to prolong the survival of heterotopic BUF heart allografts in WF recipients. Similarly, 7 day systemic (i.v.) or local (i.a.) infusion of DF (280 mg/kg/day) alone was ineffective. However, the combination of local, but not systemic, DF (280 mg/kg/day) and a subtherapeutic dose of CsA (1.0 mg/kg/day i.v.) significantly prolonged heart allograft survival to 22.8 ± 5.0 days in comparison with 6.5 ± 0.5 days in untreated controls. Thus, high intragraft

---

Table 5.1. Local immunosuppression of heart allografts[a]

CsA Dose (mg/kg)	Delivery	MST ± SD (days)	P
0	–	6.8 ± 1.2	–
2	Gavage	6.8 ± 1.3	NS
2	Systemic i.v.	13.6 ± 9.6	0.01
2	Local i.a.	40.4 ± 2.0	0.005
1	Local i.a.	11.0 ± 4.3	0.01

a. Heterotopic Buffalo (RT1^b) heart allografts were transplanted to Wistar Furth (WF; RT1^u) recipients treated systemically (i.v.) or locally (intraarterial; i.a.) with CsA infusion using a 14 day osmotic pump. Control recipients were treated with CsA delivered by oral gavage.

levels of DF potentiated the immunosuppressive effects of CsA.

Sirolimus (SRL; rapamycin), a macrolide antibiotic, prevents organ allograft rejection.[34] In the same BUF to WF rat heterotopic cardiac allograft model, systemic (i.v.) SRL therapy delivered by 14 day osmotic pump at doses of 0.08-0.8 mg/kg/day significantly prolonged the survival of heart allografts in dose-dependent fashion: 0.08 mg/kg/day to 34.0 ± 12.1 days; 0.16 mg/kg/day to 39.0 ± 8.7 days; 0.32 mg/kg/day to 55.7 ± 3.3 days; and 0.8 mg/kg/day to 86.3 ± 30.0 days, with 3/8 hearts functioning for more than 100 days. Our experiments also documented that local i.a. delivery of low-dose (0.02 mg/kg/day) SRL prolonged the survival of BUF heart allografts to 14.6 ± 1.4 days versus only 8.6 ± 2.6 days when the same dose was given i.v.,[34] suggesting that SRL does exert effects on alloimmunoresponsiveness directly at the graft site.

LOCAL IMMUNOSUPPRESSION OF LIVER AND SMALL BOWEL ALLOGRAFTS

To prevent liver or small bowel allograft rejection, recipients must be treated with high systemic doses of immunosuppressive drugs. Local delivery of CsA may reduce systemic drug exposure and toxic side effects. In recent studies, we examined the effect of delivering low-dose (2.0 mg/kg/day) CsA via the portal vein directly to the liver allograft on the survival of recipients (Table 5.2). Systemic i.v. therapy with 2.0 mg/kg/day CsA delivered for 14 days by osmotic pump mildly prolonged the survival of Lewis (RT1[l]) recipients of ACI (RT1[a]) liver allografts. In contrast, intraportal infusion of 2.0 mg/kg/day CsA extended survivals to more than 100 days, documenting that local immunosuppression may effectively block the immune response at the graft site. Local delivery also reduced systemic CsA levels. On day 7 postgrafting, i.v. CsA treatment produced mean $\pm$ SD CsA concentrations in whole blood of 302 ± 143 ng/ml, compared with levels of 73 ± 37 ng/ml during portal vein infusion.

Similar experiments were performed in Lewis rats that received PVG (RT1[c]) liver allografts treated with systemic i.v., hepatic arterial, or portal venous infusion of 15-deoxyspergualin (DSG).[35] Untreated Lewis rats rejected PVG liver allografts within 14.1 ± 2.5 days. DSG (0.32 mg/kg/day) delivered for 3 days by daily bolus injection via the penile vein did not affect the survival of liver allografts (12.0 ± 1.8 days). In contrast, 3 day DSG delivery via the hepatic artery or portal vein prolonged the survival of liver allograft recipients to 30.9 ± 4.6 days and to 24.9 ± 10.0 days, respectively. Thus, DSG suppresses liver graft rejection more effectively via the hepatic arterial or portal vein route in comparison with systemic therapy.

Recent work in our laboratory evaluated the effectiveness of i.a. infusion of CsA (2.0 mg/kg/day) on the survival of Brown Norway (BN;RT1[n]) small bowel allografts in Lewis recipients. Untreated recipients rejected orthotopic small bowel allografts within 10.6 ± 1.95 days. Intravenous CsA therapy delivered for 14 days by osmotic pump was ineffective (Table 5.3). In contrast, i.a. infusion of 2.0 mg/kg/day CsA extended graft survival to 23.0 ± 6.3 days ($P < 0.004$). Clearly, the results of local immunosuppression of rodent liver and small bowel allografts demonstrate an advantage over systemic therapy.

CONCLUSION

Intragraft immune events are the best target for blocking allograft rejection. Local drug delivery systems for heart, liver or small bowel grafts can produce continuous drug exposure with a possibility for dose adjustment to accommodate variations in the immune response. Pharmacokinetic analysis showed that local drug delivery elevates drug concentrations in the target organ and decreases systemic drug levels. However, progress in local immunosuppression requires development of new agents which do not produce toxic side effects. For example, we have recently demonstrated that antisense oligonucleotides which inhibit the expression of intracellular adhe-

Table 5.2. Local immunosuppression of liver allografts[a]

CsA dose (mg/kg)	Delivery	MST ± SD (days)	P
0	–	10.3 ± 1.8	–
2.0	Systemic i.v.	13.8 ± 3.6	NS
4.0	Systemic i.v.	35.7 ± 10.7	0.001
2.0	Local Portal Vein	> 100	0.001

a. ACI liver allografts were transplanted to Lewis recipients which remained untreated or which were treated with systemic i.v. or intraportal CsA.

Table 5.3. Local immunosuppression of small bowel allografts[a]

CsA dose (mg/kg)	Delivery	MST ± SD (days)	P
0	–	10.6 ± 2.0	–
2.0	Systemic i.v.	12.5 ± 3.0	NS
4.0	Systemic i.v.	21.4 ± 7.3	0.01
2.0	Local i.a.	23.0 ± 6.2	0.01

a. Brown Norway (BN; RT1[n]) small bowel allografts were transplanted to Lewis recipients which were untreated or treated with either i.v. or i.a. (mesenteric arterial) CsA delivered by 14 day osmotic pump.

sion molecule-1 (ICAM-1) mRNA block the rejection of heart allografts in mice.[36] Moreover, direct administration of IL-4 to heart allografts transplanted to recipients which were treated with low-dose CsA and injected once with donor blood induced long-term allograft survival.[37] Thus, modification of the immune response at the graft site by local treatment may be the best approach to use clinically for anti-rejection therapy.

REFERENCES

1. Bennett WM and Pulliam JP. Cyclosporine nephrotoxicity. Ann Int Med 1983; 99(6): 851.
2. Jolivel J, Cowan KM, Curt GA et al. The pharmacology and clinical use of methotrexate. New Engl J Med 1983; 309(18): 1094.
3. Levine LA, Jarrard DF. Treatment of cyclophosphamide induced-hemorrhagic cystitis with intravesical corboprost tromethamine. J Urology 1993; 149(4):719.
4. Kahan BD. New immunosuppressive drugs-pharmacologic approaches to alter immuno-regulation. Therapeutic Immunology 1994; 1:33.
5. Kahan BD, Tejpal N, Gibbons-Stubbers S et al. The synergistic interactions in vitro and in vivo of brequinar sodium with cyclosporine or rapamycin alone and in triple combination. Transplantation 1993; 55(4): 894.
6. Wang M, Qu X, Stepkowski SM et al. Beneficial effect of graft perfusion with anti-T cell receptor monoclonal antibodies on survival of small bowel allografts in rat recipients treated with brequinar alone or in combination with cyclosporine and sirolimus. Transplantation 1996; 61(3):458.
7. Gruber SA. The case for local immunosuppression. Transplantation 1992; 54(1):1.
8. Shoskes DA, Wood KJ. Indirect presentation of MHC antigens in transplantation. Immunol Today 1994; 15(1):32.
9. Sherman LA, Chattopadhyay S. The molecular basis of allorecognition. Annu Rev Immunol 1993; 11:385.
10. Ruth M. Antigen receptors on B lymphocytes. Annu Rev Immunol 1992; 10:97.

11. Springer TA. Adhesion receptors of the immune system. Nature 1990; 346(6283): 425.

12. Miyaijma A, Kitamura T, Harada N et al. Cytokine receptors and signal transduction. Annu Rev Immunol 1992;10:295.

13. Takahata N, Satta Y, Klein J. Polymorphism and balancing selection at major histocompatibility complex loci. Genetic 1992; 130(4):925.

14. Bjorkman PJ, Saper MA, Samraoui B et al. Structure of the human class I histocompatibility antigen, HLA-A2. Nature 1987; 329(6139):506.

15. Brown JH, Jardetzky TS, Gorga JC et al. The three-dimensional structure of the human class II histocompatibility HLA-DR1. Nature 1993; 364(6432):33.

16. Chicz RM, Urban RG, Lane WS et al. Predominant naturally processed peptides bound to HLA-DR1 are derived from MHC-related molecules and are heterogenous in size. Nature 1992; 358(6389):764.

17. Hunt DF, Michel H, Dickinson TA et al. Peptides presented to immune system by the murine class II major histocompatibility complex molecule I-A^d. Science 1992; 256(5065):1817.

18. Suciu-Foca N, Reed E, D'agati VD et al. Soluble HLA-antigens, anti-HLA antibodies and anti-idiotypic antibodies in the circulation of renal transplant recipients. Transplantation 1991; 51(3):593.

19. Watschinger B, Gallon L, Carpenter CB et al. Mechanisms of allorecognition: recognition by in vivo-primed T cells of specific major histocompatibility complex polymorphisms presented as peptides by responder antigen-presenting cells. Transplantation 1994; 57(4):572.

20. Parker KE, Dalchau R, Fowler VJ et al. Stimulation of CD4 T lymphocytes by allogeneic MHC peptides presented on autologous antigen presenting cells: evidence of the indirect pathway of allorecognition in some strain combinations. Transplantation 1992; 53(4):918.

21. Germain RN, Margulies DH. The biochemistry and cell biology of antigen processing and presentation. Annu Rev Immunol 1993; 11:403.

22. Rammensee HG, Falk K, Rotzschke. Peptides naturally presented by MHC class I molecules. Annu Rev Immunol 1993; 11:213.

23. Goldberg AL and Rock KL. Proteolysis, protosomes and antigen presentation. Nature 1992; 357(6377):375.

24. Schumacher TN, Kantesaria DV, Heemels MT et al. Peptide length and sequence specificity of the mouse TAP-1/TAP-2 translocator. J Exp Med 1994; 179(2):533.

25. Weiss A, Littman DR. Signal transduction by lymphocyte antigen receptors. Cell 1994; 76(2):263.

26. Freeman GJ, Gribben JG, Boussiotis VA et al. Cloning of B7-2: A CTLA-4 counterreceptor that costimulates human T cell proliferation. Science 1993; 262(5135):909.

27. Weiss A. Molecular and genetic insights into T cell antigen receptor structure and function. Annu Rev Genet 1991; 25:487.

28. Stepkowski SM, Goto S, Ito T et al. Prolongation of heterotopic heart allograft survival by local delivery of continuous low-dose cyclosporine therapy. Transplantation 1989; 47(1):17.

29. Jordan ML. Prostoglandins and suppression of the allograft response. Transplant Sci 1991; 1:55.

30. Strom TB, Carpenter C. Prostoglandins as an effective anti-rejection therapy in rat renal allograft recipients. Transplantation 1983; 35:279.

31. Adams MB, Enisoprost Transplant Study Group. Enisoprost in renal transplantation. Transplantation 1992; 53:338.

32. Barone D, Salvetti L, Biachi G et al. The molecular site of action of defibrotide. Pharmacol Res 1992; 25:123.

33. Ferraresso M, Rigotti P, Stepkowski SM et al. Immunosuppressive effects of defibrotide. Transplantation 1993; 56:928.

34. Stepkowski SM, Chen H, Daloze P et al. Rapamycin, a potent immunosuppressive drug for vascularized heart, kidney, and small bowel transplantation in the rat. Transplantation 1991; 51:22.

35. Yano K, Fukuda Y, Sumimoto R et al. Suppression of liver allograft rejection by administration of 15-deoxyspergualin: comparison of administration via the hepatic

artery, portal vein, or systemic circulation. Transp Int 1994; 7(3):149.

36. Stepkowski SM, Tu Y, Condon T et al. Blocking of heart allograft rejection by intracellular adhesion molecule antisense oligonucleotides alone or in combination with other immunosuppressive modalities. J Immunol 1994;153:5336.

37. Levy AE, Alexender JW. Administration of intragraft interleukin-4 prolongs cardiac allograft survival in rats treated with donor-specific transfusion/cyclosporine. Transplantation 1995; 60:405.

INHIBITION OF CARDIAC ALLOGRAFT REJECTION BY CONTINUOUS LOCAL INFUSION OF 16,16 DI-METHYL PGE$_2$

M. Wayne Flye and Samuel Yu

Previous studies have implicated prostaglandins as pivotal modulators of the immune response with special emphasis on their function as local feedback inhibitors of T lymphocyte activation in vivo and in vitro.[1] Many of the earlier studies showed that prostaglandin E$_2$ (PGE$_2$) interactions with T cells in vitro resulted in elevations of the cyclic adenosine monophosphate (cAMP) level,[2] and that such an elevated intracellular cAMP level in T cells mediated the proliferative disturbances.[3-5]

Kammer[6] presented evidence that the T cell cAMP signal activates protein kinase A by dissociating it into two regulatory and two active subunits. This, in turn, presumably leads to the inhibition of interleukin-2 (IL-2) production and mitogen-induced proliferation. The cAMP-protein kinase A pathway is also known to negatively modify the phosphoinositide-protein kinase C (PKC) pathway, Ca^{2+} fluxes, and Ca^{2+}-calmodulin metabolism in T lymphocytes.[6-8] Although a precise role of Ca^{2+} signaling in PGE$_2$-mediated suppression of T cell functions has remained controversial,[4,9,10] the finding of suppressed Ca^{2+} mobilization in T cells incubated with PGE$_2$ supports the suggestion that PGE$_2$ does directly affect Ca^{2+} signaling. Moreover, previous studies showing that increased cAMP levels correlated with decreases in phospholipase C gamma, inositol phosphate turnover,[10] and inositol triphosphate generation,[2] also implicate a role for Ca^{2+} in PGE$_2$-mediated T cell suppression.

Paliogianni et al[8] documented that PGE$_2$ and other cAMP- elevating agents can down-regulate Ca^{2+}-calmodulin-dependent calcineurin-induced

Local Immunosuppression of Organ Transplants, edited by Scott A. Gruber.
© 1996 R.G. Landes Company.

transcription of the IL-2 gene.[11] The IL-2 enhancer region is known to have sites for at least six nuclear factor (NF) proteins that are produced either constitutively (NF-IL-2A and NF-IL-2B) or after stimulation of T cells (nuclear factor of activated T cells, NF-kB, AP-1, and CD28 RC).[12,13] Thus, inhibition of IL-2 nuclear transcription by cAMP could result from either decreased production or interference with the binding and function of transcription factors necessary for IL-2 transcription. Recently, Chen and Rothenberg[14] have shown decreased levels of NF-kB and a newly described TGGGC binding factor in the nuclear extracts of T cells previously exposed to forskolin, which increases cAMP. Moreover, the reduction in NF-kB and TGGGC was found to be mediated through cAMP-dependent activation of protein kinase A.[14] These studies imply that PGE_2 may act at multiple steps to inhibit T cell functions.

Administration of PGE_1 or PGE_2 in vitro has been shown to have the following effects: (1) suppression of T lymphocyte proliferation;[15,16] (2) inhibition of the generation of lymphokines,[17] such as IL-1[18,19] and IL-2;[20,21] (3) blocking of antigen presentation;[22] (4) suppression of T lymphocyte subsets;[23-25] (5) modulation of macrophage Ia expression[26] and (6) suppression of natural killer cell activity.[27] Another important in vivo effect of PGE_2 may be to chronically depress lymphocyte traffic as measured by the output of both small and blast cells into efferent lymph.[27] While these products of the cyclooxygenase pathway suppress those of the arachidonic acid lipoxygenase pathway [e.g., leukotriene B_4 (LTB_4)],[28] defined subsets of allosensitized T lymphocytes up-regulate the in vitro and in vivo immune reactivity.

IN VIVO EFFECTS OF PGE_2

PGE_2 also interferes with in vivo interactions between monocytes and T cells, leading to suppression of antigen presentation to T cells and inhibition of monocyte expression of the class II major histocompatibility complex (MHC) antigens.[29,33]

This suggests that a defect in antigen presentation by an accessory cell also contributes to attenuated T cell activation in vivo. However, PGE_2 has also been observed to directly inhibit T cell proliferation.[30,31]

PGE_2 generated in vivo has also been implicated in the decreases in T cell proliferation, IL-2 production, IL-2 receptor expression and the shift in T cell subpopulations that follow shock, trauma and burn injury. This impairment in T cell function can then result in decreased host resistance and increased susceptibility to infection. Septic rats were observed to have a 10-fold increase in PGE_2 blood levels compared with nonseptic animals.[32] The elevated levels of PGE_2 correlated with depressed concanavalin A-stimulated lymphocyte proliferation and Ca^{2+} mobilization. However, treatment of septic rats with the cyclooxygenase inhibitor, indomethacin, permitted normal T cell proliferation and Ca^{2+} mobilization. Therefore, the adverse in vivo effects of PGE_2 appear to be due to attenuation of Ca^{2+} signaling.[32]

EFFECTS OF PGE_2 IN ORGAN TRANSPLANTATION

Although systemic immunosuppression for organ transplantation has improved considerably over the last decade, toxicity and over-immunosuppression still remain major causes of morbidity and mortality. The effective local treatment of an organ graft could possibly prevent many of these side effects. Much of the data supporting the immunosuppressive role of these prostaglandins has been indirect. For example, a cyclooxygenase blocker, such as indomethacin,[9] when given in vivo or in vitro improves the immune response.[34]

We demonstrated that the in vitro mixed lymphocyte culture (MLC) and cell-mediated cytotoxicity responses could be markedly inhibited by the addition of the PGE_2 analogue, 16,16 di-methyl (M) PGE_2 (Upjohn Co., Kalamazoo, MI).[36] Not only is proliferation in the MLC markedly inhibited, but the generation of cytolytic T lymphocytes (CTL) is also inhibited by increasing concentrations of 16,16 di-M

PGE$_2$. In addition, after CTL have matured, they can still be inhibited by the addition of 16,16 di-M PGE$_2$ as assessed in a 4 hour cytotoxicity assay (Fig. 6.1). This late effect cannot be reversed by the addition of the calcium ionophore A23187 (100 μg/ml) or 12.0 tetradecanoyl phorbol 13-acetate (5 ng/ml).

Despite this evidence indicating that cellular immunity could be inhibited in vitro, only limited attempts to demonstrate a beneficial effect of the PGE series on solid-organ allograft survival in vivo have been reported. Quagliata et al[37] increased mouse skin graft survival by 8 days when systemically-administered PGE$_1$ was combined with procarbazine, while PGE$_1$ alone had no effect. When subcutaneous PGE$_1$ was given twice daily (1 mg/kg), hamster to rat cardiac xenograft survival increased from 74 to 94 hours.[38] The limited effectiveness of PGE$_1$ and PGE$_2$ is partly due to their very short half-lives in vivo. Although these prostaglandins are metabolized locally at the injection site, they are almost totally inactivated during a single passage through the lung.[39]

In contrast, the more stable synthetic PGE$_2$ analogues have half-lives of several hours.[40] Kort et al[41] found that although oral 15(S)-15-methyl PGE$_1$ alone did not increase rat heart allograft survival, when combined with prednisolone or azathioprine, survival was increased from 8 to 25.5 and 16.5 days, respectively. Strom et al[42] found that when given twice daily intraperitoneally, 250 μg of 15(S)-15-methyl PGE$_1$ preserved normal rat renal graft function at 8 days posttransplant, even when it was begun 4 days after transplantation. Using 16,16 di-M PGE$_2$ intraperitoneally, Anderson et al[43] reported prolongation of mean skin graft survival from 13.8 to 16.7 days in mice. Treatment of rat recipients of small intestinal grafts with 16,16 di-M PGE$_2$ (100 μg/kg) twice daily plus 1 mg/kg/day of cyclosporine resulted in a delay of onset and decreased intensity of allograft rejection when compared with either agent alone.[44]

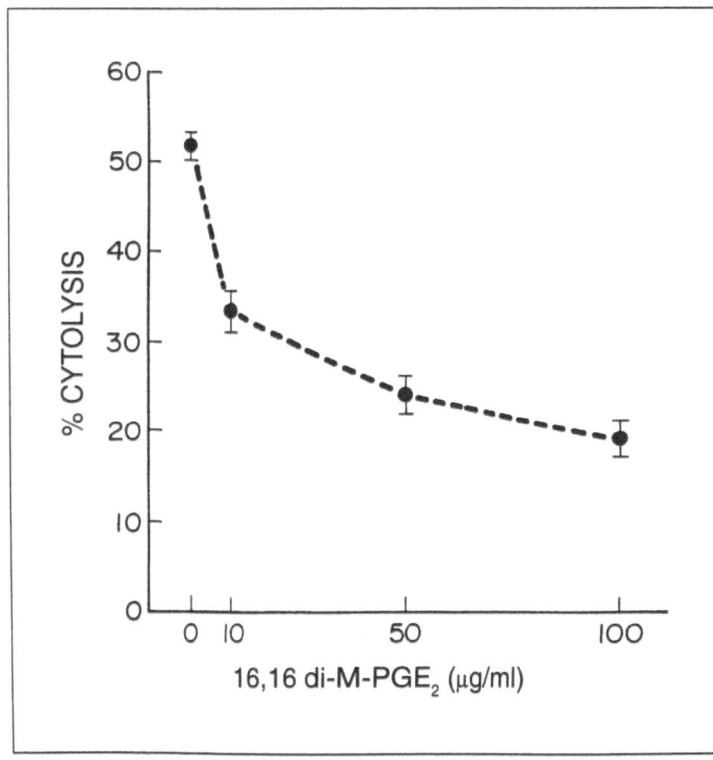

Fig. 6.1. Inhibition of lymphocyte cytotoxicity by 16,16 di-M PGE₂ is dose-dependent from 10 to 100 μg/ml.

The immunosuppressive effect of prostaglandins was shown indirectly when Scheuer et al[45] prevented tolerance induction to soluble antigen by administration of prostaglandin inhibitors. Misoprostol (200 μg 4x daily), a PGE_1 analogue with oral bioavailability, reduced the incidence of acute renal allograft rejection when compared with placebo [10 of 38 (misoprostol) versus 20 of 39 patients (placebo), P = 0.03].[46] However, generally, the potential therapeutic usefulness of the PGE series has been severely limited by very brief biologic half-life and toxic side effects associated with systemic administration.[47]

MECHANISM OF PROSTAGLANDIN INHIBITION OF T HELPER 1 (TH1) AND TH2 CELLS

The activation of $CD4^+$ T cells is an essential component in the generation of an effective and competent immune response, since the cytokines produced by these cells activate other cells required for both humoral and cell-mediated immunity.[35] The class II restricted $CD4^+$ Th cells can be identified either as Th1 cells that make IL-2 and interferon-gamma (IFN-γ) or as Th2 cells that secrete IL-4, IL-5, IL-6, and IL-10.[48] These sets of cytokines are associated with functionally distinct responses that underlie cellular versus humoral immunity.[48] In particular, IFN-γ is a potent macrophage activating factor and is critical for in vivo delayed-type hypersensitivity responses, while IL-4 and IL-5 are potent stimulants of B cell growth and differentiation.[49] IL-10 is a potent inhibitor of macrophage cytokine synthesis and antigen presentation, and many of its functions are similar to those of IL-4.[50] Finally, the cytokine products of one Th cell population can down-regulate the other Th population while amplifying its own activation.[51,52]

The two types of Th cells appear to use different pathways to transmit signals from the cell surface to the nucleus in response to activation.[53] Th2 cells are less dependent on PKC activation than are Th1 cells.[54]

Cholera toxin (CT), which ribosylates the α subunit of the G stimulatory protein, Gs, results in the accumulation of intracellular cAMP and the inhibition of IL-2 production and Th1 proliferation which normally occurs with T cell receptor (TCR) stimulation,[55] while the same doses of CT do not block IL-4 production and proliferation of Th2 cells. It is likely that the selective inhibitory effect of CT on Th1 versus Th2 cells is due to their differential sensitivity to high levels of cAMP, since administration of forskolin, a direct activator of adenylate cyclase and cAMP accumulation, leads to patterns of lymphokine secretion and proliferation in the Th1 and Th2 $CD4^+$ cells similar to that induced by CT.[55] Specifically, PGE_2 inhibits IL-2 and IFN-γ production from Th1 cells but does not inhibit IL-4 production from Th2 clones and T cell lines.[56] Therefore, PGE_2 may play an important regulatory role by inhibiting the development of a Th1 immune response and thus promoting the dominance of Th2-associated cytokines.[57] We have also demonstrated that the in vitro addition of 16,16 di-M PGE_2 to an MLC can also inhibit the generation of $CD8^+$ CTL precursors and suppress the cytolytic effect of mature committed effector cells.[83] Therefore, this agent inhibits both $CD4^+$ and $CD8^+$ T cells, and it was thought important to evaluate the in vivo effects of this agent on allograft survival.

Human cord blood naive $CD4^+$ T cells have also been shown to be influenced by PGE_2 at concentrations similar to those that inhibit IFN-γ production in Th1 clones and cell lines.[58] Katamura et al[59] demonstrated that the presence of PGE_2 and other agents (forskolin and dibutyryl cAMP) that increase cAMP during primary stimulation cause profound inhibition of IL-2 and IFN-γ, but not IL-4, production in a dose-dependent manner. These altered cytokine profiles are maintained even when subsequent antigen stimulation occurs without PGE_2 being present. Thus, the effect of PGE_2 on naive $CD4^+$ T cells is not due to transient regulation of cytokine production.

PGE$_2$ has also been shown to block macrophage functions, such as the release of tumor necrosis factor-alpha and IL-6, through an autocrine feedback mechanism involving the release of IL-10.[60] IL-10 inhibits acquisition of the ability to produce IFN-γ by naive CD4$^+$ T cells stimulated in the presence of dendritic cells.[61] Furthermore, it has been reported that PGE$_2$ can inhibit IL-12 synthesis by monocytes stimulated by LPS.[62] IL-12 strongly influences naive CD4$^+$ T cells to develop into Th1 cells. These findings show that the acute inhibitory effects of PGE$_2$ are not due to blockade of antigen recognition, but rather result from dynamic changes in cytokine production and underscore the concept that the induction of anergy is strictly an antigen-dependent response.

DEVELOPMENT OF ANERGY

At least two nonexclusive hypotheses may account for the mechanism of PGE$_2$-induced anergy. First, a substantial body of evidence has revealed that the balance between activation and anergy is respectively determined by the presence or absence of appropriate costimulatory signals.[63-65] Thus, PGE$_2$ may inhibit specialized costimulatory pathways and thereby convert an inflammatory site into an anergy-inducing microenvironment. Second, PGE$_2$ may elicit signal transduction pathways that act synergistically with antigenic signals as specific intracellular cues for expression of anergy-inducing genes. Since PGE$_2$ receptors are positively coupled to adenylate cyclase, the resulting accumulation of intracellular cAMP in lymphocytes is causally implicated in the inhibition of several different types of T cell response.[66-69]

PGE$_2$ appears to mediate a specialized role in anergy-dependent down-regulation of T cell-dependent responses. Th cell recruitment of macrophages into inflammatory sites initiates a negative-feedback loop by which macrophage-derived products such as PGE$_2$ anergize the Th cells. While PGE$_2$ inhibits Th1 cell responses and promotes Th2 cell responses,[66,71,72] Th2 cells appear resistant to the induction of aner-

gy.[63-75] For example, PGE$_2$ can induce anergy in myelin basic protein (MBP)-specific Th cells by inhibiting the production of the prototypic Th1 lymphokine, IL-2. In experimental autoimmune encephalitis, MBP-specific induction of anergy would be ensured by the requirement for concurrent recognition of PGE$_2$ and antigen. Even though anergic T cells gradually regain antigenic responsiveness in IL-2 supplemented medium in vitro, the duration of anergy may persist in vivo due to the relative lack of IL-2.[70] Hence, PGE$_2$-induced anergy represents a branchpoint in the progression of an immune response. Accordingly, T cells subjected to PGE$_2$-mediated anergy may lose their ability to produce IL-2 but may retain the ability to produce alternative autocrine growth factors, such as IL-4. While PGE$_2$ only partially inhibited MBP-stimulated proliferation, it more profoundly inhibited IL-2 than IL-4 production in T cells that transcribe mRNA for both cytokines.[76] Hence, PGE$_2$ may promote the emergence or differentiation of MBP-specific Th2 cells by inducing anergy in Th1-like cells.

SYSTEMIC VERSUS INTRAGRAFT TREATMENT OF CARDIAC ALLOGRAFT RECIPIENTS WITH 16,16 DI-M PGE$_2$

We have examined the effect of the analogue 16,16 di-M PGE$_2$ on in vivo graft rejection. Using MHC-mismatched [Lewis (LEW; RT1^l) into Buffalo (BUF; RT1^b)] rats, cardiac allografts were heterotopically placed in the abdomen. The innominate artery was cannulated with a PE-10 polyethylene tube and connected to an Alzet osmotic pump (Alza, Palo Alto, CA). 16,16 di-M PGE$_2$ was dissolved in 95% ethyl alcohol and diluted in saline to the appropriate concentration. Using the Alzet pump, drug was infused continuously for 7 (2ML1 pump) or 14 (2ML2 pump) days either into the cardiac allograft, intravenously (i.v.) via the recipient's right lumbar vein, or intraperitoneally at doses of 20, 100 or 200 µg/kg/day.[77]

Untreated BUF (group 1) recipients rejected LEW heart allografts with a mean survival time (MST ± SD) of 7.4 ± 0.5 days (n = 5) (Table 6.1). Systemic infusion of 20 µg/kg/day 16,16 di-M PGE$_2$ for 2 weeks (group 2) after transplantation did not prolong graft survival (MST = 7.0 ± 0.0, n = 3). 100 µg/kg/day i.v. (group 3) prevented rejection in two of six recipients for more than 150 days, while the other four recipients rejected their grafts at 7 days. All the recipients treated with 200 µg/day 16,16 di-M PGE$_2$ i.v. developed severe diarrhea and died with functioning grafts within 2 days after transplantation (group 4). However, intraperitoneal administration of the same dose (group 5) showed no toxic effects, and three of these recipients accepted the cardiac grafts for more than 120 days while two rejected their grafts at 7 days.

In contrast, delivery of 20 µg/kg/day 16,16 di-M PGE$_2$ directly into the graft for 2 weeks completely prevented rejection in all recipients (n = 10) (Table 6.1). All grafts functioned for more than 150 days and no recipient developed drug toxicity (group 7 versus group 1, P < 0.001). Since the same dose of intravenously administered 16,16 di-M PGE$_2$ failed to prolong graft survival (group 2), these results clearly indicate the effectiveness of local treatment in the protection of the vascularized cardiac allograft. When 20 µg/kg/day 16,16 di-M PGE$_2$ was administered for only 1 week after transplantation, 3 of 5 recipients accepted their grafts long-term (> 150 days), while the other 2 animals rejected their grafts by 14 days (group 6 versus group 1, P < 0.05). These data suggest that continuous exposure of the graft to 16,16 di-M PGE$_2$ for a 1 to 2 week period is necessary for the consistent development of tolerance.

INDUCTION OF DONOR-SPECIFIC TOLERANCE

Long-term BUF recipients bearing LEW cardiac allografts were grafted with full-thickness donor-strain LEW and third-party Wistar Furth (WF) skin to evaluate their specific immune responsiveness (Table 6.2; group 8, n = 3). All recipients accepted LEW skin grafts for more than 35 days, after which time it was difficult to differentiate the skin graft from the recipient's own skin. In contrast, WF skin grafts were rejected in 7.3 ± 0.5 days, a time period identical to that for both strains in control naive BUF rats (group 9). Following skin grafting, the cardiac allograft function remained unchanged, indicating that the rejection of third-party skin does not nonspecifically abrogate the donor-specific tolerance.

Table 6.1. Effect of 16,16 di-M PGE$_2$ treatment on LEW cardiac allograft survival in BUF recipients

| Group | 16, 16 di-M PGE$_2$ | | | Graft Survival (days) | P value[+] |
	Dosage	Route	Duration		
1		NONE		7,7,7,8,8	–
2	20 µg	IV[*]	2 wks	7,7,7	NS
3	100 µg	IV	2 wks	7,7,7,7, >150 (x2)	NS
4	200 µg	IV	2 wks	1,1,2,2,2[**]	–
5	200 µg	IP[*]	2 wks	7,7, >150 (x3)	NS
6	20 µg	IG[*]	1 wk	8,14, >150 (x3)	< 0.05
7	20 µg	IG	2 wks	>150 (x10)	< 0.001

[+] P values were compared to Group 1 by Wilcoxon rank sum test. NS = not significant.[*] IV = intravenous; IP = intraperitoneal; IG = intragraft.[**] All the recipients died within two days from drug toxicity with functioning grafts.

IMMUNOGENICITY OF THE LONG-TERM ACCEPTED CARDIAC ALLOGRAFT

One possible mechanism of graft adaptation is the loss of graft immunogenicity after transplantation to the recipient.[78] When long-term accepted LEW cardiac allografts were retransplanted into naive BUF recipients (Table 6.3; group 10), they were rejected in normal time (MST = 6.7 ± 0.5 days, n = 3), indicating that graft acceptance induced by local graft 16,16 di-M PGE₂ treatment was not due to decreased graft immunogenicity.

MONOCYTE MIGRATION

In addition, we have found that graft infusion with 16,16 di-M PGE₂ markedly inhibits monocyte influx into the interstitium but not into the glomeruli of rat renal allografts during the first 24 to 48 hours after transplantation.[79] In contrast, 16,16 di-M PGE₂ infusion has relatively little effect on the migration of leukocytes in the glomerulus or interstitium of renal isografts. These results suggest that one mechanism by which PGE₂ may inhibit host sensitization to an allograft may be suppression of migration of host monocytes

and antigen presenting cells into the allograft.

PGE₂ also induces the development of suppressor cells,[80,81] which in turn can produce PGE₂.[82] These effects may well include suppression by Th2 cells and their cytokines. Therefore, PGE₂ could act not only to locally inhibit the development of rejection, but also to maintain a systemic hyporesponsive state by inducing suppressor cells.

An appealing aspect of delivering an immunosuppressive agent directly to an organ at risk for rejection is that higher and presumably more effective concentrations of the drug can be administered while decreasing the toxic side effects that might occur from obtaining similar local levels by systemic administration. This is especially true of the natural prostaglandins, since they are almost completely cleared with one passage through the lungs,[84] thus requiring increased drug levels to achieve a therapeutic effect.

PGE₂ TOXICITY

Prostaglandins of the E series can induce diarrhea by increasing both intestinal motor activity and secretion.[85] The

Table 6.2. Donor strain LEW and third-party WF skin graft survival in BUFcardiac allograft recipients

| Group | Recipient | Skin Graft Survival (days) | |
		LEW	WF
8	Long-term BUF (16,16 di-M PGE₂)	> 35 (x3)	7,7,8
9	Naive BUF	7,7,8	7,7,8

Table 6.3. Survival of retransplanted long-surviving LEW cardiac allografts into naive BUF recipients

Group	Donor	Graft Survival (days)	MST ± SD (days)
1	Naive LEW heart	7,7,7,8,8	7.4 ± 0.5
10	Long-surviving LEW graft	6,7,7	6.7 ± 0.5

importance of drug concentration is well demonstrated by our studies, since 20 µg/kg/day 16,16 di-M PGE$_2$ delivered intravenously was ineffective, while a 10-fold higher dose given intravenously resulted in death, largely related to fluid loss from diarrhea. When given into the peritoneal cavity, the same dose of 16,16 di-M PGE$_2$ (200 µg/kg/day) was not terribly effective in preventing rejection (group 5) but also did not result in noticeable side effects. One-tenth the dose (20 µg/kg/day) given directly into the graft was uniformly effective in inducing graft acceptance without any side effects.

CONCLUSION

Our most remarkable finding is that no other treatment is necessary to prevent subsequent rejection after 16,16 di-M PGE$_2$ is discontinued. The nature of the "tolerant" state apparently induced is currently being examined. The recipient's second graft (skin graft) acceptance is donor-specific, while there is no change in the immunogenicity of retransplanted long-surviving cardiac grafts. Although the exact mechanisms responsible for the demonstrated permanent engraftment are unknown, the potential benefit of short-term local treatment with 16,16 di-M PGE$_2$ after transplantation merits careful examination in other species, including man.

REFERENCES

1. Goodwin JS, Webb DR. Regulation of the immune response by prostaglandins. Clin Immunol Immunopath 1980; 15:106.
2. Rincon M, Tugores A, Lopez-Rivas A et al. Prostaglandin E$_2$ and the increase of intracellular cAMP inhibit the expression of interleukin 2 receptors in human T cells. Eur J Immunol 1988; 18:1791.
3. Baker PE, Fahey JV, Munck A. Prostaglandin inhibition of T cell proliferation is mediated at two levels. Cell Immunol 1981; 61:52.
4. Lingk DS, Chan MA, Gelfand EW. Increased cyclic adenosine monophosphate levels block progression but not initiation of human T cell proliferation. J Immunol 1990; 145:449.
5. Munoz E, Zubiaga AM, Merrow M et al. Cholera toxin discriminates between T helper 1 and 2 cells in T cell receptor-mediated activation: role of cAMP in T cell proliferation. J Exp Med 1990; 172:95.
6. Kammer GM. The adenylate cyclase-cAMP protein kinase A pathway and regulation of the immune response. Immunol Today 1988; 9:222.
7. Bauman GP, Bartik MM, Brooks WH et al. Induction of cAMP-dependent protein kinase (PKA) activity in T cells after stimulation of PGE$_2$ or the beta-adrenergic receptors: relationship between PKA activity and inhibition of anti-CD3 monoclonal antibody-induced T cell proliferation. Cell Immunol 1994;158:182.
8. Paliogianni F, Kincaid RL, Boumpas DT. Prostaglandin E$_2$ and other cyclic AMP elevating agents inhibit interleukin 2 gene transcription by counteracting calcineurin-dependent pathway. J Exp Med 1993; 178:1813.
9. Chouaib S, Robb RJ, Welte K et al. Analysis of prostaglandin E$_2$ effect on T lymphocyte activation: abrogation of prostaglandin E$_2$ inhibitory effect by the tumor promoter 12.0 tetradecanoyl phorbol-13 acetate. J Clin Invest 1987; 80:333.
10. Lerner A, Jacobson B, Miller RA. Cyclic AMP concentrations modulate both calcium flux and hydrolysis of phosphotidylinositol phosphates in mouse T lymphocytes. J Immunol 1988; 140:936.
11. Clipstone NA, Crabtree GR. Identification of calcineurin as a key signalling enzyme in T lymphocyte activation. Nature (London) 1992; 357:695.
12. Crabtree GR. Contingent genetic regulatory events in T lymphocyte activation. Science 1989; 243:355.
13. Ulman KS, Northrop JP, Verweij CL et al. Transmission of signals from the lymphocyte antigen receptor to the genes responsible for cell proliferation and immune function: the missing link. Annu Rev Imunol 1990; 8:421.
14. Chen D, Rothenberg EV. Interleukin-2 transcription factors as molecular targets of cAMP inhibition: delayed inhibition kinetics and combinatorial transcription roles. J Exp Med 1994; 179:931.

15. Leung KH, Mihich E. Prostaglandin modulation of development of cell-mediated immunity in culture. Nature 1980; 288:597.

16. Bowes LG, Dumble LJ, Pollak R et al. Prostaglandin E₁ and E₂ suppression of in vitro lymphoid responses to alloantigen. Transpl Proc 1989; 21:369.

17. Gordon D, Bray MA, Morley J. Control of lymphokine secretion by prostaglandins. Nature 1976; 262:401.

18. Kunkel SL, Chensue SW, Phan SH. Prostaglandins as endogenous mediators of interleukin 1 production. J Immunol 1986; 136:186.

19. Knudsen PJ, Dinarello CA, Strom TB. Prostaglandins post-transcriptionally inhibit monocyte expression of interleukin 1 activity by increasing intracellular cyclic adenosine monophosphate. J Immunol 1986; 137:3189.

20. Chouaib S, Fradelizi D. The mechanism of inhibition of human IL-2 production. J Immunol 1982; 129:2463.

21. Baker PE, Fahey JV, Munck A. Prostaglandin inhibition of T-cell proliferation is mediated at two levels. Cell Immunol 1981; 61:52.

22. Stephan RN, Conrad PJ, Saizawa M et al. Prostaglandin E₂ depresses antigen-presenting cell function of peritoneal macrophages. J Surg Res 1988; 44:733.

23. Jordan ML, Hoffman RA, Debe EF et al. Prostaglandin E₂ mediates subset-specific effects on the functional responses of allosensitized T lymphocyte clones. Transplantation 1987; 43:117.

24. Makoul GT, Robinson DR, Bhalla AK et al. Prostaglandin E₂ inhibits the activation of cloned T cell hybridomas. J Immunol 1985; 134:2645.

25. Honda M, Steinberg AD. Effects of prostaglandin E₂ on responses of T-cell subsets to mitogen and autologous non-T-cell stimulation. Biol Immunol 1984; 33:111.

26. Snyder DS, Beller DI, Unanue ER. Prostaglandins modulate macrophage Ia expression. Nature 1982; 299:163.

27. Garcia-Penarrubia P, Bankhurst AD, Koster FT. Prostaglandins from human T suppressor/cytotoxic cells modulate natural killer antibacterial activity. J Exp Med 1989; 170:601.

28. Jordan ML, Carlson A, Hoffman RA et al. Lipoxygenase pathway inhibition impairs the allograft response. Surgery 1987; 102:248.

29. Stephan RN, Conrad PJ, Saizawa M et al. Prostaglandin E₂ depresses antigen presenting cell function of peritoneal macrophages. J Surg Res 1988; 44:733.

30. Goodwin JS, Bankhurst AD, Messner RP. Suppression of human T cell mitogenesis by prostaglandin: existence of a prostaglandin-producing suppressor cell. J Exp Med 1977; 146:1719.

31. Minakuchi R, Walkholtz MC, Davis LS et al. Delineation of the mechanism of inhibition of human T cell activation by PGE₂. J Immunol 1990; 145:2616.

32. Choudhry MA, Ahmad S, Sayeed MM. Role of Ca²⁺ in PGE₂ T lymphocyte proliferative suppression in sepsis. Infection and Immunity 1995; 63:3101.

33. Snider ME, Fertel RH, Zwilling BS. Prostaglandin regulation of macrophage function: Effect of endogenous and exogenous prostaglandins. Cell Immunol 1982; 74:234.

34. Latter DA, Tchervenkov JI, Nohr CW et al. The effect of indomethacin on burn-induced immunosuppression. J Surg Res 1987; 43:246.

35. Powrie F, Coffman RL. Cytokine regulation of T cell function: potential for therapeutic intervention. Immunol Today 1993; 14:270-274.

36. Flye MW, Yu S. Inhibition of cell-mediated cytotoxicity by 16,16-dimethyl PGE₂. Transplant Proc 1989; 21:1156.

37. Quagliata F, Lawrence VJW, Philips-Quagliata JM. Prostaglandin E₁ as a regulator of lymphocyte function. Cell Immunol 1973; 6:457.

38. Kakita A, Blanchard J, Fortner JG. Effectiveness of prostaglandin E₁ and procarbazine hydrochloride in prolonging the survival of vascularized cardiac hamster-to-rat xenograft. Transplantation 1975; 20:439.

39. Piper PJ, Vane JR, Wyllie JH. Inactivation of prostaglandins by the lungs. Nature 1970; 225:600.

40. Weeks JR, Ducharme DW, Magee WE et al. The biological activity of the 15(S)-15-methyl analogues of prostaglandins E₂ and F2α. J Pharmacol Exp Ther 1983; 186:67.

41. Kort WJ, Bonta IL, Adolfs MJP et al. Synergism of 15(S)-15-methyl prostaglandin E_1 with either azathioprine or prednisolone on the survival of heart allografts in rats. Prostaglandins Leukotrienes and Med 1982; 8:661.

42. Strom TB, Carpenter CB. Prostaglandin as an effective antirejection therapy in rat renal allograft recipients. Transplantation 1983; 35:279.

43. Anderson CB, Jaffee BM, Graff RJ. Prolongation of murine skin allografts by prostaglandin E. Transplantation 1977; 23:444.

44. Koh IHJ, Kim PCW, Chung SW et al. The effects of 16,16 dimethyl Prostaglandin E_2 therapy alone and in combination with low dose cyclosporine on rat small intestinal transplantation. Transplantation 1992; 54:592.

45. Scheuer WV, Hobbs MV, Weigle WO. Interference with tolerance induction in vivo by inhibitors of prostaglandin synthesis. Cell Immunol 1987; 104:409.

46. Moran M, Mozes MF, and Maddux MS. Prevention of acute graft rejection by the Prostaglandin E_1 analogue Misoprostol in renal transplant recipients treated with cyclosporine and prednisone. New Eng J Med 1990; 322:1183.

47. Bakhle YS, Jancar S, Whittle BJR. Uptake and inactivation of prostaglandin E_2 and its 15(S) methyl and 16, 16 dimethyl analogues in rat isolated lung. Bibl Anat 1977; 16:390.

48. Mosmann TR, Coffman RL. Th1 and Th2: different patterns of lymphokine secretion lead to different functional properties. Annu Rev Immunol 1989; 7:145.

49. Croft M, Swain SL. B cell response to T helper cell subsets. II. Both the stage of T cell differentiation and the cytokines secreted determine the extent and nature of helper activity. J Immunol 1991; 147:3679.

50. Fiorentino DF, Ztotnik A, Vieira P et al. IL-10 acts on the antigen presenting cell to inhibit cytokine production by Th1 cells. J Immunol 1991; 146:3444.

51. Gajewski TF, Joyce J and Fitch FW. Antiproliferative effects of IFN-γ in immune regulation. III. Differential selection of Th1 and Th2 murine helper T lymphocyte clones using recombinant IL-2 and recombinant IFN-γ. J Immunol 1989; 143:15.

52. Parronchi P, DeCarli M, Manetti R. IL-4 and IFN (α and γ) exert opposite regulatory effects on the development of cytolytic potential by Th1 or Th2 human T cell clones. J Immunol 1992; 149:2977.

53. Gajewski TF, Schell SR, Fitch FW. Evidence implicating utilization of different T cell receptor associated signaling pathways by Th1 and Th2 clones. J Immunol 1990; 144:4110.

54. Janeway Jr CA, Carding S, Jones B. CD4+ T cells: specificity and function. Immunol Rev 1988; 101:39.

55. Munoz E, Zubiaga AM, Marrow M et al. Cholera toxin discriminates between T helper 1 and 2 cells in T cell receptor mediated activation: Role of cAMP in T cell proliferation. J Exp Med 1990; 172:951.

56. Betz M, Fox BS. Prostaglandin E_2 inhibits production of Th1 lymphokines but not of Th2 lymphokines. J Immunol 1991; 146:108.

57. Phipps RP, Stein SH, Roper RL. A new view of prostaglandin E regulation of the immune response. Immunol Today 1991; 12:349.

58. Hilkens CMU, Vermeulen H, Neerven RJ et al. Differential modulation of T helper type 1 (Th1) and T helper type 2 (Th2) cytokine secretion by prostaglandin E_2 critically depends on IL-2. Eur J Immunol 1995; 25:59.

59. Katamura K, Shintaku N, Yamauchi Y et al. Prostaglandin E_2 at priming of naive CD4+ T cells inhibits acquisition of ability to produce IFN-γ and IL-2, but not IL-4 and IL-5. J Immunol 1995; 155:4604.

60. Strassman G, Patil-Koota V, Fikelman F et al. Evidence for the involvement of IL-10 in the differential deactivation of murine peritoneal macrophages by PGE_2. J Exp Med 1994; 180:2365.

61. Hsieh CS, Heimberger AB, Told JS et al. Differential regulation of T helper phenotype development by interleukins 4 and 10 in an α/β T cell receptor transgenic system. Proc Natl Acad Sci 1992; 89:6065.

62. Kraan TC, Boeije LCM, Smeenk RJT et al. PGE is a potent inhibitor of human IL-12 production. J Exp Med 1995; 181:775.

63. Lafferty KJ, Prowse SJ, Simeonovic CJ et al. Immunobiology of tissue transplantation:

A return to the leukocyte concept. Annu Rev Immunol 1983; 1:143.

64. Mueller DL, Jenkins MK, Schwartz RH. Clonal expansion versus functional clonal inactivation: A costimulatory signalling pathway determines the outcome of T cell antigen receptor occupancy. Annu Rev Immunol 1989; 7:445.

65. Mannie MD. Immune discrimination of self and nonself: A unified theory for the induction of self tolerance among thymocytes and mature peripheral T cells. Med Hypotheses 1993; 40:105.

66. Roper RL, Conrad KH, Brown DM et al. Prostaglandin E2 promotes IL-4-induced IgE and IgG1 synthesis. J Immunol 1990; 145:2644.

67. Anastassiou ED, Paliogianni F, Balow JP et al. Prostaglandin E2 and other cyclic AMP-elevating agents modulate IL-2 and IL-2R alpha gene expression at multiple levels. J Immunol 1992; 148:2845.

68. Hofmann B, Nishanian P, Nguyen T et al. Human immunodeficiency virus proteins induce the inhibitory cAMP/protein kinase A pathway in normal lymphocytes. Proc Natl Acad Sci USA 1993; 90:6676.

69. Paliogianni F, Kincaid RL, Boumpas DT. Prostaglandin E2 and other cyclic AMP elevating agents inhibit interleukin-2 gene transcription by counteracting calcineurin-dependent pathways. J Exp Med 1993; 178:1813.

70. Gutierrez-Ramos JC, Moreno de Alboran I, Martinez C. In vivo administration of interleukin-2 turns on anergic self-reactive T cells and leads to autoimmune disease. Eur J Immunol 1992; 22:2867.

71. Phipps RP, Stein SH, Roper RL. A new view of prostaglandin E regulation of the immune response. Immunol Today 1991; 12:349.

72. Betz M, Fox B. Prostaglandin E2 inhibits production of Th1 lymphokines but not of Th2 lymphokines. J Immunol 1991; 146:108.

73. Gilbert KM, Hoang KD, Weigle WO. Th1 and Th2 clones differ in their response to a tolerogenic signal. J Immunol 1990; 144:2063.

74. Williams ME, Shea CM, Lichtman AH et al. Antigen receptor-mediated anergy in resting T lymphocytes and T cell clones. Correlation with lymphokine secretion patterns. J Immunol 1992; 149:1921.

75. Peterson JD, Karpus WJ, Clatch RJ et al. Split tolerance of Th1 and Th2 cells in tolerance to Theiler's murine encephalomyelitis virus. Eur J Immunol 1993; 23:46.

76. Mannie MD, Morrison-Plummer J, McConnell TJ. Differentiation of encephalitogenic T cells confers resistance to an inhibitory anti-CD4 monoclonal antibody. J Immunol 1993; 151:7293.

77. Kamei T, Callery MP, Flye MW. Intragraft delivery of 16,16-Dimethyl PGE₂ induces donor specific tolerance in rat cardiac allograft recipients. Transplantation 1991; 51:242.

78. Lechler RI, Batchelor JR. Restoration of immunogenicity to passenger cell-depleted kidney allografts by the addition of donor strain dendritic cells. J Exp Med 1982; 155:31.

79. Schreiner GF, Kamei T, Lefkowith J et al. Modulation of the kinetics of the initial leukocyte migration into renal allografts by 16, 16 dimethyl PGE₂. Transplantation 1993; 56:417.

80. Webb DR, Nowowiejski I. Control of suppressor cell activation via endogenous prostaglandin synthesis: The role of T cells and macrophages. Cell Immunol 1981; 63:321.

81. Webb DR, Nowowiejski I. Nitrogen-induced changes in lymphocyte prostaglandin levels: A signal for the induction of suppressor cell activity. Cell Immunol 1978; 41:72.

82. Penarrubia PG, Bankhurst AD, Koster FT. Prostaglandins from human T suppressor/cytotoxic cells modulate natural killer antibacterial activity. J Exp Med 1989; 170:601.

83. Foegh ML, Alijani MR, Helfrich GB et al. Eicosanoids and organ transplantation. Ann Clin Res 1984; 16:318.

84. Piper PJ, Vane JR, Wyllie JH. Inactivation of prostaglandins by the lung. Nature 1970; 225:600.

85. Field M, Musch MW, Stoff JS. Role of prostaglandins in the regulation of intestinal electrolyte transport. Prostaglandins 1981; 21:73.

========= CHAPTER 7 =========

INTRARENAL ADMINISTRATION OF ANTI T CELL-MONOCLONAL ANTIBODY

Norio Yoshimura, Chol Joo Lee and Takahiro Oka

Although the actual immunological events developing within the allograft remain poorly understood, it is widely accepted that T lymphocytes play an important role in acute rejection. Indeed, many reports have described the accumulation of T cells in rejecting grafts.[1,2] Recently, OKT3 has been used clinically to reverse acute allograft rejection.[3] However, limitations to its usefulness include systemic side effects such as pulmonary edema, infection, and allergic reactions. Despite these limitations, a number of factors suggest that appropriate use of anti-T cell monoclonal antibody (MoAb) might allow for more specific alterations of the immune system that could be useful clinically. The postulated local regulation of the immune response within the graft makes the transplanted organ a favorable object for local immunosuppressive therapy. Therefore, we investigated the efficacy of local administration of anti-T cell MoAb via the renal artery in a rat kidney transplant model, with the hope of increasing its antirejection effect and decreasing toxicity.

EXPERIMENTAL MODEL OF LOCAL INTRAARTERIAL INFUSION OF MoAB

Inbred male rats weighing 250-350 g were used in all experiments, Lewis rats (LEW, RT-1^l) as recipients, and Brown-Norway rats (BN, RT-1^n) as donors. These rats were obtained from Seiwa Experimental Animal Farm (Fukuoka, Japan).

Local Immunosuppression of Organ Transplants, edited by Scott A. Gruber.
© 1996 R.G. Landes Company.

PRODUCTION AND PREPARATION OF MoAb (OX-19)

Hybridoma cells secreting the antibody OX-19 were obtained as a gift from Dr. Alan Williams (Oxford, UK). Hybridoma cells were injected intraperitoneally into pristane-primed BALB/C mice for the production of ascites. OX-19 was purified by passage of the ascites over an affigel protein A column (Biorad, Richmond, CA),[4,5] was retitrated using protein levels for antibody, and its absorbance at 280 nm measured for determination of monoclonal immunoglobulin levels.

RENAL TRANSPLANTATION AND ADMINISTRATION OF OX-19

Heterotopic renal transplantation was performed from BN to LEW using microsurgical techniques. All recipients were bilaterally nephrectomized at the time of transplantation.[6,7] Ureters were anastomosed end-to-end over a fine polyethylene internal stent. Ischemic time was approximately 30 minutes. OX-19 was given by continuous intrarenal (RA-treated group), continuous intravenous (i.v.-treated group), or bolus intravenous (one-shot i.v. group) infusion. For continuous intrarenal arterial infusion, a catheter was introduced into the abdominal aorta at the bifurcation of the iliac artery and its tip located at the take-off of the transplanted renal artery (Fig. 7.1). A catheter was introduced into the femoral vein for continuous intravenous infusion. After patency was checked, the catheter was immediately connected to an osmotic minipump (Alzet 2MLI, Alza Corporation, CA)[8,9] filled with OX-19 in normal saline. The pump was implanted subcutaneously on the abdominal wall of the recipient, and several doses of OX-19 (19, 37.5, 75, 300 µg/kg/day) were delivered continuously via the RA or i.v. route for 7 days after transplantation. Bolus intravenous injection of OX-19 (75 µg/kg/day) once a day from day 0 to day 7 was also performed. Moreover, for the treatment of ongoing rejection, administration of OX-19

was started on day 4 after grafting for 7 days. Rejection was determined by death of the recipient and confirmed by histological examination.

EFFECT OF LOCAL TREATMENT WITH MoAb ON RENAL ALLOGRAFT SURVIVAL

Untreated LEW hosts rejected BN grafts at 7.8 ± 0.2 (SEM) days (n = 10, Fig. 7.2). A single bolus intravenous injection of OX-19 (75 µg/kg/day) for 7 days did not prolong the survival of BN grafts (mean survival time [MST] = 7.0 ± 0.2 days, n = 5, P = NS). Continuous administration of OX-19 (75 µg/kg/day) for 7 days via the femoral vein (i.v.-treated group) caused a slight, but not significant, prolongation of BN graft survival to 8.8 ± 0.9 days (n = 5, P = NS, Fig. 7.2). On the other hand, continuous intrarenal infusion of OX-19 (75 µg/kg/day) for 7 days remarkably prolonged BN graft survival in LEW hosts (MST = 16.8 ± 1.3 days, n = 8, P < 0.01). Continuous intrarenal infusion of normal saline for 7 days did not prolong graft survival (MST = 7.8 ± 0.2, n = 8, Fig. 7.2).

In order to assess the optimal dose of MoAb, serial doses (19, 37.5, 75 and 300 µg/kg/day) of OX-19 were continuously administered via the RA or i.v. route into LEW recipients. Systemic administration of 19, 37.5 and 75 µg/kg/day of OX-19 via the femoral vein did not affect graft survival times, with MST values of 7.2 ± 0.3 days (n = 5), 8.2 ± 0.4 days (n = 5) and 8.8 ± 0.9 days (n = 5), respectively. In contrast, local administration of 19, 37.5 and 75 µg/kg/day of OX-19 yielded mean survival times of 8.0 ± 0.3 days (n = 5), 9.4 ± 0.6 days (n = 5) and 16.8 ± 1.3 days (n = 8), respectively. Thus, increasing doses of OX-19 prolonged graft survival proportionately with an optimum of 75 µg/kg/day (P < 0.05) in the RA-treated group. Although 300 µg/kg/day of OX-19 prolonged graft survival (MST = 15.3 ± 0.7 days in the RA-treated group and MST = 14.8 ± 2.0 days in the i.v.-treated group) to the same degree as

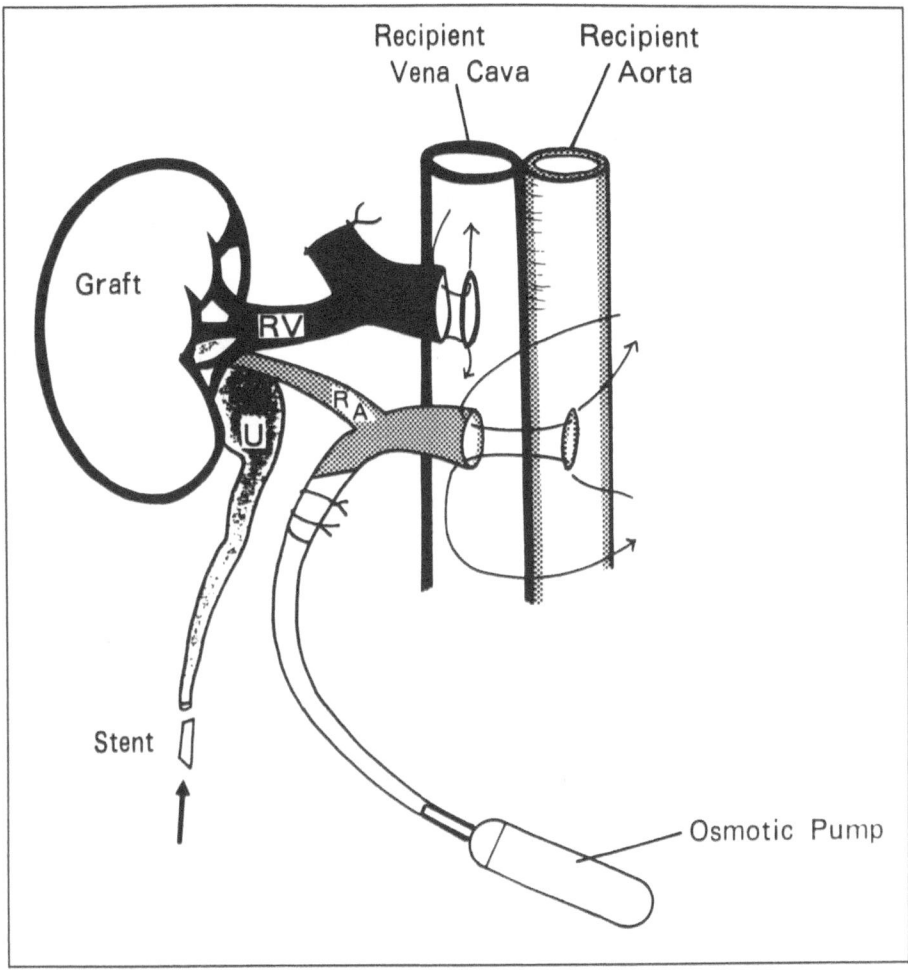

Fig. 7.1. Local treatment with MoAb OX-19 using osmotic minipump in a rat renal transplant model. RV = renal vein; U = ureter. Reproduced with permission from Lee CJ et al, Clin Exp Immunol 1993; 91:362.

75 μg/kg/day delivered locally, some recipients in the high-dose group died from abdominal infection without any sign of rejection.

Continuous local infusion of OX-19 (75 μg/kg/day), even from day 4 after renal grafting, produced a significant prolongation of graft survival (MST = 11.4 ± 0.8 days, n = 8) compared with the untreated control group (MST = 7.8 ± 0.2 days, n = 10, P < 0.01). On the other hand, continuous systemic infusion of OX-19 from day 4 after grafting did not prolong graft survival (MST = 7.6 ± 0.2 days, n = 5) compared with untreated controls (P = NS).

HISTOLOGICAL EXAMINATION OF RENAL ALLOGRAFTS

The transplant kidneys from untreated (Fig. 7.3A) or i.v.-treated (Fig. 7.3B) hosts on day 6 after grafting demonstrated a dense interstitial mononuclear cell infiltrate around the artery with a disappearance or degeneration of glomeruli. On the other hand, transplant kidneys from RA-treated hosts demonstrated mild tubular necrosis, but no mononuclear cell infiltration or interstitial edema (Fig. 7.3C).

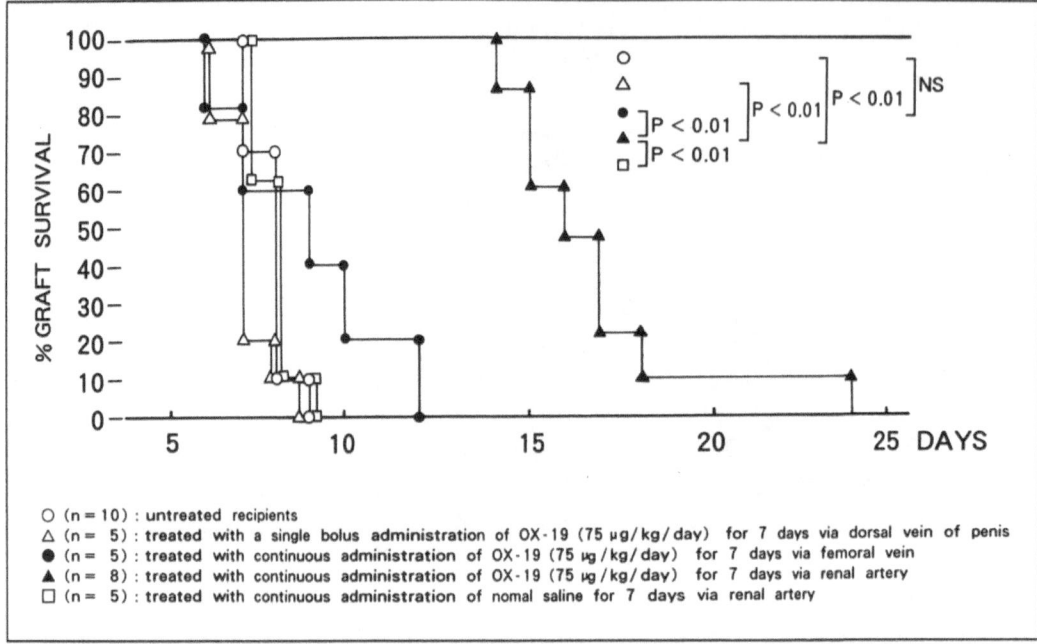

Fig. 7.2. The effect of local administration of OX-19 on LEW hosts bearing BN renal grafts: group 1 = untreated control (O–O); group 2 = i.v. bolus administration of OX-19 (Λ–Λ); group 3 = continuous i.v. infusion (●–●); group 4 = continuous RA infusion (▲–▲); group 5 = treated solely with normal saline via RA route (□–□). Reproduced with permission from Lee CJ et al, Clin Exp Immunol 1993; 91:362.

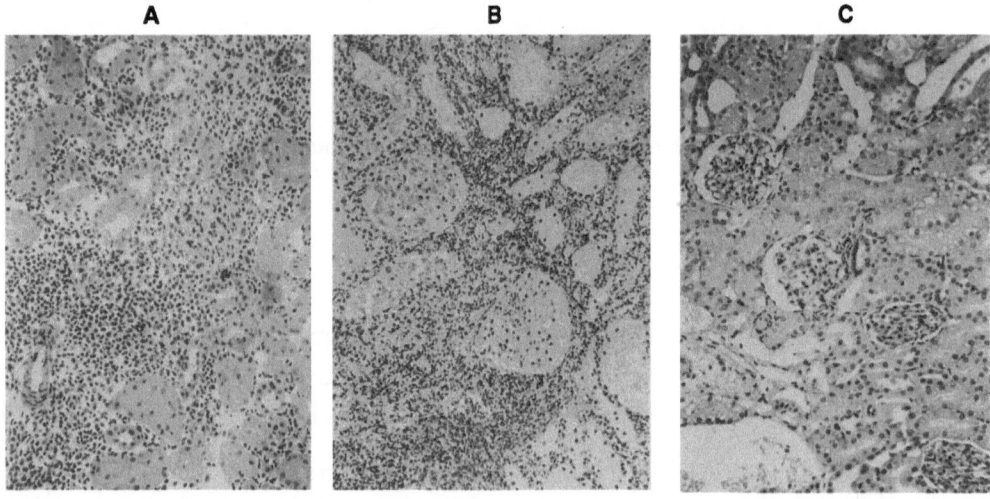

Fig. 7.3. Histological findings. (A) Untreated kidney graft at day 6 after transplantation. (B) Graft from an i.v.-treated host at day 6. (C) Graft at day 6 which received OX-19 continuously via the renal artery. (H&E stain; original magnification x100). Reproduced with permission from Lee CJ et al, Clin Exp Immunol 1993; 91:362.

IMMUNOLOGICAL EVENTS WITHIN THE GRAFT AND SPLEEN

The total number of graft infiltrating cells (GICs) from RA-treated hosts was much less ($1 - 3 \times 10^6$/graft) than that from untreated control hosts ($10 - 20 \times 10^6$/graft) or i.v.-treated hosts ($5 - 10 \times 10^6$/graft). The results of flow cytometry analysis of GICs from LEW recipients are shown in Figure 7.4. GICs obtained from RA-treated hosts on day 6 postgrafting displayed a significantly lower proportion of OX-19 positive ($8.5 \pm 3.5\%$, n = 5) and OX-8 positive ($12.1 \pm 0.9\%$, n = 5) cells when compared with those from untreated control hosts ($67.8 \pm 4.8\%$ and $39.4 \pm 3.7\%$, respectively, n = 5, $P < 0.01$) or from i.v.-treated hosts ($26.4 \pm 2.0\%$ and $22.5 \pm 2.6\%$, respectively, n = 5, $P < 0.01$). The proportion of W3/25 positive cells from RA-treated hosts ($4.8 \pm 0.4\%$) was significantly lower than that from untreated controls ($35.8 \pm 1.3\%$, $P < 0.01$), but not statistically different from that of i.v.-treated hosts ($3.4 \pm 0.7\%$, P = NS).

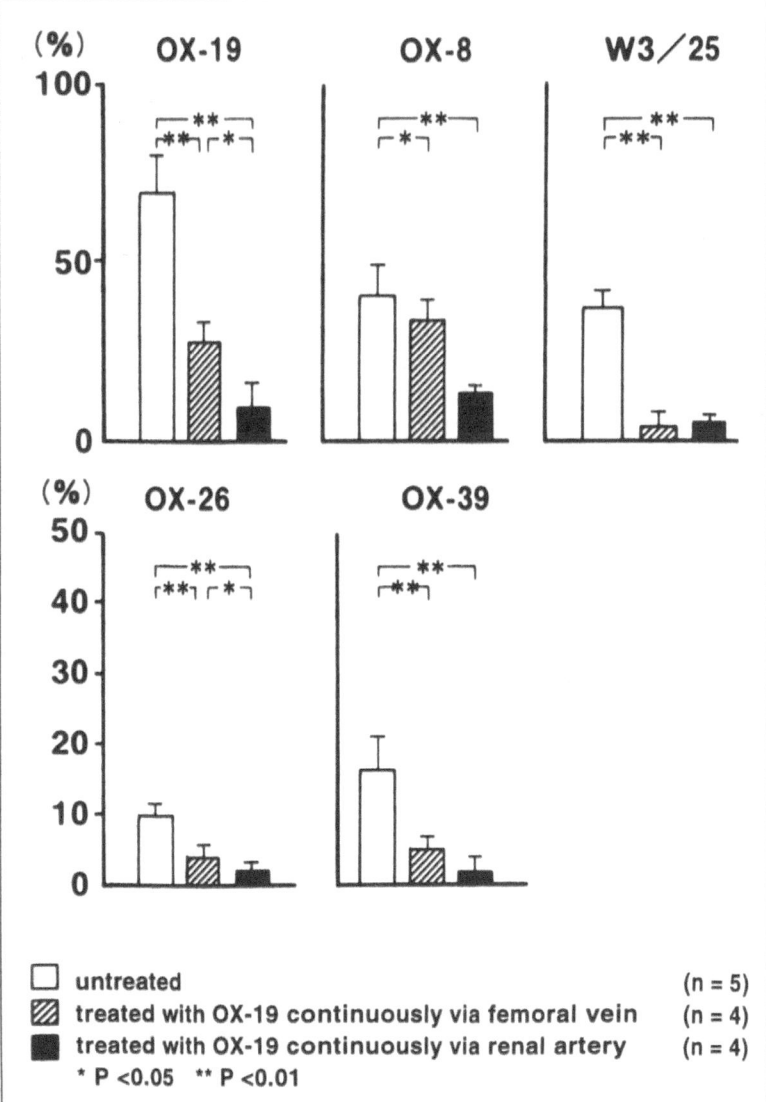

Fig. 7.4. Percentage of graft infiltrating cells from LEW recipients treated with MoAbs on postoperative day 6 (donor: BN). GICs incubated with MoAbs were further incubated with goat anti-mouse IgG (FITC- conjugated) and examined by FACS. The negative control was obtained by using only FITC-goat anti-mouse IgG (absence of mouse anti-rat MoAb). Those were less than 1%. All numerical values represent mean ± SEM (%). Statistical evaluation was performed using Student's t-test.

□ untreated (n = 5)
▨ treated with OX-19 continuously via femoral vein (n = 4)
■ treated with OX-19 continuously via renal artery (n = 4)
* P <0.05   ** P <0.01

Moreover, the expression of activated T cell markers was also tested (Fig. 7.4). GICs from RA-treated hosts displayed a significantly lower proportion of OX-26 (transferrin receptor) positive cells (1.3 ± 0.8%, n = 5) when compared with those from untreated control hosts (9.6 ± 0.4%, n = 5, P < 0.01) or from i.v.-treated hosts (3.6 ± 0.6%, P < 0.05). The proportion of OX-39 (interleukin-2 [IL-2] receptor) positive cells from RA-treated hosts (1.6 ± 0.7%, n = 5) was significantly lower than that from untreated controls (15.9 ± 2.4%, n = 5, P < 0.01) and from i.v.-treated hosts (4.3 ± 1.0%, n = 5, P < 0.05).

The spleens of RA-treated hosts on day 6 postgrafting also contained a significantly lower proportion of OX-19 (7.1 ± 2.4%), W3/25 (15.1 ± 2.4%), OX-26 (14 ± 0.6%), and OX-39 (0.1 ± 0.1%) positive cells when compared with those of untreated control hosts (62.8 ± 2.6%, 44.7 ± 4.2%, 5.3 ± 0.4% and 5.6 ± 0.1%, respectively, P < 0.01, Fig. 7.5). The percentages in the RA-treated hosts were also lower than those in the i.v.-treated hosts (4.4 ± 2.9%, 8.9 ± 2.0%, 1.6 ± 1.2% and 0.6 ± 0.4%, respectively), but the difference did not reach statistical significance.

CYTOKINE RELEASE FROM SPLENOCYTES

The amount of IL-2 produced from spleen cells in i.v.-treated hosts on day 6 postgrafting was significantly less (11.9 ± 0.4 U/ml, n = 5) than that in untreated control hosts (29.2 ± 0.3 U/ml, n = 5, P < 0.01) and in RA-treated hosts (20.1 ± 0.4 U/ml, n = 5, P < 0.01) (Fig. 7.6). Interferon-gamma (IFN-γ) production by spleen cells in i.v.-treated hosts was significantly less (23.4 ± 5.3 IU/ml, n = 5) than that in untreated control hosts (39.7 ± 8.3 IU/ml, n = 5, P < 0.05) and in RA-treated hosts (38.6 ± 8.3 IU/ml, n = 5, P < 0.05) (Fig. 7.6).

DISCUSSION

Local events within the transplant kidney play an important role during the afferent, as well as the efferent, phase of the immune response. When selective administration of immunosuppressive drugs to renal allografts interferes with these processes, allograft rejection may be manipulated locally. This approach to immunosuppressive therapy offers interesting perspectives because reduced systemic drug levels lead to fewer systemic side effects of the immunosuppressive agents used. Previously-studied agents for intraarterial administration to renal transplants, including methotrexate,[10] actinomycin D,[11] corticosteroids,[12] prostaglandin E_2,[13,16] 6-mercaptopurine[14] and cyclosporine A,[15] are chemically-synthesized materials, and show no specificity in immunosuppressive action. It is now universally accepted that T cells play an important role in acute rejection and that T cell infiltration within the graft is strongly related to rejection crises. Taking this into consideration, local administration of monoclonal anti-T cell antibody may be advantageous when compared with conventional systemic treatment on the basis of specificity and selectivity.[17,18]

Gruber et al[19] proposed several advantages of selective intraarterial infusion of drug when compared with intravenous infusion. First, the drug concentration within the target organ can be maintained at a high level for a longer period of time. Second, systemic drug concentrations may be reduced by local infusion as a result of the first-pass extraction of drug by the target organ.[20] Thus, local drug infusion produces a more selective presence of drug at its primary site of action. Indeed, our study clearly showed that the graft survival time was significantly prolonged in the group receiving selective administration of OX-19 via the renal artery when compared with the group receiving systemic therapy. These results were supported by histologic examination of the rejecting grafts.

Phenotypic characterization of GICs and spleen cells and functional assessment of spleen cells from MoAb-treated hosts were performed in this study in order to compare the effects of local and systemic administration of OX-19 on immunological events in the host. The percentage of

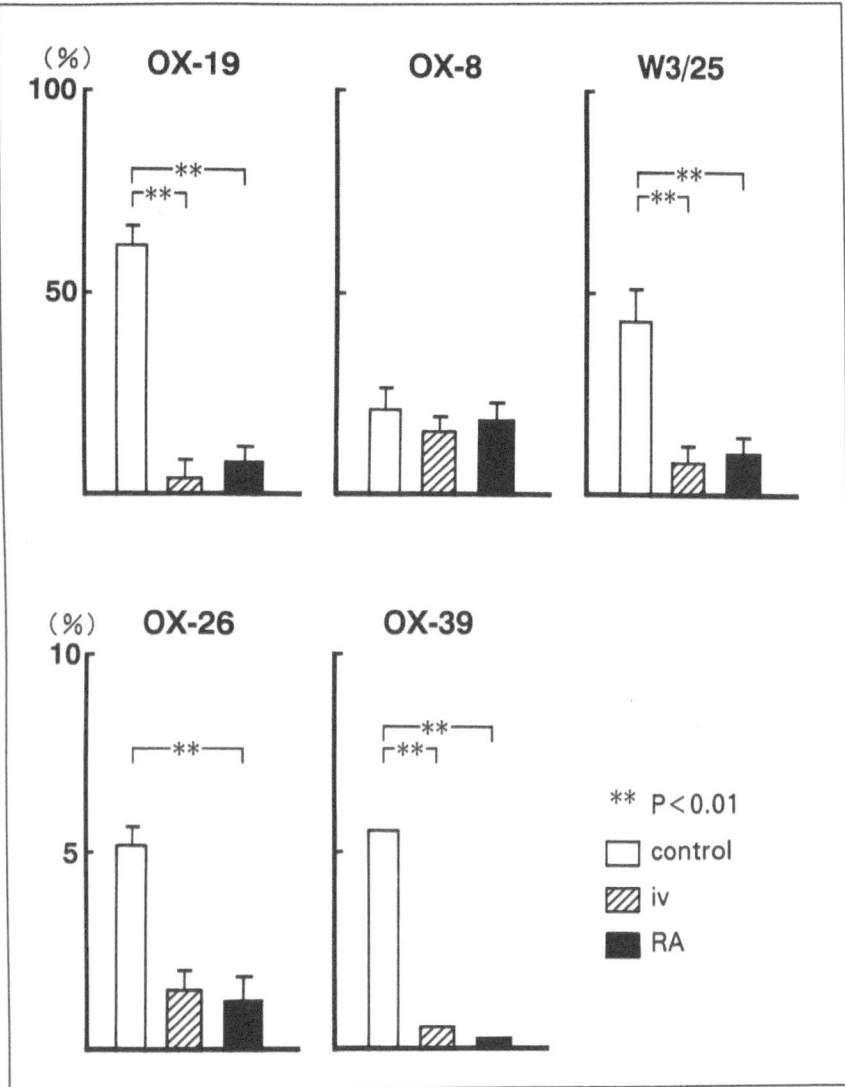

Fig. 7.5. Percentage of spleen cells from LEW recipients treated with MoAbs on postoperative day 6. Spleen cells incubated with MoAbs were further incubated with goat anti-mouse IgG (FITC-conjugated) and examined by FACS. The negative control was obtained by using only FITC-goat anti-mouse IgG (absence of mouse anti-rat MoAb). Those were less than 1%. All numerical values represent mean ± SEM (%). Statistical evaluation was performed using Student's t-test.

OX-19 positive or OX-8 positive cells within the graft was significantly less than that in untreated controls or i.v.-treated hosts. The percentage of antigen-activated cells, namely IL-2 receptor positive and transferrin receptor positive cells, within the graft was also significantly less than that in the other groups. These data sug-

gested that local, but not systemic, administration of OX-19 effectively suppressed T cell function within the graft and are in agreement with the results of Ruers et al.[21] The Dutch group showed that continuous intrarenal infusion of prednisolone decreased major histocompatibility complex (MHC) class II and IL-2 receptor expres-

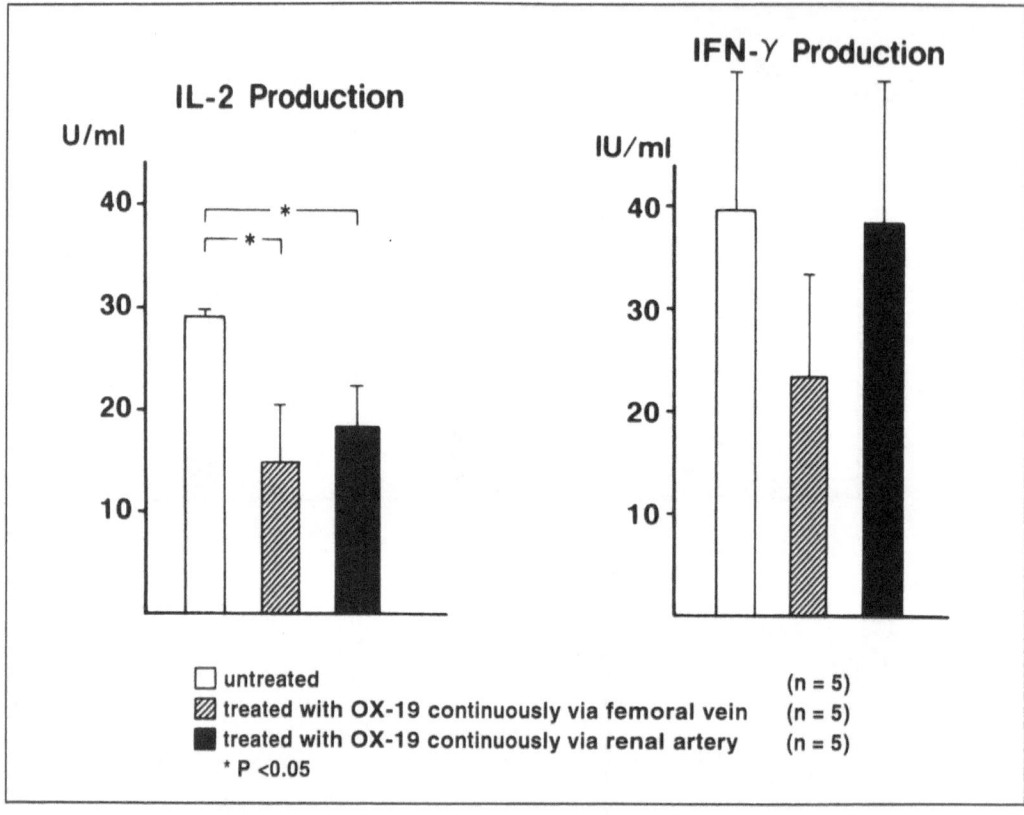

Fig. 7.6. Cytokine production of con A-stimulated spleen cells harvested from LEW recipients with an engrafted BN kidney on postoperative day 6. 2 x 10⁶/ml spleen cells were stimulated with con A (10 μg/ml) for 48 hrs, and supernatants were quantitated by using a dependent cell line for each cytokine (CTLL-2 for IL-2 assay, L929 for IFN-γ assay). All values represent mean ± SEM. Statistical evaluation was performed by Student's t-test.

sion on the grafted tissue by immunohistochemical study when compared with same-dose systemic administration.

Although phenotypic differences in the spleen were not detected between the RA-treated hosts and i.v.-treated hosts, lymphokine production was significantly decreased in the latter. A cascade of lympokines is involved in the process of T cell activation.[22,23] IL-1 activates helper T cells to produce IL-2, and IL-2 induces the production of IFN-γ or macrophage activating factor as well as the generation of cytotoxic T cells and natural killer cells[24-26] (Fig. 7.7). Therefore, the remarkable impairment of cytokine generation in the spleen caused by systemic administration of OX-19 reflects an overall disturbance of immune function in the hosts

which in contrast, might be preserved in RA-treated recipients.

Because the goal of transplantation is to induce specific tolerance without affecting overall immune function, our model of intrarenal delivery of monoclonal anti-T cell antibody may afford localized immunosuppression of certain grafts such as kidney or liver with reduction of morbidity in transplant patients and in this way would open new perspectives in clinical immunosuppressive therapy.

SUMMARY

We compared the efficacy of continuous intraarterial versus intravenous infusion of monoclonal anti-T cell antibody in a rat renal transplant model with regard to overall survival, histologic severity of rejection,

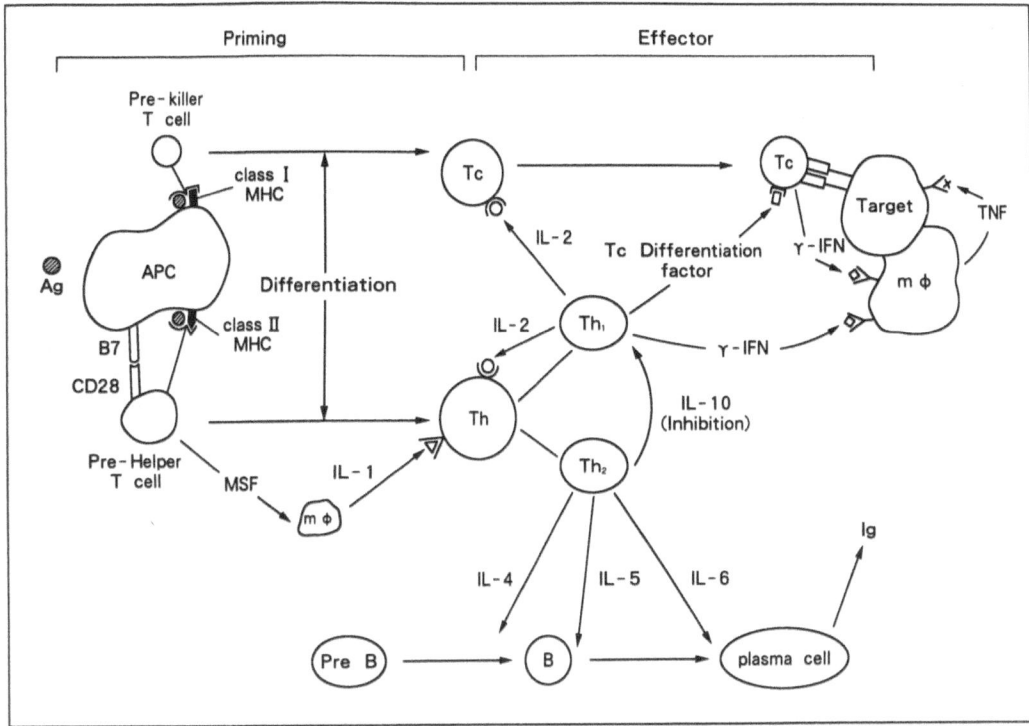

Fig. 7.7. The role of cytokines in transplantation immunology. mφ = macrophage; Th = T helper cell; Tc = T cytotoxic cell; TNF = tumor necrosis factor; APC = antigen presenting cell; MSF = macrophage stimulating factor.

subsets of infiltrating lymphocytes and activity of lymphokine production from splenic cells. Local delivery of a monoclonal anti-T cell antibody can effectively prolong graft survival with reduced T cell infiltration into the graft and reduced lymphokine production from the spleen.

REFERENCES

1. Strom TB, Tilney NL, Carpenter CB et al. Cellular components of allograft rejection. J Immunol 1977; 118:2020.

2. Loveland BE, Hograth PH, McKenzie IFC et al. Cells mediating allograft rejection in the mouse. J Exp Med 1977; 153:1044.

3. Cosimi AB, Colvin R, Burton R et al. Use of monoclonal antibodies to T-cell subsets for immunologic monitoring and treatment in recipients of renal allografts. N Engl J Med 1981; 305:308.

4. Weyand CM, Goronzy J, Swarztrauber K et al. Immunosuppression by anti-CD4 treatment in vivo. Transplantation 1989; 47:1034.

5. Herbert J, Roser B. Strategies of monoclonal therapy that induce permanent tolerance of organ transplants. Transplantation 1988; 46:128.

6. Lee S. An improved technique of renal transplantation in the rat. Surgery 1967; 61:771.

7. Yoshimura N, Matsui S, Hamasima T et al. The effects of perioperative portal venous inoculation with donor lymphocytes on renal allograft survival in the rat. Transplantation 1990; 49:167.

8. Tilney NL, Kupiec-Weglinski JW, Heideke CD et al. Mechanisms of rejection and prolongation of vascularized organ allografts. Immunological Rev 1983; 77:185.

9. Sprent J, Miller JFAP. Fate of H-2 activated T lymphocytes in syngeneic hosts. II. Residence in recirculating lymphocyte pool and capacity to migrate to allografts. Cell Immunol 1976; 21:303.

10. Miura T, Shah S, Khazei AM. Continuous chronometric infusion of immunosuppressive drugs into the arterial blood supply of

a transplanted kidney. Lahey Clin Bull 1964; 13:136.

11. Retik AB, Dubernard J-M, Hester WJ et al. A study of the effects of intraarterial immunosuppressive drug therapy on canine renal allografts. Surgery 1966; 60:1242.

12. Laupacis A, Keown PA, Rankin RN et al. Intraarterial methylprednisolone and heparin (IAT) for the treatment of refractory renal transplant rejection episodes. Transplant Proc 1982; 14:693.

13. Campbell D, Wiggins R, Kunkel S et al. Constant intrarenal infusion of PGE into a canine renal transplant using a totally implantable pump. Transplantation 1984; 38:209.

14. Gruber SA, Hrushesky WJM, Cipolle RJ et al. Local immunosuppression with reduced systemic toxicity in a canine renal allograft model. Transplantation 1989; 48:936.

15. Stepkowski S, Goto S, Reynolds K, Ito T et al. Induction of unresponsiveness after local low-dose cyclosporine administration. Transplant Proc 1989; 21:1120.

16. Kamei T, Callery MP, Flye MW. Intragraft Delivery of 16, 16-Dimethyl PGE Induces Donor-Specific Tolerance in Rat Cardiac Allograft Recipients. Transplantation 1991; 151:242.

17. Lee CJ, Yoshimura N, Shiho O et al. Local immunosuppression therapy with monoclonal anti-T cell antibody on renal allograft survival in the rat. Clin Exp Immunol 1993; 91:362.

18. Yoshimura N, Lee CJ, Shiho O et al. Local immunosuppressive therapy with monoclonal anti-T cell antibody on renal allograft survival in the rat. II. Phenotypic and functional assessment of spleen cells. Transplant Proc 1995; 27:390.

19. Gruber SA, Canafax DM, Cipolle RJ et al. Local immunosuppression of the vascularized graft. Surgery 1990; 107:209.

20. Gruber SA, Erdmann GR, Burke BA et al. Mizoribine pharmacokinetics and pharmacodynamics in a canine renal allograft model of local immunosuppression. Transplantation 1992; 53:12-19.

21. Ruers TJM, Buurman WA, Van Der Linden CJ et al. Immunohistological observations in rat kidney allografts after local steroid administration. J Exp Med 1987; 166:1205.

22. Kasahara T, Hooks JJ, Dougherty SF et al. Interleukin 2-mediated immune interferon (IFN-γ) production by human T cells and cell subsets. J Immunol 1983; 130:1784.

23. Kern DE, Gillis S, Okada M et al. The role of interleukin 2 (IL-2). in the differentiation of cytotoxic T cells: the effect of monoclonal anti-IL-2 antibody and absorption with IL-2 dependent cell lines. J Immunol 1981; 127:1323.

24. Wanger H, Rollinghoff M. T-T-cell interactions during in vitro cytotoxic allograft responses:I. Soluble products from activated Ly1+T cells trigger autonomously antigen-primed Ly2, 3+T cells to cell proliferation and cytotoxic activity. J Exp Med 1978; 148:1523.

25. Kaieda T, Okada M, Yoshimura N et al. A human helper T cell clone secreting both killer helper factor(s) and T cell-replacing factor(s). J immunol 1982; 129:46.

26. Arenzana-Sesdedos F, Virelizier JL, Fiers W. Interferons as macrophage-activating factors. J Immunol 1985; 134:2444.

CHAPTER 8

Intraportal Delivery of Immunosuppressants to Intrahepatic Islet Allografts

Donald C. Dafoe and Edward J. Alfrey

INTRODUCTION

For many years, the prevailing schema of alloreactivity made local immunosuppression illogical.[1] The understanding was that a vascularized allograft was recognized by the host through peripheral sensitization. Host immune cells circulating through the graft were exposed to nonself histocompatibility antigens. Subsequent proliferation of responder cells occurred in the spleen or lymph nodes. The effector response was mediated by sensitized lymphoid cells returning to the graft and destroying cells bearing foreign histocompatibility antigens. Nonspecific immunosuppressive agents, such as azathioprine and steroids, interfered with proliferating cells in the spleen and other lymphoid depots. Given this schema, the value of immunosuppression at the graft site was doubtful.

The cascade of events following allografting has undergone constant review and revision. Recently, the importance of the local environment has been recognized. The sponge matrix allograft model and others have advanced the understanding of intragraft events.[2,3] This has resulted in a conceptual change in the schema of alloreactivity. Inflammation or systemic immunization in the vascularized allograft attracts a variety of cells, including specifically reactive cells against donor histocompatibility antigens. Secondary to changes in local vascular permeability and the elaboration of chemotactic agents, the allograft is infiltrated primarily by nonspecific immune cells, but also by some specific cells. Cytokines are

Local Immunosuppression of Organ Transplants, edited by Scott A. Gruber.
© 1996 R.G. Landes Company.

produced by sensitized specific T-helper cells (Th) supporting maturation and expansion of specific cytotoxic T cells (Tc).

The significant conclusions of these studies are that effector cells differentiate and mature in the allograft and this process is dependent upon locally produced lymphokines. Based on these conclusions, local immunosuppression merits re-evaluation.

Intraarterial delivery of immunosuppressive agents to vascularized allografts has been shown to prolong allograft survival in several experimental models.[4-7] The dual blood supply to the liver—hepatic artery and portal vein—presents a unique opportunity for local delivery of immunosuppressive agents intraportally. This approach had not been previously investigated. In a review of local immunosuppression, Gruber[8] characterized the ideal immunosuppressive agent as cleared rapidly outside of and/or highly extracted by the target organ to produce a regional advantage (increased efficacy) and/or systemic advantage (decreased toxicity). In theory, local delivery of the ideal agent could establish high levels in the allograft and low levels systemically. We selected the agents budesonide, cyclosporine and FK506 that are metabolized or avidly bound by the liver to evaluate the effect of local immunosuppression by intraportal delivery on intrahepatic islet allograft survival.[9,10]

THE MODEL: INTRAPORTAL DELIVERY OF IMMUNOSUPPRESSANTS TO INTRAHEPATIC ISLET ALLOGRAFTS IN RATS

In the model chosen for study, isolated rodent islets were inoculated into the portal vein of diabetic recipients. Rats were selected as the experimental animal because of our experience with islet transplantation in this species as well as the availability of inbred strains allowing transplantation across well-defined histocompatibility barriers.

The intraportal islet allograft model has several advantages. Islet allografting

rapidly reverses experimental diabetes in rats (usually within 24 hours). The strong immunogenicity of islets consistently leads to early acute rejection which is readily identified by recurrent hyperglycemia. A large experimental background with islet transplantation in rats has been reported in the immunobiology literature.[11-13]

Intraportal infusion was easily accomplished in the rat utilizing implantable osmotic minipumps. The minipump imbibes fluid from surrounding tissue through a semipermeable membrane, resulting in compression of a reservoir filled with the agent of interest.[14] The minipumps were tested with each of the agents studied, and the agents were found to be stable and biocompatible with the minipump. In preliminary work, the subcutaneous space of the back was noted to be a better site for minipump placement than the peritoneal cavity. The splenic vein was the vessel most suitable for access to the portal vein. The pump catheter was inserted into the splenic vein and secured in place, with a ligature placed on the spleen side of the splenic vein. This did not result in splenic infarction—an unwanted consequence that would confound the experimental model—presumably because of collateral drainage via the short gastric vessels.

The intraportal route offered several advantages. Intraarterial introduction of immunosuppressive agents has been studied, but carries with it the risk of thrombosis with graft loss. Although this potential risk is shared by the intraportal route, cannulation of a venous branch (e.g., draining into the superior mesenteric vein) and the high flow portal system may protect against thrombosis. Intraportal infusion by minipump will constantly deliver high doses of immunosuppressive agents into the microenvironment of transplanted islets that lodge in the distal hepatic venules and sinusoids. Within 2 weeks, an arterial blood supply develops according to Andersson and co-workers.[15] That is, intrahepatically transplanted islets are initially nourished by portal blood; then approximately 14 days after transplantation, the islets no longer are exposed primarily to agents in portal venous blood, but rather to systemic blood constituents via the newly-formed arterial blood supply.

Intrahepatic islets are also exposed to lymphoid cells trafficking through the liver. The intrahepatic site may be a particularly hostile environment to allografted islets because of proximity to immunocompetent cells, such as macrophages and natural killer cells.[16] Our experimental design using the intrahepatic site constituted a discriminating model because of the formidable barrier to successful transplantation.

The intrahepatic site also offers physiological and endocrinological benefit.[17] Better glucose tolerance is effected by hepatic insulin extraction. Insulin extraction by the liver avoids detrimental peripheral hyperinsulinism that ensues from systemic venous drainage of pancreas or islet grafts (e.g., in the renal subcapsular transplant site). Intriguingly, delivery of alloantigen into the liver has been noted by a number of investigators to favor immunological tolerance.[18,19] Kupffer cells, the unique macrophages that line the hepatic sinusoids, appear to be pivotal in the response to alloantigen. The Kupffer cell population is accessible to manipulation via portal venous delivery of various agents. In man and large animals, embolization of islet autografts and allografts into the portal vein has been successful, making this model clinically relevant.[20-22]

In a provocative study of intrahepatic islet allografts, Kamei and Yasunami[23] described "local unresponsiveness" that appears to be dependent on immunomodulation of the intrahepatic environment. Streptozotocin-induced diabetes was reversed in rats by intraportal inoculation of allogeneic islets and 3 days of cyclosporine treatment. This regimen allowed permanent survival of islets in the liver, but only modest prolongation of islet allograft survival in the renal subcapsular space in another group of animals. If diabetes was re-induced in the "tolerant" rats by streptozotocin treatment, new donor-strain islets could be successfully transplanted to

the liver (but not the renal subcapsule) without any additional immunosuppression. These findings appear to be at variance with extensive studies by Reece-Smith et al[24] which indicated that survival of islet allografts is more easily induced in the renal subcapsular site than in the intrahepatic site in rats. However, in contrast to Kamei and Yasunami,[23] Reece-Smith and co-workers[24] administered a brief course of antilymphocyte serum rather than cyclosporine. Furthermore, Kamei and Yasunami[23] also noted that without cyclosporine, intrahepatic islets were rejected more rapidly than renal subcapsular islets. This suggests that cyclosporine may favor the induction of suppressor cells in the vicinity of the intrahepatic islets. The effect did not appear to be a systemic one since skin allografts were rejected by recipients of established intrahepatic islets. The relative contribution of various factors, including cyclosporine, islets, T cells, antigen presenting cells and Kupffer cells, in the microenvironment of the hepatic sinusoids to the production of "local unresponsiveness" has not been determined.

Recipients were male Wistar-Furth (RT-1u) rats weighing 200-250 grams that were rendered diabetic (blood glucose > 300 mg/dl) with a single intravenous injection of streptozotocin (80 mg/kg; Zanosar, Upjohn, Kalamazoo, MI). Blood glucose determinations were done by tail bleeding using a Glucometer (Ames Co, Miles Laboratories, Elkhart, IN). While awaiting transplantation, diabetic rats received long-acting protamine zinc insulin (Eli Lilly, Indianapolis, IN) in doses of 2-4 U/day depending on blood glucose determinations to prevent weight loss and general debility. After islet transplantation, recurrent diabetes was defined as blood glucose > 250 mg/dl on two consecutive daily determinations. Rats had free access to standard chow and water. Surgery was performed and animal care administered in accordance with the policies of the Institutional Animal Care and Use Committee at Stanford University Medical Center.

Islets were isolated from four to six Lewis (RT-1l) rats using standard techniques of collagenase digestion (Type V, Sigma, St. Louis, MO), passage through a nylon filter, and density gradient separation using Ficoll.[25] Between 1000 and 1500 islets were slowly injected intraportally in a 1 ml suspension of Hank's solution. The immunosuppressant (budesonide, cyclosporine or FK506) was placed in an implantable osmotic minipump (Alzet, Palo Alto, CA) that continuously delivered the drug for either 14 or 28 days. The proximal splenic vein was cannulated for intraportal delivery as described above and the jugular vein was cannulated for systemic delivery using a polyethylene catheter (PE 50, Clay Adams, Parsippany, NJ) from the minipump placed subcutaneously on the back. The minipumps were checked by laparotomy for proper position and flow on the 7th day after implantation. Depending on the experimental protocol, the minipump was removed 14 or 28 days after implantation to assure that the reservoir was empty.

Tissue specimens for microscopic examination were processed after adequate fixation in Bouin's solution. Sections were stained with hematoxylin and eosin. Aldehyde fuchsin staining was used to demonstrate insulin granules.

Statistical analysis was carried out using the Statworks software program (Cricket Software, Philadelphia, PA). To assess differences in nonparametric mean survival time (MST) data between experimental groups, the Wilcoxon signed rank test was used. Mean values were expressed with standard deviations ($\pm$ SD). Categorical differences were analyzed by chi-square test. A $P < 0.05$ was considered significant.

This model has potential for immediate clinical application. Just as implantable pumps have been employed to selectively deliver cancer chemotherapeutic agents, continuous portal vein or hepatic artery infusion of immunosuppressive agents would be readily applicable to human islet and liver transplantation. Furthermore, it is conceivable that percutaneous trans-

hepatic catheterization of the portal vein could provide intensive local therapy for refractory rejection.

IMMUNOSUPPRESSIVE AGENTS

STEROIDS

Local immunosuppression with intra-arterial prednisolone has been shown to significantly prolong graft survival in a rat renal allograft model.[5] In theory, this prolongation was mediated by inhibition of gamma-interferon and interleukin-2 (IL-2) production resulting in decreased donor major histocompatibility complex (MHC) class II antigen presentation to Th and decreased proliferation of Tc, respectively. Allograft cells were found to have reduced expression of MHC class I molecules serving as recognition targets for class I-restricted effector cells. Local immunosuppression depressed the efferent limb of alloreactivity by inhibiting cytokine production. Local delivery of steroids may also blunt the afferent limb of alloreactivity by limiting IL-1 production by macrophages. IL-1 is considered an important soluble second signal necessary for activation of alloreactivity following antigen-specific T cell receptor triggering of Th by foreign MHC class II molecules.

In our trials of intraportal delivery, we used the steroid budesonide. Budesonide is a nonhalogenated glucocorticoid with potent local anti-inflammatory properties.[26] It is used topically in the clinical treatment of asthma and dermatological disease. Its pharmacokinetics are characterized by high hepatic clearance. More than 80% of the active parent compound is biotransformed during one pass through the liver. The metabolites have greatly reduced glucocorticoid potency. For example, the major metabolite, 6-beta-hydroxy-budesonide, has less than 1% of the receptor binding affinity and biological activity of budesonide. Ruers and colleagues[6] used an inventive model to study the effect of local delivery of budesonide (chapter 4). Cardiac allografts were transplanted heterotopically into the abdomen with portal venous drainage, and budesonide was infused via the aorta into graft coronary arteries. As anticipated, levels of budesonide were high in coronary artery blood and myocardium of the graft, while systemic levels of the agent remained low because of clearance by the liver. Due to the fact that myocardial tissue selectively binds budesonide, systemic administration of budesonide also resulted in high tissue levels in the heart graft. Since allograft tissue levels of budesonide were similar with local and systemic administration, it was not surprising that median allograft survival was comparable with local and systemic immunosuppression. However, systemic delivery produced high systemic steroid levels and was associated with serious toxicity, while the local immunosuppression caused much less toxicity. We reasoned that the results with intrahepatic islets would be different in that budesonide is not selectively bound by liver; in fact, it is actively metabolized by the liver. Thus, we thought use of budesonide in our islet transplantation model was likely to result in a greater disparity in allograft survival between the systemic and local delivery groups.

In the experiment by Ruers et al,[6] local and systemic administration of budesonide was studied using 40, 90 and 120 μg/kg/day. With escalating doses, the MST increased from 7 days in untreated controls to 13, 16 and 20 days, respectively. The systemic dose of budesonide was limited by toxicity (loss of body, spleen, thymus and adrenal weight), and steroid-induced lymphocytolysis was apparently responsible for spleen and thymus weight loss. Most likely, this lymphocytolytic effect also contributed to improved allograft survival.

Budesonide also has powerful anti-inflammatory effects, such as attenuation of changes in vascular permeability associated with inflammation. These anti-inflammatory effects may protect the allograft by suppression of the delayed-type hypersensitivity component of alloreactivity.

In our trials, budesonide was obtained through the generosity of the Astra Pharmaceutical Production AB, Lund, Sweden. Based on the work of Ruers and co-workers,[6] the doses of budesonide selected for minipump delivery were 240 and 360 μg/kg/day for 14 days. Despite these 2- to 3-fold higher doses, budesonide delivered intraportally did not significantly prolong the MST of islet allografts over that of untreated controls (Table 8.1). Failure due to rejection from inadequate dosing is unlikely, and it is possible that high-dose budesonide prevented engraftment of or damaged engrafted islets.

CYCLOSPORINE

Cyclosporine is a fungal metabolite widely used in experimental and clinical immunosuppression.[27] Although the ratio of hepatic clearance from blood is only 0.3, the liver is the major depot for cyclosporine metabolism. After first-pass extraction by the hepatic cytochrome P-450 system, further metabolism may occur during enterohepatic circulation.

Cyclosporine has been used in several different protocols in the rat allograft model. Local delivery of low-dose cyclosporine (2 mg/kg/day) into the coronary artery of heterotopic cardiac allografts was compared with administration by gavage or intravenous infusion.[4] A finite period of local cyclosporine delivery resulted in high

Table 8.1. Graft survival after intrahepatic transplantation of islet allografts: Intraportal budesonide versus no treatment

Treatment	Daily Dose	N	MST ± SD (days)
None		7	7 ± 1 (5,6,6,7,8,8,9)
Budesonide	240 μg/kg	4	4 ± 1 (3,4,4,5)
Budesonide	360 μg/kg	4	7 ± 5 (4,5,6,14)

drug levels in the graft tissue and markedly prolonged graft survival. Allospecific T cells were present in recipient lymph nodes and spleen. Both Tc activity toward donor targets and delayed-type hypersensitivity were also attenuated. We studied intraportal low-dose cyclosporine infusion in the intrahepatic islet allograft model. One drawback is that cyclosporine inhibits insulin secretion and may interfere with insulin synthesis.[28] Therefore, high local levels of cyclosporine may be toxic to islet allografts, but these effects are dose-related and reversible.

The intravenous formulation of cyclosporine (Sandimmune, Sandoz Corp., Basel, Switzerland) was administered intraportally with the minipump. Two doses, 2 and 4 mg/kg/day, were utilized based on prior work in the rat cardiac allograft model.[4] Cyclosporine infused at 2 mg/kg/day in two rats established mean peripheral blood cyclosporine levels of 306 ng/ml, 220 ± 68 ng/ml and 368 ± 1 ng/ml at 24 hours, 48 hours and 14 days, respectively. In six recipients of cyclosporine at 4 mg/kg/day, levels were determined on portal and peripheral venous blood 7 days after transplantation. Levels were not significantly different in portal vein blood (508 ± 374 ng/ml) when compared with peripheral blood (771 ± 467 ng/ml); that is, there was not a significant cyclosporine gradient across the liver. Finally, there was no significant increase in the MST of cyclosporine-treated islet allograft recipients over that of untreated controls (Table 8.2).

FK506

FK506 is a macrolide with potent immunosuppressive properties (10-100x that of cyclosporine).[29] It is a lipophilic agent that is absorbed by the gut, distributed extensively in tissues, and metabolized completely, primarily by the liver.[30] The first-pass hepatic extraction of FK506 has not been studied. In high doses, FK506 may be toxic to islets.[31,32]

FK506 was provided by Fujisawa Pharmaceutical Company, Osaka, Japan. The agent was dissolved in propylene glycol. Based on the dose used in experimental and clinical reports,[29,33] we selected 0.16 mg/kg/day. Serum FK506 levels were determined 14 days after transplantation employing a two-step competitive binding immunoassay.[34]

Results are summarized in Table 8.3. Immunosuppression with FK506, either via the intraportal or intravenous route, significantly extended islet allograft survival when compared with nonimmunosuppressed recipients (or recipients immunosuppressed with intraportal budesonide or cyclosporine). Intraportal delivery of FK506 for 14 and 28 days of treatment was superior to intravenous delivery in prolonging survival of islet allografts. Only 1 of 14 recipients (7%) became hyperglycemic due to rejection of the islet allograft while maintained on intraportal FK506 compared with 4 of 14 (29%) receiving intravenous FK506, but this difference did not achieve statistical significance. In the intravenous FK506 group, rejection uniformly occurred either during infusion or within 14 days of discontinuation. After completion of intraportal FK506 infusion, 14 normoglycemic recipients remained so for a mean of 42 ± 25 days (range: 9 to > 100 days) in the 14 day treatment group and 46 ± 15 days (range: 30 to > 100 days) in the 28

Table 8.2. Graft survival after intrahepatic transplantation of islet allografts: Intraportal cyclosporine versus no treatment

Treatment	Daily Dose	N	MST ± SD (days)
None		7	7 ± 1 (5,6,6,7,8,8,9)
Cyclosporine	2 mg/kg	8	17 ± 29 (5,5,5,5,6,9,9,88)
Cyclosporine	4 mg/kg	5	13 ± 18 (3,4,6,8,45)

day treatment group. The delay in rejection may reflect a gradual dissipation of high FK506 levels in tissue depots or a residual immunosuppressive effect secondary to high local levels.

Histological study of the liver from normoglycemic recipients demonstrated healthy islets in the sinusoidal space. To rule out FK506-induced islet toxicity as the cause of recurrent hyperglycemia, three recipients with recurrent hyperglycemia were studied histologically and found to have acute rejection, manifested as an infiltrate of mononuclear cells in the portal triad where degranulated islets were also seen.

In general, local FK506 administration prevented islet allograft rejection. Intraportal FK506 (0.16 mg/kg/day) for 14 days significantly lengthened MST when compared with untreated controls (49 ± 29 versus 7 ± 1 days, $P < 0.01$) and intravenous FK506 (17 ± 7 days, $P < 0.01$). A longer course of intraportal FK506, 28 days, also demonstrated the superiority of intraportal versus intravenous delivery. MSTs were 81 ± 32 and 34 ± 4 days, respectively, for the intraportal and intravenous routes ($P < 0.01$). Importantly, mean systemic FK506 levels on the 14th day of a 28 day infusion were significantly lower in the intraportal group than in the intravenous group (1.3 ± 0.6 versus 3.5 ± 0.9 ng/ml, respectively; $P < 0.02$). Although these blood levels were in the low range according to clinical practice,[33] the prevention of rejection in intraportal FK506-treated recipients suggests that intrahepatic FK506 levels were in the therapeutic range. Taken altogether, the data are consistent with hepatic extraction by metabolism of FK506. Regarding systemic toxicity, 4 days after transplantation, there was a significant difference in mean body weight between the two groups; the intravenous FK506 group lost 9.4 grams, while the intraportal group lost only 0.3 grams ($P < 0.05$). Thereafter, the intravenous group gained weight rapidly and matched the intraportal group. Other than the crude index of mean body weight, specific renal or other toxicities were not investigated. There was no mortality in any of the experimental groups. It is logical to assume that lower systemic drug levels would translate into less systemic toxicity.

As an extension of the study, we noted that three of seven recipients treated for 28 days with intraportal FK506 became hyperglycemic many days after discontinuation of FK506 presumably due to rejection. To study the phenomenon of sensitization following intraportal FK506 immunosuppression, retransplantation was carried out using Lewis, donor-specific, islets and no immunosuppression. Normoglycemia was established in each animal before recurrent hyperglycemia occurred 4, 14 and 19 days after transplantation (MST 12.3 ± 8 days). In comparison,

---

Table 8.3. Graft survival after intrahepatic transplantation of islet allografts: Intraportal FK506 versus no treatment

Treatment	Duration	N	Route	MST ± SD (days)	
None		7		7 ± 1	(5,6,6,7,8,8,9)
FK506	14	7	IPO*	49 ± 29	(9,23,49,50,52,59,>100)
FK506	14	7	IV**	17 ± 7	(8,10,11,19,24,24,25)
FK506	28	7	IPO	81 ± 32	(58,62,68,68,72,92,>100)
FK506	28	7	IV	34 ± 4	(28,32,33,34,36,36,42)

* IPO = intraportal **IV = intravenous
Significantly prolonged islet allograft survival in: untreated vs. all FK506 groups, $P < 0.01$; FK506 14 days IPO versus 7 days (not shown), $P < 0.01$; FK506 IPO versus IV at 14 and 28 days, $P < 0.01$. P values determined using the Wilcoxon signed rank test.

two untreated recipients of Lewis islet regrafts that were not immunosuppressed at the time of either the initial islet allograft or regraft developed recurrent hyperglycemia very rapidly after 3 and 4 days (MST 3.5 days). This pilot experiment suggests that a prior course of intraportal FK506 confers a degree of protection from second-set intrahepatic islet allograft rejection in the absence of additional immunosuppression.

DISCUSSION

These experimental trials of local immunosuppression were unique with regard to the use of intraportal delivery of immunosuppressive agents to nonvascularized intrahepatic islet allografts. Most investigations have employed intraarterial delivery of immunosuppressants to vascularized allografts.[4-7]

The ideal immunosuppressive agent for local delivery should have high first-pass metabolism by the target organ or rapid clearance outside the target organ.[8] This will result in high allograft drug levels and low systemic drug levels. Tissue binding characteristics are also important, since selective allograft tissue binding with early saturation kinetics may have the undesirable effect of equalizing efficacy of local and systemic delivery.

In our studies, three agents were investigated: budesonide, cyclosporine and FK506. We found that neither intraportal budesonide nor cyclosporine in the doses studied significantly prolonged the MST of islet allografts over that of untreated controls. On the other hand, survival of islet allografts was enhanced in recipients of FK506 intraportally, compared with untreated animals or those that received intravenous FK506. The goal of local immunosuppression was achieved, since this survival advantage occurred in the setting of significantly lower systemic FK506 levels in the intraportal group.[9,10]

In a pilot trial, we found that intraportal FK506-treated recipients that rejected islet allografts enjoyed freedom from early second-set rejection upon retransplantation even in the absence of additional

immunosuppression. These findings raise the intriguing possibility of intraportal delivery of immunosuppressive agents in association with donor antigen in an effort to immunomodulate the intrahepatic transplant site and induce allograft acceptance.

Intraportal delivery of immunosuppressants could find application in the clinical arena. It is entirely feasible to implant a pump and deliver immunosuppressive agents into the portal vein in islet or liver transplant recipients. It is conceivable that resistant acute rejection could be reversed with intraportal delivery of immunosuppressants via transhepatic access to the portal vein, obtained by percutaneous puncture or through transjugular cannulation of the hepatic veins, thereby providing high local concentrations of the agent and avoiding systemic toxicity. Continued investigation may establish the scientific and practical foundation for clinical trials.

ACKNOWLEDGEMENT

This work was supported by the philanthropic sorority Beta Sigma Phi and the Juvenile Diabetes Foundation International. Dr. A.M. Alak, Fujisawa Pharmaceutical Company, Chicago, performed the FK506 assays.

REFERENCES

1. Ascher NL, Hoffman R, Hanto DW et al. Cellular events within the rejecting allograft. Transplantation 1983; 35:193.
2. Hayry P Intragraft events in allograft destruction. Transplantation 1984; 38:1.
3. Orosz CG, Bishop DK, Ferguson RM. In vivo mechanisms of alloreactivity. Transplantation 1989; 48:818.
4. Stepkowski SM, Goto S, Ito T et al. Prolongation of heterotopic heart allograft survival by local delivery of continuous low-dose cyclosporine therapy. Transplantation 1989; 47:17.
5. Ruers TJM, Buurman WA, Smits JFM et al. Local treatment of renal allografts, a promising way to reduce the dosage of immunosuppressive drugs. Transplantation 1986; 41:156.
6. Ruers TJM, Daeman MJAP, Thijssen HHW et al. Sensitivity of graft rejection in rats to

local immunosuppressive therapy. Transplantation 1988; 46:820.

7. Gruber SA, Canafax DM, Cipolle RJ et al. Local immunosuppression of the vascularized graft. Surgery 1990; 107:209.

8. Gruber SA. The case for local immunosuppression. Transplantation 1992; 54:1.

9. Wang X, Berezniak R, Tafra L et al. Intraportal FK506 improves intrahepatic islet allograft survival. Transplant Proc 1991; 23:3211.

10. Wang X, Alfrey EJ, Posselt A et al. Intraportal delivery of immunosuppression to intrahepatic islet allograft recipients. Transplant Int 1995; 8:268.

11. Reckard CR, Barker CF. Transplantation of isolated pancreatic islets across strong and weak histocompatibility barriers. Transplant Proc 1973; 5:761.

12. Naji A, Silvers WK, Plotkin SA et al. Successful islet transplantation in spontaneous diabetes. Surgery 1979; 86:218.

13. Groth CG, ed. Pancreas and Islet Transplantation. Diabetes 1989; 38(suppl):1.

14. Theeuwes F, Yum SI. Principles of design and operation of generic osmotic pumps for the delivery of semisolid and liquid drug formulations. Ann Biomed Eng 1976; 4:343.

15. Andersson A, Korsgren O, Jansson L. Intraportally transplanted pancreatic islets revascularized from hepatic arterial system. Diabetes 1989; 38(suppl):192.

16. Nash JR, Bell PRF. Islet transplantation - synergism between antilymphocyte and antimacrophage agents. J Surg Res 1984; 36:154.

17. Gray DWR, Morris PJ. Developments in isolated pancreatic islet transplantation. Transplantation 1987; 43:321.

18. Qian J, Kokudo S, Sato S et al. Tolerance induction of alloreactivity by portal venous inoculation with allogeneic cells followed by the injection of cyclophosphamide. Transplantation 1987; 43:538.

19. Mattingly JA, Waksman BH. Immunologic suppression after oral administration of antigen. J Immunol 1978; 121:1878.

20. Dubernard JM, Sutherland DER. International Handbook of Pancreas Transplantation. Dordrecht, the Netherlands: Kluwer Academic Publishers, 1989.

21. Van Der Vliet JA, Kaufman DB, Meloche RM et al. A simple method of canine pancreatic islet isolation and intrahepatic transplantation. J Surg Res 1989; 46:126.

22. Alejandro R, Cutfield R, Shienvold FL et al. Successful long-term survival of pancreatic islet allografts in spontaneous or pancreatectomy-induced diabetes in dogs. Diabetes 1985; 34:825.

23. Kamei T, Yasunami Y. Demonstration of donor specific unresponsiveness in rat islet allografts: importance of transplant site for induction by cyclosporin A and maintenance. Diabetologia 1989; 32:779.

24. Reece-Smith H, Dutoit DF, McShane P et al. Prolonged survival of pancreatic islet allografts transplanted beneath the renal capsule. Transplantation 1981; 31:305.

25. Ziegler MM, Reckard CR, Barker CF. Long term metabolic and immunological considerations in transplantation of pancreatic islets. J Surg Res 1974; 16:575.

26. Edsbacker S, Andersson P, Lindberg C et al. Metabolic acetal splitting of budesonide. Drug Metab Disp 1987; 15:403.

27. Kahan BD. Cyclosporine. N Engl J Med 1989; 321:1725.

28. Hahn HJ, Laube F, Lucke S et al. Toxic effects of cyclosporine on the endocrine pancreas of wistar rats. Transplantation 1986; 41:44.

29. Peters DH, Fitton A, Plosker GL et al. Tacrolimus. Drugs 1993; 46:746.

30. Jain AB, Ventakaramanan R, Cadoff E et al. Effect of hepatic dysfunction and T-tube clamping on FK506 pharmacokinetics and trough concentrations. Transplant Proc 1990; 22:57.

31. Hirano Y, Fujihira S, Ohara K et al. Morphological and functional changes of islets of langerhans in FK506-treated rats. Transplantation 1992; 53:889.

32. Ohara K, Billington R, James RW et al. Toxicologic evaluation of FK506. Transplant Proc 1990:22:83.

33. Venkataramanan R, Jain A, Cadoff E, at al. Pharmacokinetics of FK506. Transplant Proc 1990; 22:52.

34. Tamura K, Kobayashi M, Hoshimoto K. A highly sensitive method to assay FK506 levels in plasma. Transplant Proc 1987; 19:23.

SECTION C:
PUMP-BASED LOCAL INFUSION IN CANINE ALLOGRAFT MODELS

LOCAL HEPARIN, 6-MERCAPTOPURINE, PREDNISOLONE, AND MIZORIBINE DELIVERY IN A CANINE RENAL ALLOGRAFT MODEL

Scott A. Gruber, Shengguang Xiao and Stephen E. Hughes

RATIONALE FOR AND FEASIBILITY OF THE CANINE MODEL

Although the rat models described in the previous section elegantly demonstrate the efficacy of local immunosuppression, they have several limitations when one considers the potential for eventual clinical application. The osmotic pumps utilized for drug delivery are inaccessible within the abdomen, cannot be emptied of and refilled with drug, and can only infuse drug for a 2 week interval. As a result, long-term considerations such as pump compatibility, drug stability and catheter-induced thrombosis and infection cannot be evaluated. Furthermore, repeated blood sampling to assess regional and systemic pharmacokinetics is not practical. Despite the generalized species simililarity which exists in the pharmacokinetic advantage of regional drug delivery,[1] the results obtained from these models may not be entirely relevant to higher animals and man in view of significant species differences in drug disposition and pharmacologic activity, a point well illustrated by the corticosteroids.[2-6] Finally, heterotopic placement of the transplanted organ to

Local Immunosuppression of Organ Transplants, edited by Scott A. Gruber.

increase the pharmacokinetic advantage achievable from local infusion of a particular drug is not clinically feasible.

In view of these limitations and with an eye towards direct clinical application, we developed a canine renal allograft model of local immunosuppression utilizing implantable, programmable infusion pumps and biocompatible catheters to investigate the pharmacokinetic parameters and pharmacodynamic effects of intraarterial (i.a.) drug delivery to the transplanted kidney.[7,8] This model more closely resembles the situation in man anatomically and physiologically, and could be applied directly to man with little modification. Briefly, mon-

grel dogs, 16-25 kg in weight, undergo bilateral nephrectomy and autografting or exchange renal allografting of one kidney to the right iliac fossa via end-to-end renal-external iliac artery and end-to-side renal-external iliac vein anastomoses. A soft, flexible silicone 4 Fr arterial infusion catheter (Model 8702 Drug Administration Catheter, Medtronic, Inc., Minneapolis, MN) is inserted into the aorta with its tip in the iliac artery and its proximal end tunneled subcutaneously to a "pump pocket" in the lateral chest wall (Fig. 9.1). In autotransplants, a second, venous sampling catheter may be placed with its tip in the iliac vein just proximal to the anas-

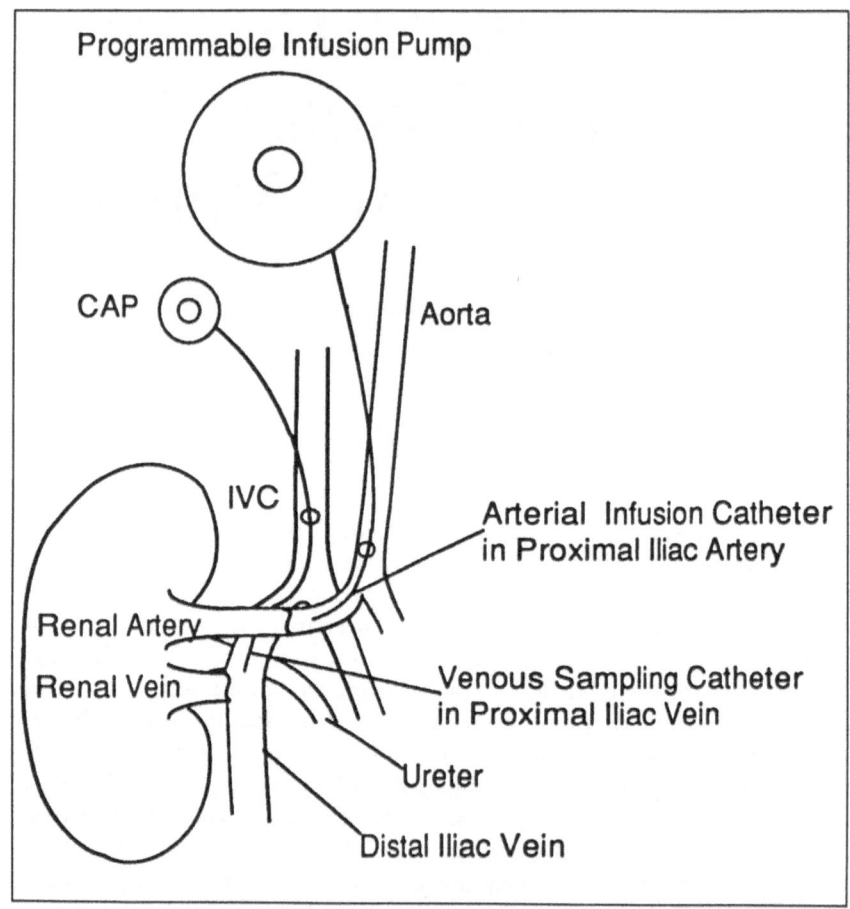

Fig. 9.1. Location of arterial infusion pump/catheter system and optional venous sampling catheter at the completion of canine renal transplantation. The SynchroMed® Infusion Pump and catheter access port (CAP) are located in separate subcutaneous pockets on the right lateral chest wall. IVC = inferior vena cava. Reproduced with permission from Gruber SA et al, Transplantation 1989; 48:928.

tomosis and connected to a subcutaneously-placed catheter access port. This catheter has permitted repeated determination of drug concentrations in the renal effluent during local infusion of immunosuppressive agents.

The SynchroMed Infusion Pump (Model 8610H SynchroMed Infusion Pump, Medtronic, Inc.) contains a collapsible 18 ml drug reservoir and can be externally programmed by telemetry utilizing a Physician Programmer (Model 8800M, Medtronic, Inc.) and programming wand (Fig. 9.2). At surgery, the pump is filled with a solution containing the immunosuppressive agent to be administered (if any) together with 1000 units/ml heparin (Upjohn Co., Kalamazoo, MI) and may be programmed to deliver the desired dose by continuous infusion at a constant flow rate (0.009-0.9 ml/hr), by time-qualified bolus injections, or any combination of the two (Fig. 9.3). Postoperatively, the pump can be reprogrammed and percutaneously emp-

tied of and refilled with solution as necessary using sterile technique. Patency of the catheter access port is maintained with daily percutaneous flushes of 3 ml heparinized saline (1000 units/ml).

Eighteen autotransplanted dogs with arterial catheter placement received intrarenal heparin saline at 1-2 ml/day; 16 were sacrificed from 19 to 250 days postoperatively. Serum creatinine (Cr) became elevated in only one animal, found to have severe pyelonephritis and catheter-tip perforation of the iliac artery on day 42. No other dogs demonstrated significant vessel wall reaction to the indwelling catheters. Minimal to mild interstitial nephritis was found in eight specimens. Although the presence of cortical petechiae in two dogs and cortical scarring with dystrophic calcification in a third might be suggestive of embolic "showering" of the kidney, there was no evidence of thrombus on gross examination of the catheter and iliac/renal arterial wall nor of embolus on histologic

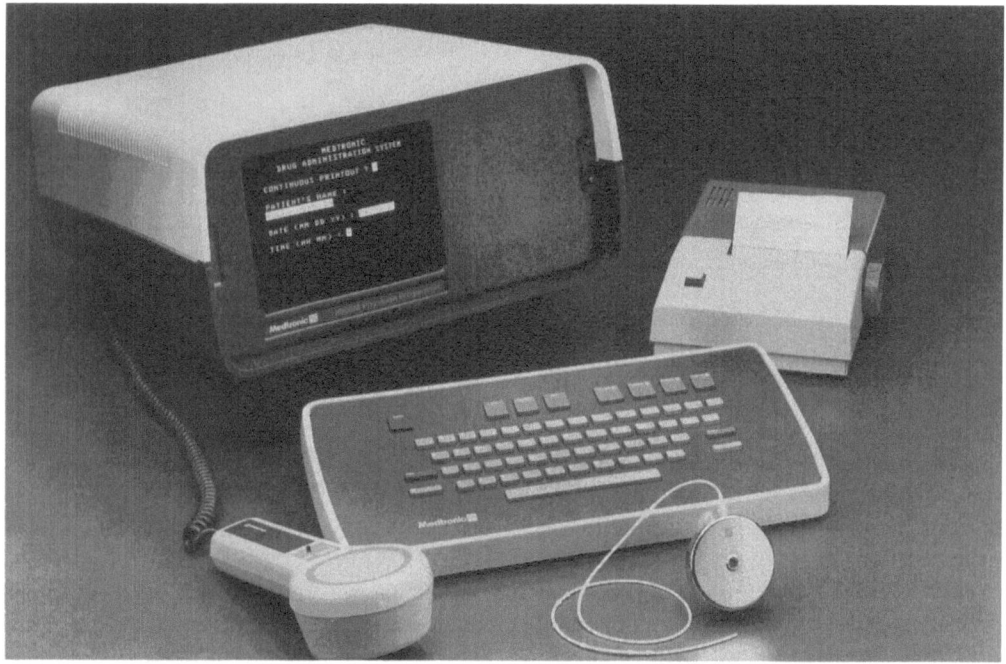

Fig. 9.2. The SynchroMed® Infusion System, consisting of the Physician Programmer, printer, and programming wand. The programming wand is used to noninvasively program the infusion pump by two-way radio communication (telemetry).

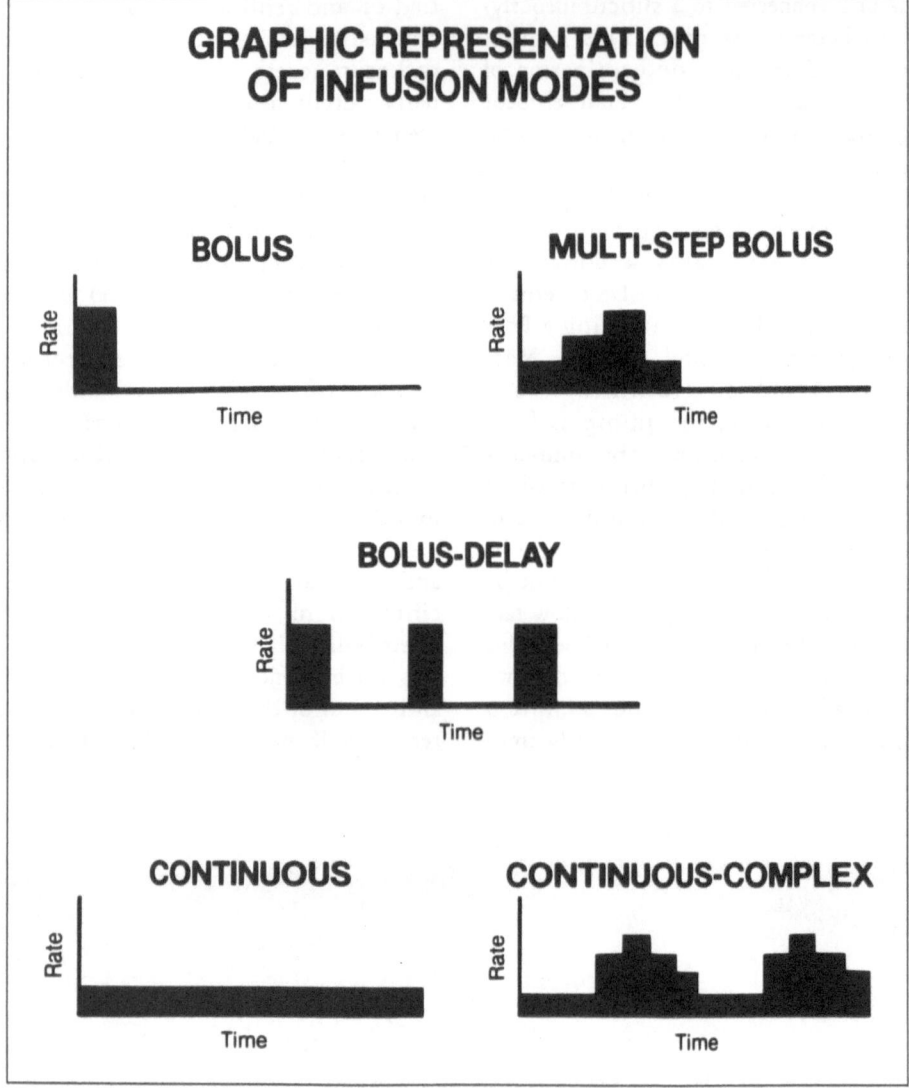

Fig. 9.3. Graphic representation of the five different infusion modes of the SynchroMed® Infusion Pump.

examination of the renal parenchyma in these animals. There were no cases of renal/iliac artery thrombosis, presumably due to the continuous presence of high local concentrations of heparin, and the two dogs that were not sacrificed survived beyond 2 years with normal Cr and urine analyses. Therefore, long-term arterial catheter implantation appears technically feasible and does not compromise renal function or histologic integrity.

PHARMACOKINETIC ADVANTAGE OF LOCAL 6-MERCAPTOPURINE (6-MP) INFUSION

Seven autotransplanted dogs with arterial catheter and catheter access port implantation underwent intraoperative renal blood flow measurement.[8] On the third postoperative day, simultaneous iliac vein and systemic (jugular vein) concentrations of 6-MP, the major immunosuppressive metabolite of azathioprine, were determined during a continuous 24-hr i.a. infusion (10 mg/kg/24 hr). The gradient between regional and systemic 6-MP concentrations was maximal initially when the pump was turned on, continuously decreased until steady-state was reached, and disappeared immediately after the pump was turned off.[7] Following termination of the infusion, 10 mg/kg 6-MP was administered to the same dogs as an intravenous (i.v.) bolus, and systemic drug concentrations were determined. Mean ($\pm$ SE) total body clearance (TBC) and elimination half-life ($T_{1/2}$) were 887 ± 159 ml/min and 1.4 ± 0.2 hr, respectively, in the i.v. bolus study, indicating that 6-MP is rapidly cleared from the systemic circulation. In addition, the kidney removed as much as 60-95% (mean extraction = 83%) of locally infused 6-MP, reducing the amount of drug entering the systemic circulation to 5-40% of that which would be present during an i.v. infusion of the same dose. Consequently, high-dose intrarenal 6-MP infusion produced both a 4-fold increase in local drug concentration (regional advantage) and an 80% decrease in systemic drug delivery (systemic advantage) to create an overall renal-to-systemic concentration gradient (selectivity) of 30-fold. These studies demonstrate that one can temporally and spatially regulate drug delivery with a rapid effect on local drug concentrations and represent a first attempt to validate the principles governing the pharmacokinetic advantage of target-aimed drug delivery in a large-animal model.

PHARMACODYNAMICS OF LOCAL HEPARIN INFUSION

Heparin must be added to all pump solutions to prevent catheter-induced arterial thrombosis and has demonstrated immunosuppressive activity both in vitro and in vivo.[9-11] Moreover, a significant fraction of heparin may be excreted unchanged in the urine following high-dose i.v. injection.[12-14] We therefore utilized our canine model to: (1) estimate the first-pass renal extraction of locally-infused heparin and

delineate the systemic consequences of intrarenal heparin delivery in autografts and (2) examine the effect of i.a. heparin infusion on the histologic features of rejection and overall survival of allograft recipients.[15]

In the autotransplant i.v. bolus study, $T_{1/2}$ ranged from 0.26 to 1.91 hr, with a 3-fold variation in TBC of heparin activity among the four animals studied. Systemic activated coagulation time (ACT) values rose linearly with i.a. heparin dose over the range of infusion rates tested in all four autotransplanted dogs (r > 0.9), and there was little or no first-pass renal extraction of heparin effect by the transplanted kidney. In the allograft study, the dose rate was adjusted daily via the programmable pump to continuously infuse as much heparin as possible intrarenally, but still maintain the systemic ACT close to but not exceeding 125% of the preoperative baseline value. The mean heparin dose delivered over the survival period ranged from 5.64 to 21.56 units/kg/hr in the nine dogs studied. There was no difference in survival by life-table analysis between the heparin-treated dogs (median survival time [MST] = 7 days) and a group of 14 untreated controls (MST = 7 days), and there was no significant correlation between the mean heparin dose received and either survival time or histologic severity of tubulo-interstitial (TI) rejection. However, the severity of the vascular component of rejection appeared to decrease with increasing mean heparin dose, and vascular rejection was significantly more intense in the heparin-treated group as a whole, with a greater percentage of kidneys demonstrating thrombosis, necrosis and transmural inflammation.

LOCAL VERSUS SYSTEMIC 6-MP INFUSION

To determine whether the pharmacokinetic advantage of i.a. 6-MP infusion could be utilized to therapeutic benefit in our canine model, we compared the efficacy of continuous i.a. versus i.v. 6-MP infusion in allotransplanted animals with regard to overall survival, incidence of systemic and renal toxicity and systemic drug exposure.[16] Table 9.1A-D summarizes the survival and toxicity data. A dose of 0.5 mg/kg/day 6-MP did not prolong survival over heparin-treated or untreated controls when administered either locally or systemically. All dogs died with elevated Cr values and evidence of rejection on renal pathologic examination, with the exception of one systemically-treated animal that was sacrificed on postoperative day 13 with a septic picture despite normal laboratory values. Systemic exposure to 6-MP, assessed by the plasma concentration of its inactive, renally-excreted metabolite, 6-thiouric acid (6-TU), was significantly less in the locally treated than in the systemi-

cally-treated dogs when serum Cr concentrations were normal or moderately elevated, but not when renal function became severely impaired (Fig. 9.4).

0.75 mg/kg/day 6-MP i.a. significantly prolonged survival over both untreated and heparin-treated controls, with all dogs eventually dying of rejection. However, 0.75 mg/kg/day i.v. failed to prolong survival over controls ($P > 0.1$) and produced death from systemic toxicity, characterized by leukopenia, thrombocytopenia, hepatotoxicity and sepsis in three animals, with the remainder dying early of rejection. Figure 9.5A,B contrasts the postoperative courses of the two longest-surviving dogs receiving 0.75 mg/kg/day 6-MP, one treated locally and one systemically,

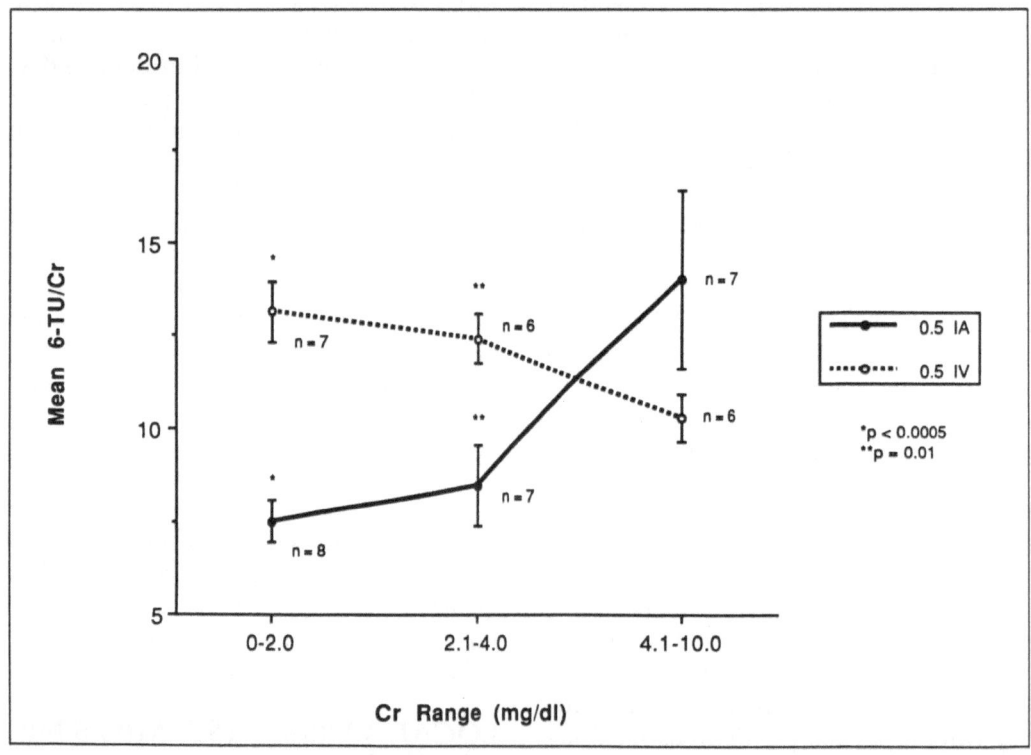

Fig. 9.4. *Variation of mean systemic 6-TU/Cr concentration ratio with increasing renal dysfunction in canine renal allograft recipients treated with 0.5 mg/kg/day 6-MP by continuous i.a. or i.v. infusion. Systemic 6-MP exposure remained relatively constant in dogs receiving the drug intravenously irrespective of renal function, and was significantly less in the locally-treated than in the systemically-treated dogs when renal function was normal or moderately depressed, but not when renal function was severely impaired. Values plotted are mean ± SE, with the number of animals possessing at least one 6-TU value in the each Cr range indicated (maximum n = 9 for both i.a. and i.v. groups). Reproduced with permission from Gruber SA et al, Transplantation 1989; 48:936.*

Table 9.1. Survival data of canine renal allograft recipients treated with 6-MP infusion

6-MP Dose (mg/kg/d)	Cause of Death (n)[a]		Survival [Time to Systemic Toxicity] (days)	MST (days)	Survival vs Control
A. Control	R	(14)	3; 3; 4; 4; 5; 6; 6; 7; 8; 8; 9; 10; 11; 13	7	—
	ST	(0)			
	N	(0)			
Heparin 5000 U/d i.a.	R	(7)	6; 6; 7; 7; 8; 9; 20	7	P = 0.41
	ST	(0)			
	N	(0)			
B. 0.5 i.a.	R	(9)	6; 6; 6; 7; 8; 8; 10; 10; 20	8	P = 0.28
	ST	(0)			
	N	(0)			
0.5 i.v.	R	(8)	6; 6; 7; 7; 7; 8; 26; 32	7	P = 0.17
	ST	(1)	13 [13]		
	N	(0)			
C. 0.75 i.a.	R	(7)	8; 8; 10; 20; 28; 29; 31	20	P = 0.007
	ST	(0)			
	N	(0)			
0.75 i.v.	R	(4)	6; 6; 7; 7	7	P = 0.14
	ST	(3)	16 [16]; 21 [16]; 30 [18]		
	N	(0)			
D. 2.0 i.a.	R	(1)	8[b]	12	P = 0.01
	ST	(0)			
	N	(7)	7; 8[b]; 10; 12; 13; 17; 21		
2.0 i.v.	R	(2)	5; 5	12	P = 0.02
	ST	(5)	12 [9]; 12 [10]; 17 [14]; 17 [7]; 19 [7]		
	N	(0)			

[a] R = rejection; ST = systemic toxicity; N = nephrotoxicity.
[b] Concomitant rejection (2+) and nephrotoxicity (3+).
Reproduced with permission from Gruber SA et al, Transplantation 1989; 48:936.

with regard to laboratory evidence of rejection and drug toxicity, respectively. By day 18, the systemically-treated animal had already developed evidence of significant 6-MP-induced marrow suppression, which would have required marked dosage reduction or drug discontinuation under clinical circumstances. On the other hand, rejection did not become clinically manifest in the dog receiving i.a. 6-MP until day 27, and could conceivably have been treated at this point by increasing the 6-MP dose without fear of systemic toxicity.

Six of seven dogs receiving 2.0 mg/kg/day 6-MP i.a. developed azotemia secondary to drug-induced nephrotoxicity, characterized by thrombotic glomerulopathy, thrombotic vasculopathy with predominant involvement of the arcuate and interlobular arteries and ischemic-based lesions, including cortical and medullary infarction and acute tubular necrosis. Mononuclear cell infiltrates suggestive of TI or vascular rejection were conspicuously absent. The remaining animal died from concomitant rejection and nephrotoxicity. Two additional autotransplanted control dogs treated

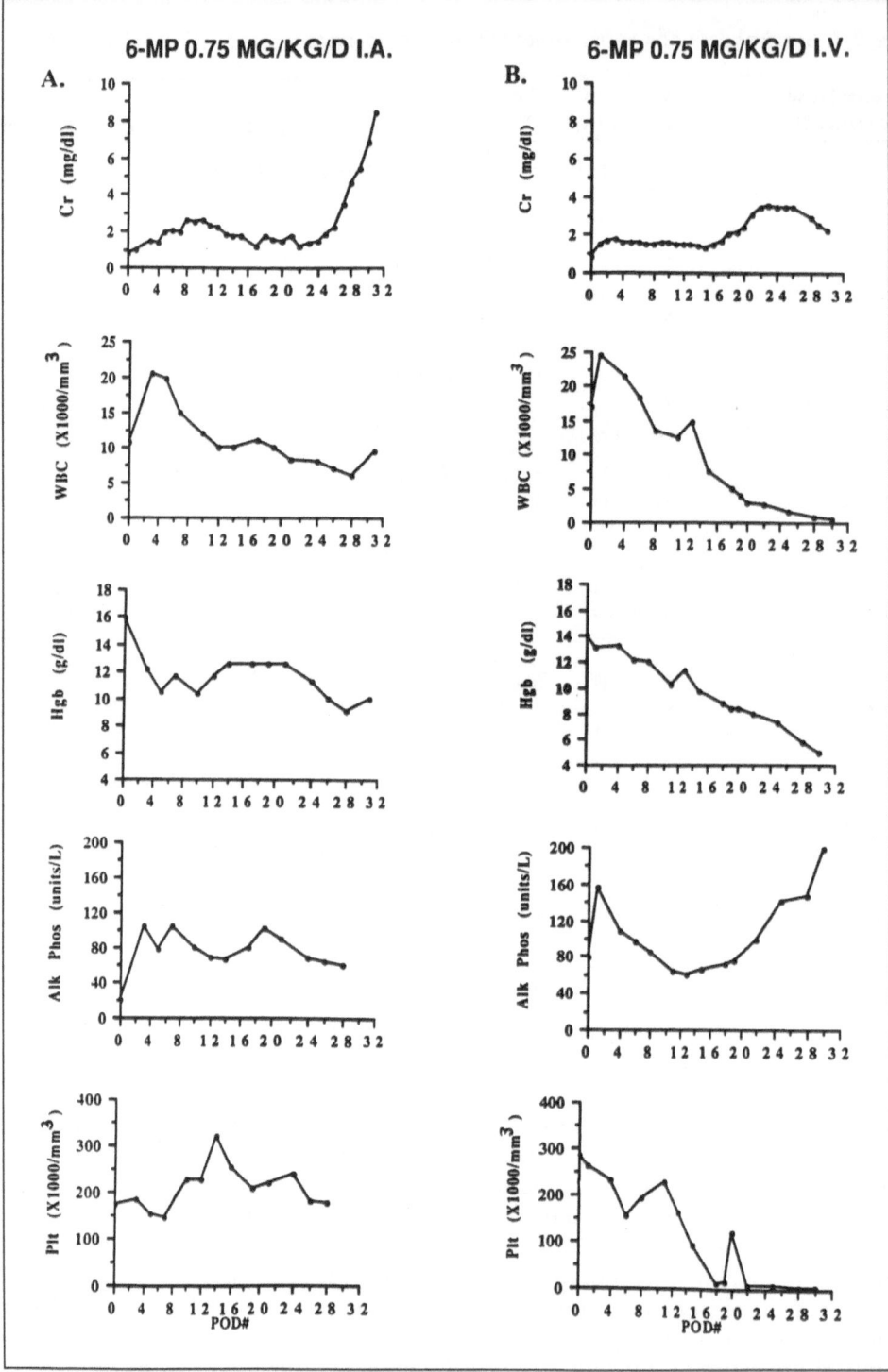

Fig. 9.5. Postoperative course of canine renal allograft recipients treated with 0.75 mg/kg/day 6-MP locally (A) and systemically (B). Changes in Cr, white blood count (WBC), hemoglobin (hgb), alkaline phosphatase (alk phos), and platelet count (Plt) are shown during the survival period of each animal. Rejection did not become clinically manifest in the dog receiving i.a. 6-MP until day 27, while by day 18, the systemically-treated animal had already developed evidence of significant 6-MP-induced bone marrow suppression.

with this dose also died of renal insufficiency in the same period of time and with identical findings on renal pathologic examination. Of seven animals receiving 2.0 mg/kg/day i.v., five died from early, severe systemic drug toxicity and two from early rejection. Figure 9.6A,B contrasts the postoperative courses of representative dogs receiving 2.0 mg/kg/day 6-MP i.a. and i.v. with regard to laboratory evidence of renal and systemic toxicity, respectively.

Of five animals treated with an intermediate 6-MP dose of 1.0 mg/kg/day (MST = 10 days), three died from rejection and the other two demonstrated mixed renal pathology (evidence of both nephrotoxicity and rejection) on histologic examination. Finally, all three dogs receiving 6-MP 1.5 mg/kg/day i.a. died on days 12, 18 and 21 with evidence of moderate to severe nephrotoxicity and concomitant mild rejection.

In contrast to the early failures of regional azathioprine and 6-MP therapy,[17,18] we found that continuous i.a. infusion of 10-fold lower doses of 6-MP demonstrated an antirejection effect equivalent or superior to that of i.v. therapy with reduced systemic drug exposure and toxicity. Our ability to identify a spectrum of lesions histologically distinguishable from rejection in both allo- and autotransplanted dogs receiving doses as low as 1.0-2.0 mg/kg/day 6-MP i.a. suggests that the ineffectiveness of high-dose (5-10 mg/kg/day) local 6-MP infusion noted by Terz et al[18] was in fact due to the production of early, severe nephrotoxicity mistakenly interpreted as severe rejection. In addition, the administration of very high intrarenal doses of 6-MP by early investigators presumably injured and/or overwhelmed the efficient renal extraction mechanism, allowing enough drug to enter the systemic circulation to produce leukopenia. Although these studies represent the first demonstration of the efficacy of local immunosuppressive therapy in a large-animal model, 6-MP may not be an ideal agent for clinical use because of its undesirable physicochemical properties (requiring pH > 10 to maintain solubility) and nephrotoxicity at high doses.

LOCAL VERSUS SYSTEMIC PREDNISOLONE INFUSION

Unfortunately, the impressive results obtained with local steroid administration alone in a rat transplant model[19,20] (chapter 4) have not been achieved in previous canine renal allograft studies with local[18,21,22] or systemic[23] administration. Moreover, clinically successful use of intrarenal steroid infusion to reverse early rejection episodes has been limited to bolus administration of methylprednisolone in combination with other agents against a background of multimodality immunosuppression[24,25] (chapter 3). We therefore investigated the effect of supplemental i.a. or i.v. prednisolone infusion on overall survival and systemic toxicity of canine renal allograft recipients treated with a background of oral azathioprine (2 mg/kg/day).[6] Local administration of increasing doses of i.a. or i.v. prednisolone failed to prolong overall survival compared with control dogs receiving oral azathioprine and i.a. heparin (Table 9.2A-D). This was due to a shift in the cause of death from rejection alone in the control group to rejection and systemic toxicity in the steroid-treated groups. Steroid-induced toxicity was characterized by the development of abdominal wound infection, cellulitis and dehiscence, peritonitis, pump pocket abscess, upper gastrointestinal bleeding and generalized sepsis. Thus, in contrast to 6-MP, which undergoes high first-pass renal elimination, immunosuppressive efficacy and systemic toxicity remained inseparable during intrarenal steroid infusion in the dog. These results are in agreement with previous studies in the dog and contrast with impressive results recently obtained in rat models. Species differences in corticosteroid pharmacodynamics[2-5] are undoubtedly of major importance in explaining these discordant observations, and will determine whether effective local immunosuppression can be achieved without systemic toxicity in a particular experimental model.

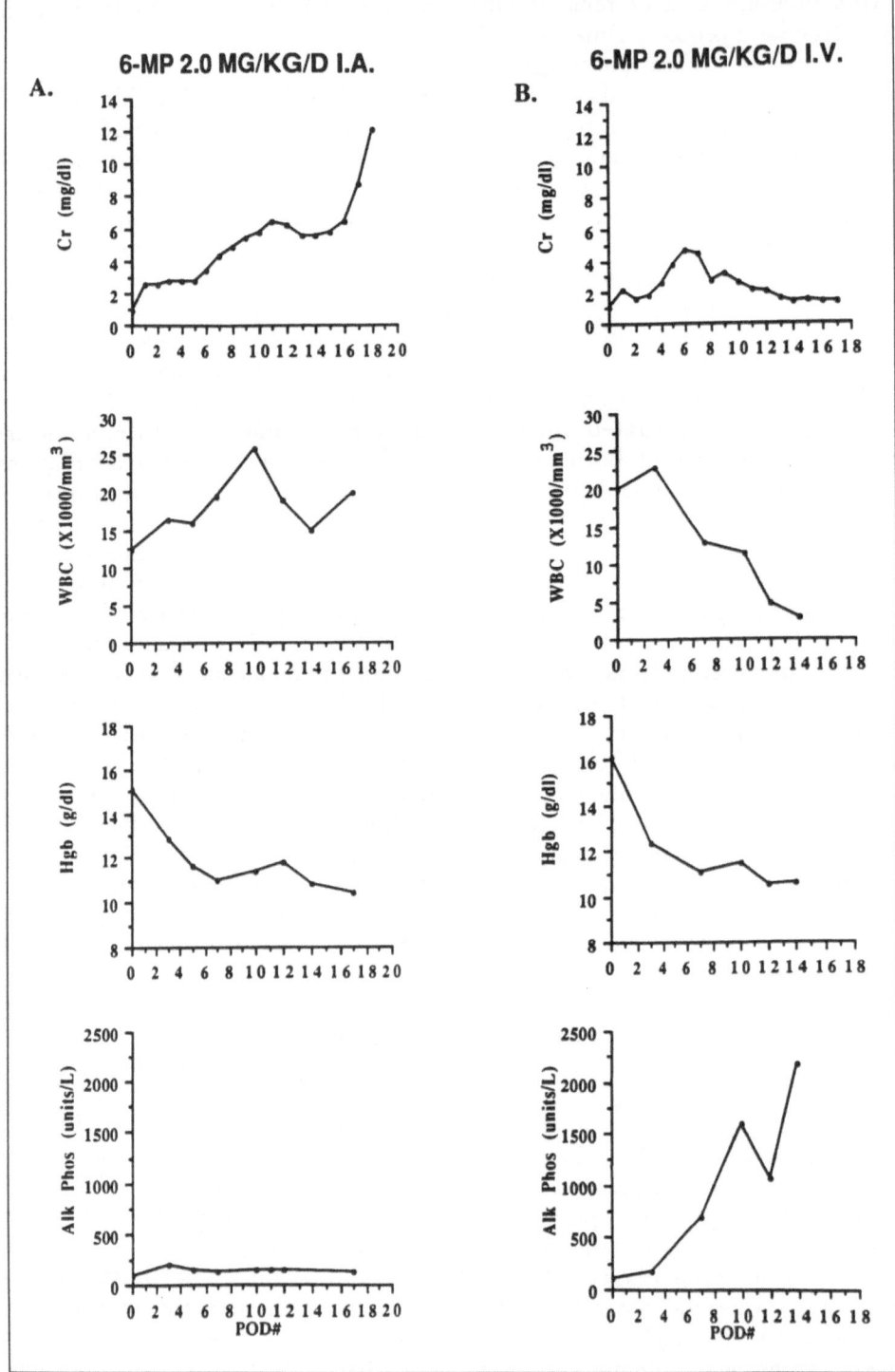

Fig. 9.6. Postoperative course of canine renal allograft recipients treated with 2.0 mg/kg/day 6-MP locally (A) and systemically (B). Changes in Cr, WBC, hgb, and alk phos are shown during the survival period of each animal. The dog receiving i.a. 6-MP demonstrated thrombotic vasculopathy and glomerulopathy, cortical infarction, and acute tubular necrosis with no evidence of rejection on renal histologic examination, while the systemically-treated animal developed leukopenia and hepatotoxicity in the same time frame.

Table 9.2. *Survival data of canine renal allograft recipients treated with oral azathioprine (2 mg/kg/d) and local or systemic prednisolone infusion*

Oral therapy	Infusion therapy Drug	Dose (mg/kg/d)	n	Cause of death (n)[a]		Survival (days)	MST (days)
A. None	None	–	14	R	(14)	3; 3; 4; 4; 5; 6; 6; 7; 8; 8; 9; 10; 11; 13	7
Aza[b]	Heparin	2000 units/d	9	R	(9)	7; 8; 9; 9; 11; 14; 21; 24 ; 25	11
B.				R	(6)	8; 8; 8; 9; 11; 18	
Aza	Pred[b]	0.5 i.a.	9	ST	(2)	20; 20	11
				O	(1)	41[c]	
Aza	Pred	0.5 i.v.	5	R	(3)	12[d]; 12; 17	14
				ST	(2)	14; 24	
C. Aza	Pred	1.0 i.a.	3	R	(2)	10; 12	
				ST	(1)	20	
Aza	Pred	1.0 i.v.	4	R	(4)	9; 11; 11; 14	
D.				R	(2)	14; 14	
Aza	Pred	2.0 i.a.	8	ST	(5)	8; 11; 14; 14; 19	14
				O	(1)	22[e]	

[a] R = rejection; ST = systemic toxicity (no R); O = other (no ST or R).
[b] Aza = azathioprine; Pred = prednisolone.
[c] Acute and chronic pyelonephritis, Cr 8.1 mg/dl.
[d] Pump stopped on day 8, Cr 2.2 mg/dl.
[e] Small bowel intusseception, Cr 2.3 mg/dl.
Reproduced with permission from Gruber SA et al, Transplantation 1989; 48:1072.

PHARMACOKINETICS AND PHARMACODYNAMICS OF INTRARENAL MIZORIBINE (MZB) INFUSION

Our experience with the agents heparin, 6-MP, and prednisolone enabled us to establish a set of desirable physicochemical and pharmacokinetic characteristics that a new immunosuppressive drug should possess to be utilized in our model of regional drug delivery to therapeutic advantage. These include compatibility with heparin and pump components, solubility and long-term stability at high concentration, absence of nephrotoxicity, readily available assay for the drug and its metabolites and rapid clearance outside of or highly extracted by the kidney. MZB is a renally-eliminated antimetabolite which competitively inhibits the same enzyme in the purine biosynthetic pathway as mycophenolate mofetil (inosine 5'-monophosphate dehydrogenase), has been used increasingly in Japan since 1978 in place of azathioprine as part of multiple drug regimens for clinical renal transplantation, is currently undergoing Phase II clinical trials in Europe, and meets all of the above criteria.[26-32] Although it is neither myelosuppressive nor hepatotoxic, MZB produces survival-limiting gastrointestinal toxicity, characterized by severe anorexia, vomiting and diarrhea, when given orally to dogs in therapeutic doses.[33,34]

We therefore hypothesized that local administration of MZB to canine renal allograft recipients would prolong graft and animal survival with reduced systemic toxicity as a result of high, first-pass renal elimination of the drug. First, we determined the systemic pharmacokinetics and renal extraction of MZB in autotransplanted dogs. Second, we compared the efficacy and toxicity of continuous i.a. versus i.v. MZB infusion in allotransplants at several doses, with and without a background of oral cyclosporine A (CsA) administration.

Five autotransplanted mongrel dogs were given MZB by both i.v. bolus (5 mg/kg) and i.a. infusion (5.0 mg/kg/day).[35] Mean ± SD elimination half-life was 3.02 ± 0.81 hr, and the transplanted kidney removed as much as 47-59% (mean 56%) of locally infused MZB. With increasing local and systemic MZB delivery in a single autografted dog undergoing both i.a. and i.v. pump/catheter placement, renal extraction decreased from at least 47% (5.0 mg/kg/day) to 33% (7.5 mg/kg/day), and finally to 18% (10.0 mg/kg/day).

Table 9.3A-D gives the survival and toxicity data of canine renal allograft recipients treated with continuous MZB infusion. A dose of 3.0 mg/kg/day MZB did not significantly prolong survival of renal allograft recipients over that of untreated controls when administered either locally or systemically. All dogs receiving 4.0 mg/kg/day MZB i.a. died from rejection, and a survival advantage was still not realized. In contrast, 4.0 mg/kg/day i.v. prolonged survival over controls but not when directly compared with the i.a. group, and pro-

duced death from severe debility (anorexia, emesis, diarrhea, weight loss) in five of seven animals with significantly higher mean systemic MZB levels. Four of six dogs receiving 5.0 mg/kg/day MZB i.a. and two of four dogs receiving 5.0 mg/kg/day i.v. died from severe debility, though survival in both groups was prolonged over control values.

Increasing the i.a. MZB dose further to 7.5 mg/kg/day merely produced rapid death from systemic toxicity in three of four dogs and one death from rejection (MST = 8 days), without prolonging survival compared to controls (P = 0.58). Finally, six additional dogs receiving 4.5 mg/kg/day i.a. (MST = 10 days) all died from rejection without any evidence of systemic drug toxicity preceding Cr elevation, and survival was still not prolonged when compared with the control group (P = 0.16).

The overall mean steady-state systemic MZB concentration during the period of normal renal function (Cr ≤ 2.0 mg/dl) was significantly higher in dogs dying from debility/infection than from rejection (Fig. 9.7). Although there was no change in systemic drug levels when increasing the intrarenal MZB dose from 3.0-4.0 mg/kg/day, further dose increments (4.0-7.5 mg/kg/day) produced a sharp linear increase in overall mean steady-state plasma drug concentrations (Fig. 9.8).

Table 9.3. Survival data of canine renal allograft recipients treated with MZB infusion

MZB dose (mg/kg/d)		Cause of death[a]			Overall mean [MZB]		Survival (days)		Survival P value	
	n	R	D	I	(µg/ml)	(n)	Median	(range)	vs control	i.a. vs i.v.
A. Control	12	12	0	0	—	—	8	(4-13)	—	—
B. 3.0 i.a.	5	5	0	0	0.69±0.25	(5)	9	(7-13)	0.19	
3.0 i.v.	5	5	0	0	0.76±0.62	(2)	12	(5-15)	0.06	0.34
C. 4.0 i.a.	7	6	0	1	0.69±0.22[b]	(7)	7	(6-28)	0.44	
4.0 i.v.	7	2	5	0	1.17±0.41[b]	(6)	14	(7-36)	0.03	0.30
D. 5.0 i.a.	6	2	4	0	1.20±0.34	(6)	14	(7-19)	0.01	
5.0 i.v.	4	2	2	0	1.40±0.25	(4)	14	(7-15)	0.05	0.67

[a] R = rejection; D = debility; I = infection.

[b] P = 0.02.

Reproduced with permission from Gruber SA et al, Transplantation 1992; 53:12.

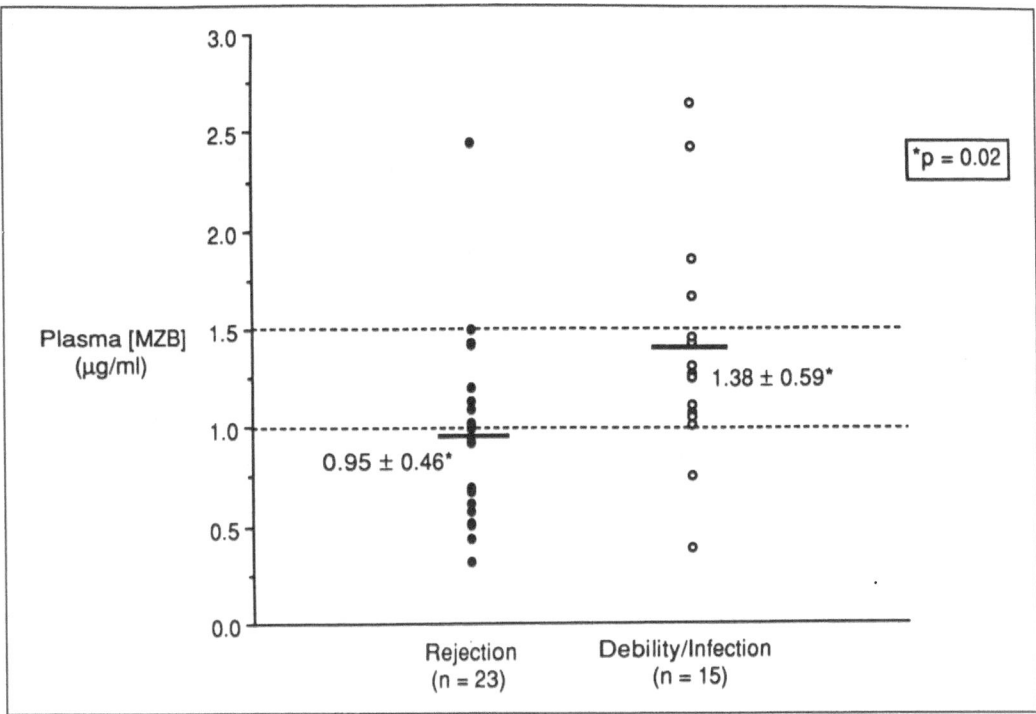

Fig. 9.7. Scatter plot of mean steady-state MZB concentrations for canine renal allograft recipients dying primarily from rejection (●; n = 23) and from debility or infection (○; n = 15). Horizontal bars represent overall mean values, which are expressed as mean ± SD. Reproduced with permission from Gruber SA et al, Transplantation 1992; 53:12.

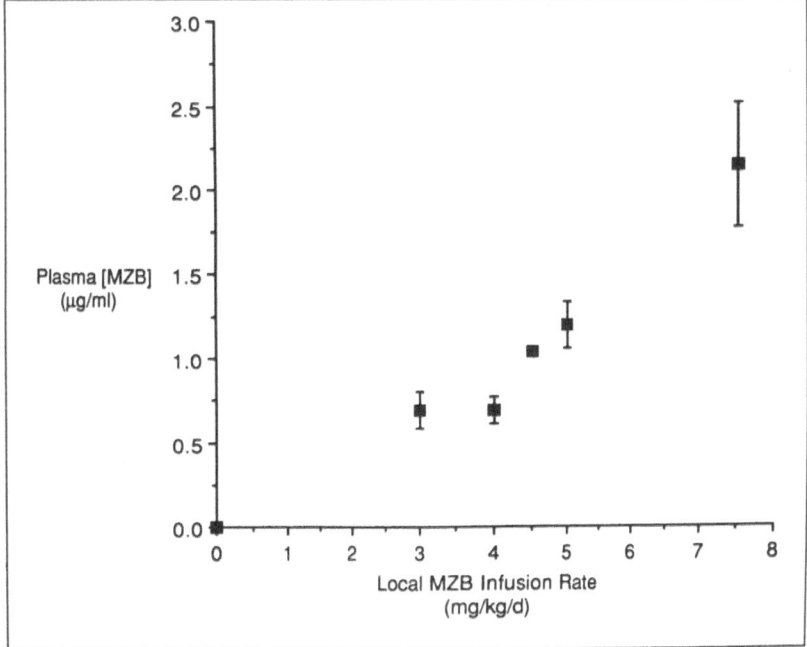

Fig. 9.8. Overall mean ± SE steady-state systemic MZB concentrations for groups of dogs receiving MZB by continuous i.a. infusion from 3.0 to 7.5 mg/kg/d. Reproduced with permission from Gruber SA et al, Transplantation 1992; 53:12.

Table 9.4. Survival data of canine renal allograft recipients treated with combination oral CsA (5 mg/kg/d) and MZB infusion (4.0 mg/kg/d)

Regimen	n	Cause of death[a] R	D	I	Overall mean [MZB] (µg/ml)	(n)	Survival (days) Median	(range)	Survival P value vs control	i.a. vs i.v.
Control	12	12	0	0	—	—	8	(4-13)	—	—
CsA	8	8	0	0	—	—	9	(5-10)[b,c]	0.85	—
MZB i.a.	7	6	0	1	0.69±0.22[d]	(7)	7	(6-28)[e]	0.44	0.30
MZB i.v.	7	2	5	0	1.17±0.41[d]	(6)	14	(7-36)	0.03	
MZB i.a. + CsA	9	6	3	0	0.84±0.33	(9)	23	(10-49)[b,e]	0.002	0.04
MZB i.v. + CsA	8	3	4	1	1.09±0.41	(8)	11	(7-27)[c]	0.02	

[a]R = rejection; D = debility; I = infection.
[b]$P = 0.002$.
[c]$P = 0.02$.
[d]$P = 0.02$.
[e]$P = 0.01$.
Reproduced with permission from Gruber SA et al, Transplantation 1992; 53:12-19.

Coadministration of a subtherapeutic dose of oral CsA (5 mg/kg/day) significantly prolonged the overall survival of dogs receiving MZB 4.0 mg/kg/day i.a. but not i.v., so that a significant difference in overall survival between the combined MZB i.a. + CsA and MZB i.v. + CsA groups was now realized in favor of the former. The addition of CsA did not significantly alter the overall mean steady-state MZB concentrations for the MZB i.a. or i.v. groups ($P = 0.33$ and $P = 0.73$, respectively), although the difference between the combined groups was no longer statistically significant ($P = 0.18$). In the combined MZB + CsA groups, one-third of the i.a.-treated and one-half of the i.v.-treated dogs died from debility, and one other systemically-treated animal died from severe pneumonia.

In summary, infusion of MZB directly into the kidney transplant produces lower systemic drug levels than same-dose i.v. administration, in agreement with pharmacokinetic studies in autografts. However, at local doses required to achieve immu-nosuppression, the transplanted kidney was not able to extract enough drug to prevent death from systemic toxicity, presumably as a result of saturation of renal elimination mechanisms, so that an overall survival benefit was not realized. Combination of a subtherapeutic dose of oral CsA with i.a., but not i.v., MZB infusion conferred a survival advantage with lower systemic MZB concentrations, suggesting mediation via a local immunosuppressive effect.

CONCLUSION

Our preliminary single-agent studies in a canine renal allograft model represent a foundational step in the design of multi-drug local immunosuppressive regimens which ideally will prevent rejection of the allotransplanted kidney with minimal systemic side effects. The two major ingredients for clinical application, namely, (1) programmable, implantable, biocompatible, pump/catheter drug-delivery systems and (2) relatively nonspecific immunosuppressive agents with appropriate pharmacokinetic properties, are presently available or easily developed using current technology. In addition, pharmacodynamic (regional toxicity), pharmaceutical (drug solubility, stability and compatibility) and fluid mechanical (inhomogeneous drug distribution) considerations also need attention (chapter 2).

REFERENCES

1. Dedrick RL. Interspecies scaling of regional drug delivery. J Pharm Sci 1986; 75:1047.
2. Clayman HN. Corticosteroids and lymphoid cells. New Eng J Med 1972; 287:388.
3. Shewell J, Long DA. A species difference with regard to the effect of cortisone acetate on body weight, gamma-globulin and circulating antitoxin levels. J Hyg 1956; 54:452.
4. Clayman HN, Moorhead JW, Benner WH. Corticosteroids and lymphoid cells in vitro. I. Hydrocortisone lysis of human guinea pig, and mouse thymus cells. J Lab Clin Med 1971; 78:499.
5. Fauci AS, Dale DC, Balow JE. Glucocorticosteroid therapy: mechanisms of action and clinical considerations. Ann Int Med 1976; 84:304.
6. Gruber SA, Hrushesky WJM, Canafax DM et al. Local prednisolone infusion of canine renal allografts. Transplantation 1989; 48:1072.
7. Gruber SA, Cipolle RJ, Canafax DM et al. An implantable pump for intrarenal infusion of immunosuppressants in a canine autotransplant model. Pharm Res 1988; 12:781.
8. Gruber SA, Canafax DM, Erdmann GR et al. The pharmacokinetic advantage of local 6-mercaptopurine infusion in a canine renal transplant model. Transplantation 1989; 48:928.
9. Martz E, Benacerraf B. Inhibition of immune cell-mediated killing by heparin. Clin Immunol Immunopath 1973; 1:533.
10. Cohen S, Benacerraf B, McCluskey RT et al. Effect of anticoagulants on delayed hypersensitivity reactions. J Immunol 1967; 98:351.
11. MacDonald A, Busch GJ, Alexander JL et al. Heparin and aspirin in the treatment of hyperacute rejection of renal allografts in presensitized dogs. Transplantation 1970; 9:1.
12. Piper J. The fate of heparin in rabbits after intravenous injection. Filtration and tubular secretion in the kidneys. Acta Pharmacol (Copenh) 1947; 3:373.
13. McAllister BM, Demis DJ. Heparin metabolism: isolation and characterization of uroheparin. Nature 1966; 212:293.
14. Boneu B, Caranobe C, Cadroy Y et al. Pharmacokinetic studies of standard unfractionated heparin, and low molecular weight heparins in the rabbit. Semin Thromb Hemost 1988; 14:18.
15. Gruber SA, Cipolle RJ, Canafax DM et al. Pharmacodynamics of local heparin delivery in a canine renal allograft model. J Pharmacol Exp Ther 1990; 252:733.
16. Gruber SA, Hrushesky WJM, Cipolle RJ et al. Local immunosuppression with reduced systemic toxicity in a canine renal allograft model. Transplantation 1989; 48:936.
17. Retik AB, Dubernard J-M, Hester WJ et al. A study of the effects of intraarterial immunosuppressive drug therapy on canine renal allografts. Surgery 1966; 60:1242.
18. Terz JJ, Crampton R, Miller D et al. Regional infusion chemotherapy for prolongation of kidney allografts. J Surg Res 1969; 9:13.
19. Ruers TJM, Buurman WA, Smits JFM et al. Local treatment of renal allografts, a promising way to reduce the dosage of immunosuppressive drugs. Transplantation 1986; 41:156-61.
20. Ruers TJM, Daeman MJAP, Thijssen HHW et al. Sensitivity of graft rejection in rats to local immunosuppressive therapy. Transplantation 1988; 46:820.
21. Ackerman RW, Barnard CN. The effect of direct infusions of cortisone into the renal artery of a transplanted kidney. S A Med J 1966; 40:83.
22. Dougherty JC, Nehlsen SL, Minick R et al. Failure of regional immunosuppressive therapy to modify renal allograft rejection. Transplantation 1968; 6:554.
23. Homan WP, French ME, Fabre JW et al. The interaction of cyclosporin A with other immunosuppressive agents in dog recipients

of renal allografts. Transplant Proc 1980; 12:287.

24. Kountz SL, Cohn RB. Initial treatment of renal allografts with large intrarenal doses of immunosuppressive drugs. Lancet 1969; 1:338.

25. Laupacis A, Keown PA, Rankin RN et al. Intraarterial methylprednisolone and heparin (IAT) for the treatment of refractory renal transplant rejection episodes. Transplant Proc 1982; 14:693.

26. Mizuno K, Tsujino M, Takada M et al. Studies on bredinin I. isolation, characterization and biological properties. J Antibiot (Tokyo) 1974; 27:775.

27. Koyama H, Tsuji M. Genetic and biochemical studies on the activation and cytotoxic mechanism of bredinin a potent inhibitor of purine biosynthesis in mammalian cells. Biochem Pharmacol 1983; 32:3547.

28. Kokado Y, Ishibahi M, Jiang H et al. Low-dose ciclosporin, mizoribine and prednisolone in renal transplantation: a new triple-drug therapy. Clin Transplantation 1990; 4:191.

29. Mita K, Akiyama N, Nagao T et al. Advantages of mizoribine over azathioprine in combination therapy with cyclosporine for renal transplantation. Transplant Proc 1990; 22:1679.

30. Erdmann GR, Gruber SA, McGuiggan MM et al. Determination of mizoribine in plasma using ion pair high performance liquid chromatography. J Chromatogr 1989; 494:354.

31. Murase J, Mizuno K, Kawai K et al. Absorption, distribution, metabolism, and excretion of bredinin in rats. Pharmacometrics 1978; 15:829.

32. Lee HA, Slapak M, Venkatraman G et al. Mizoribine as an alternative to azathioprine in triple therapy. Immunosuppressive regimens in cadaveric renal transplantation: two successive studies. Tranplant Proc 1995; 27:1050.

33. Uchida H, Yokota K, Akiyama N et al. Effectiveness of a new drug, bredinin, on canine kidney allotransplant survival. Transplant Proc 1979; 11:865.

34. Gregory C, Gourley I, Haskins S et al. Effects of mizoribine on canine renal allograft recipients. Amer J Vet Res 1988; 49:305.

35. Gruber SA, Erdmann GR, Burke BA et al. Mizoribine pharmacokinetics and pharmacodynamics in a canine renal allograft model of local immunosuppression. Transplantation 1992; 53:12.

CHAPTER 10

INTRAPORTAL CYCLOSPORINE A IN CANINE LIVER TRANSPLANTATION

Saiho Ko, Yoshiyuki Nakajima and Hiroshige Nakano

INTRODUCTION

Although the application of cyclosporine (CsA)-based immunosuppressive regimens in the early 1980s provided dramatic improvements in the results of liver transplantation[1], early postoperative complications such as acute rejection and infection are still the major causes of morbidity and mortality.[2] In addition, adverse effects of immunosuppressants such as nephrotoxicity due to CsA and deterioration of systemic immune function restrict the permissible dosage of these drugs.[1]

Local immunosuppression by direct infusion of immunosuppressive drugs into the graft is a possible way to prevent rejection and reduce systemic adverse effects simultaneously.[3,4] Excellent studies on local immunosuppression in kidney and heart transplantation models have been reported by some investigators,[5-9] but to the best of our knowledge, we are the first to evaluate the effect of local immunosuppression with portal venous infusion of CsA in liver transplantation.[10,11] In this chapter, the efficacy of intraportal infusion of CsA in preventing hepatic allograft rejection is documented in a canine model.

IMMUNOSUPPRESSIVE EFFECTS OF INTRAPORTAL CsA

Healthy young adult mongrel dogs of both sexes weighing 12-18 kg were used as donors and recipients, and orthotopic liver transplantation was performed. Animals were divided into the following groups according to the method of immunosuppression: group I, controls, no immunosuppression; group II, 3 mg/kg/day of intravenous CsA was administered continuously; group III, 3 mg/kg/day of CsA was administered

Local Immunosuppression of Organ Transplants, edited by Scott A. Gruber.

locally into the portal vein continuously. Intravenous administration of CsA was performed via a urokinase coated silastic catheter (Thrombolyte® 16G, Sherwood Japan, Tokyo, Japan) placed in the left jugular vein. Intraportal administration of CsA was performed via a peripheral branch of the splenic vein. The catheter was passed through the abdominal wall and was fixed on the back of the dog. Infusion of CsA was performed with an automatic micro-infusion pump. CsA administration in each group was started on the day of transplantation and discontinued on the 14th day. Survival time, blood chemical analyses, and histological findings of the graft were evaluated in each group. For histological examination, open liver biopsies were performed on the 14th day in surviving recipients. In animals sacrificed before day 14, autopsy specimens were used for histological evaluation. Microscopic findings

of acute rejection were assessed according to Kemnitz's criteria by hematoxylin and eosin staining.[12]

Table 10.1 gives the survival time and cause of death of the recipients in each group. Survival time in group III was significantly prolonged compared with groups I and II, although survival time in group II was no different from that in group I. All animals in group I, and four out of five in group II died of acute rejection. In group III, four out of eight recipients died of other complications and the histological examination in these recipients at autopsy did not show any findings of acute rejection. The longest survival time was 85 days in group III, despite discontinuation of CsA on day 14. Serum bilirubin, AST, and ALT levels of the dogs in group III were stable and significantly lower than those in the other groups (Figs. 10.1-10.3).[10] Histological examination revealed that acute rejec-

Table 10.1. Survival time and causes of death in canine liver transplant recipients

Group	Cyclosporine A Dose (mg/kg/day)	Survival (days)	Cause of Death
I (n = 7)	none	6	Rejection
		7	Rejection
		7	Rejection
		7	Rejection
		10	Rejection
		12	Rejection
		13	Rejection
II (n = 5)	3 intravenous for 14 days	6	Rejection
		7	Rejection
		7	Rejection
		8	Rejection
		10	Malnutrition
III (n = 8)	3 intraportal for 14 days	10	Intussusception
		13	Rejection
		15	Unknown
		16	Malnutrition
		20	Perforation of duodenal ulcer
		20	Rejection
		20	Rejection
		85	Rejection

Recipients in group III had significantly longer survival than those in groups I and II (P < 0.025)
Reproduced with permission from Transplantation 1994; 57:1818.

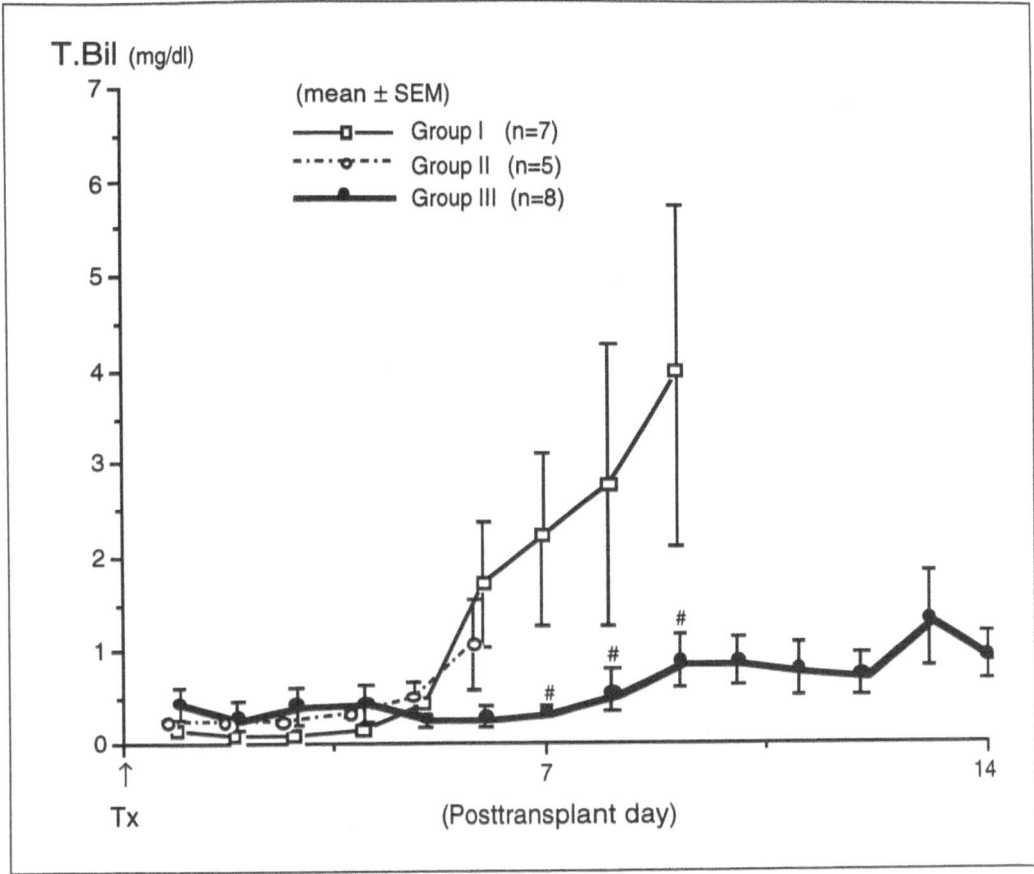

Fig. 10.1. Serum total bilirubin (T.Bil) levels in each group. The values in group III were stable and lower for 14 days posttransplantation in comparison with the other groups. (#) shows the significant difference versus group I (P < 0.05).

tion was effectively suppressed by the 14th day in group III, while marked rejection patterns were observed in group I and group II (Table 10.2, Fig. 10.4).

These results demonstrated the efficacy of local immunosuppression with low-dose intraportal CsA in preventing hepatic allograft rejection in comparison with systemic immunosuppressive treatment.

INFLUENCE OF INTRAPORTAL CsA ON SYSTEMIC SIDE EFFECTS

The most common side effect of CsA is nephrotoxicity, which is often a dose limiting factor. In our canine transplantation model, renal function tests including blood urea nitrogen and serum creatinine levels were measured in each recipient. No

abnormal elevation of these tests was observed in groups II and III. In addition, no histological findings of nephrotoxicity at autopsy and no infectious complications were observed in groups II and III. These results might be attributed to the low dose of CsA utilized in this series.

PHARMACOLOGICAL PROFILE OF INTRAPORTAL CsA IN CANINE LIVER TRANSPLANTATION

Peripheral whole blood levels of CsA and tissue levels of CsA in the liver, pancreas, kidney, and spleen were measured in groups II and III using a monoclonal radioimmunoassay kit (Cyclo-Trac®, Baxter, Tokyo, Japan). For determination of tissue levels of CsA, tissue samples were homog-

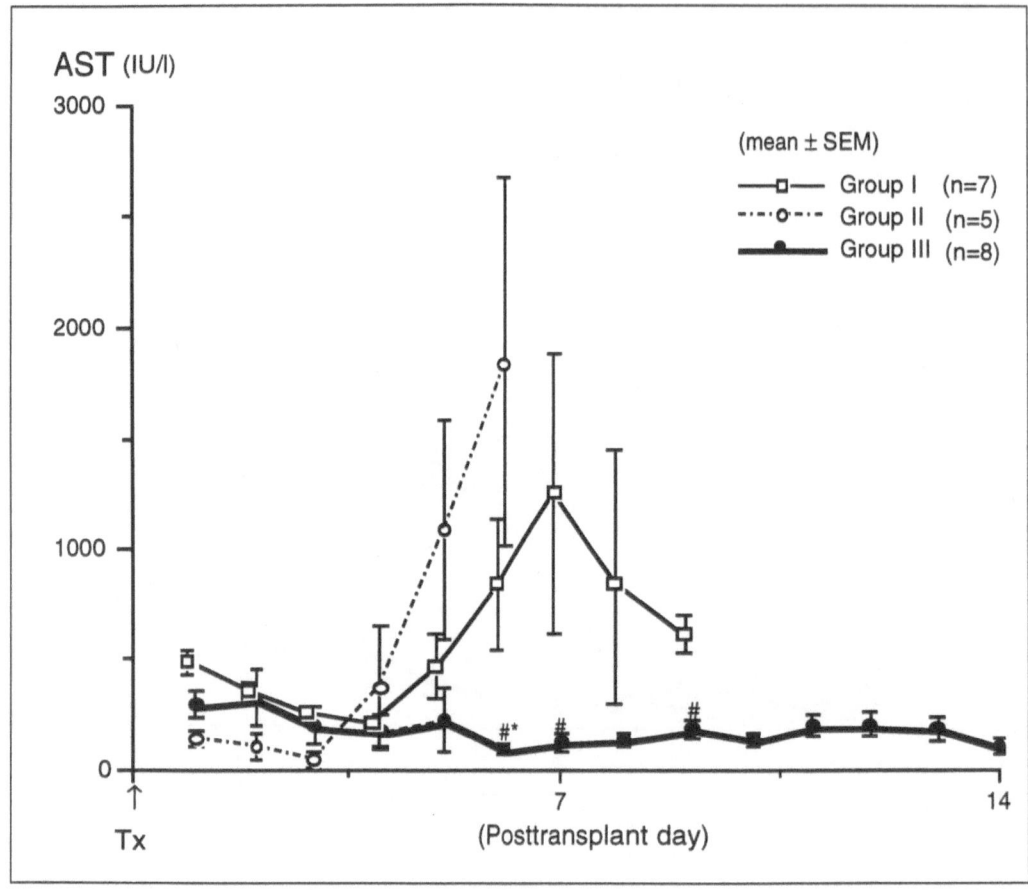

Fig. 10.2. Serum AST levels in each group. The values in group III were stable for 14 days posttransplantation, and lower than in the other groups after the 6th or 7th day. (#) and (*) show the significant difference versus groups I and II, respectively (P < 0.05). Reproduced with permission from Transplantation 1994; 57:1818.

enized in saline and centrifuged. CsA levels of the supernatant were measured, and tissue CsA levels were calculated as the amount of CsA per gram of tissue.

Peripheral whole blood levels of CsA until the 5th day were compared between groups II and III during continuous infusion. Although allograft rejection was effectively suppressed in group III, CsA levels in group III were significantly lower than those in group II, in which four of five animals died of rejection (Fig. 10.5). Tissue levels were measured from autopsy specimens of the recipient who died within 14 days, because CsA was discontinued on day 14. Tissue CsA levels varied greatly among recipients even in the same group, probably because CsA levels are significantly influenced by liver function.[13] However, tissue CsA levels in the liver were relatively higher than those in other organs in group III, while tissue CsA levels in the liver were relatively lower than those in other organs in group II (Table 10.3).

Reduction of peripheral blood levels of CsA by intraportal administration was attributed to the first-pass extraction of CsA by the transplanted liver. Takada et al[14] reported that 35% of CsA directly infused into the portal vein was extracted by the liver in a rat model. Low blood .levels of CsA during local immunosuppression would alleviate systemic adverse effects such as nephrotoxicity and opportunistic infection.[1,2,15] In addition, high tissue levels of CsA in the grafted liver would contribute to the effective prevention of hepatic allograft rejection.

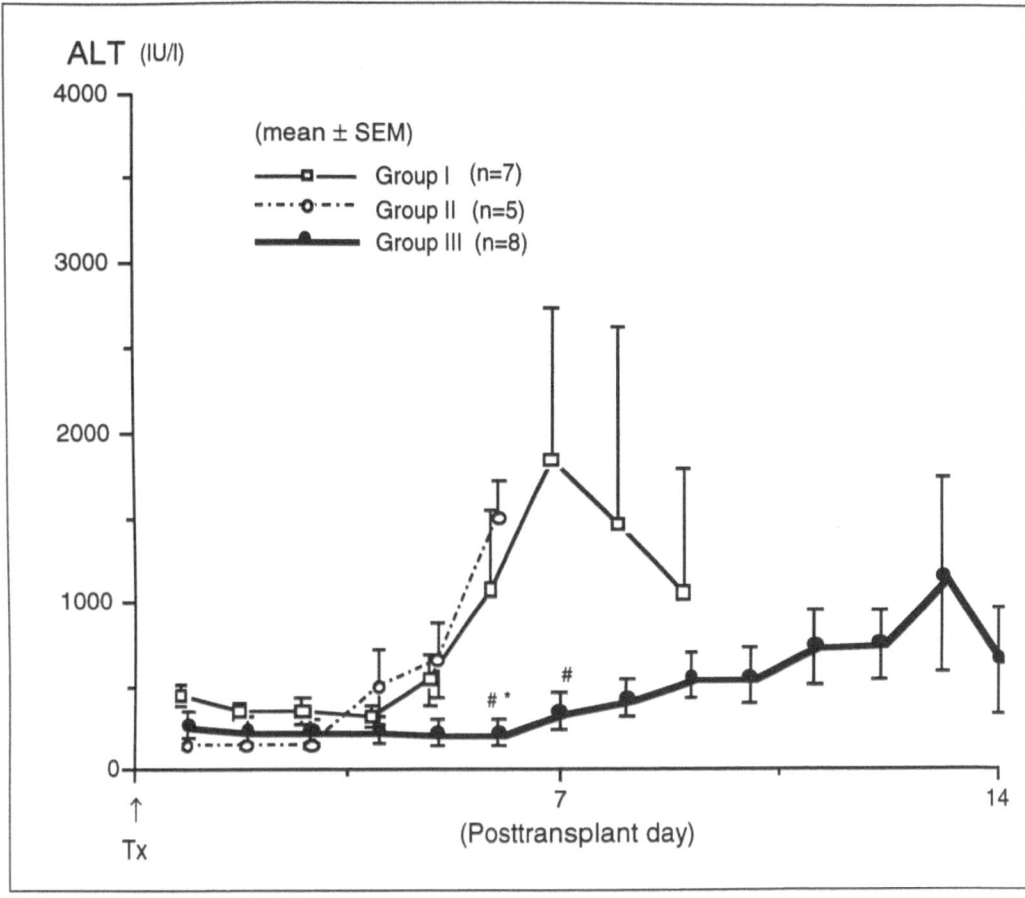

Fig. 10.3. Serum ALT levels in each group. The values in group III were stable for 14 days posttransplantation, and lower than in the other groups after the 6th or 7th day. (#) and (*) show the significant difference versus groups I and II, respectively (P < 0.05). Reproduced with permission from Transplantation 1994; 57:1818.

MECHANISM OF LOCAL IMMUNOSUPPRESSION

Recent studies in transplantation immunology have revealed that acute allograft rejection is largely regulated locally in the graft rather than systemically.[16-19] The mechanism of the effect of local immunosuppression may be explained by the actions of various cytokines. Cytokines are well known to play a central role in rejecting allografts.[20] Expression of major histocompatibility complex (MHC) antigens and induction of adhesion molecules on the graft, recruitment of lymphocytes to the graft, and maturation of cytotoxic T-lymphocytes within the graft may be promoted by cytokines such as interleukin-2 (IL-2), interferon-gamma (IFN-γ),

IL-1, and tumor necrosis factor-alpha (TNF-α).[20-25] Since the cytokines exert most of their actions in a paracrine fashion rather than systemically,[21] inhibition of cytokine production within the graft could prevent the endothelial activation which leads to destruction of the vascularized allograft.[21-24] CsA could produce its effect not only by the inhibition of cytokine release such as IL-2 and IFN-γ from T- lymphocytes, but also by the inhibition of IL-1 and TNF-α from macrophages.[26-28] Therefore, it is suggested that a high intragraft CsA concentration obtained by direct intraportal infusion could effectively suppress the production of cytokines in the graft, which would result in prevention of graft endothelial activation and allograft rejection.

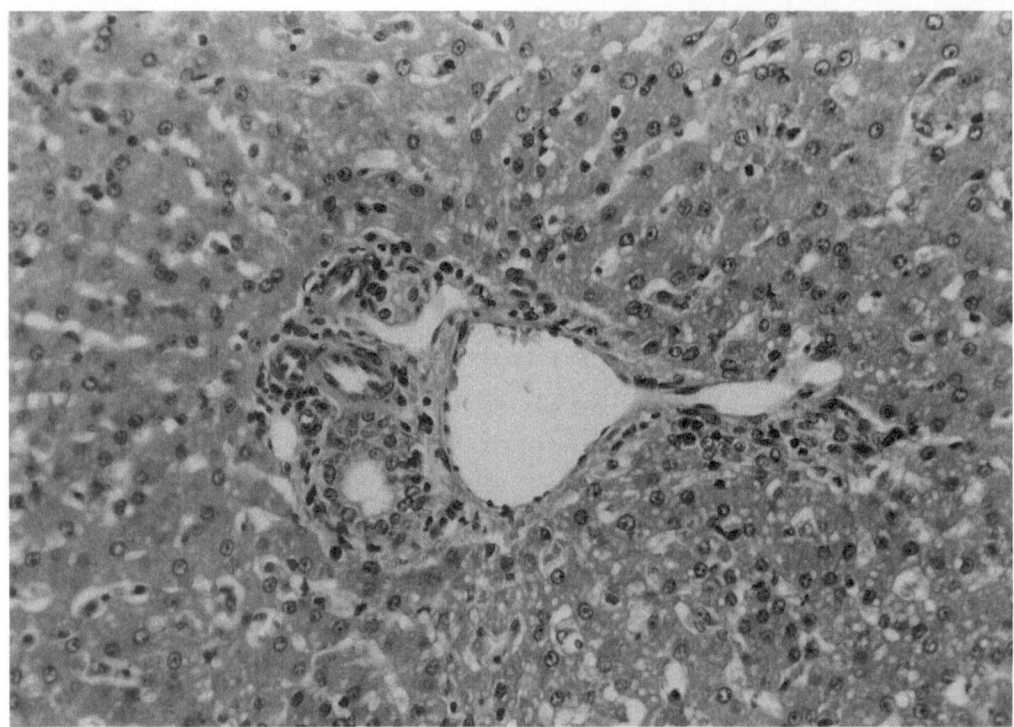

Fig. 10.4. Histology of the hepatic allograft on the 14th day after transplantaion in a recipient who was treated with 3 mg/kg/day of intraportal CsA. Mononuclear infiltration of the portal tract is minimal, and no bile duct damage is seen.

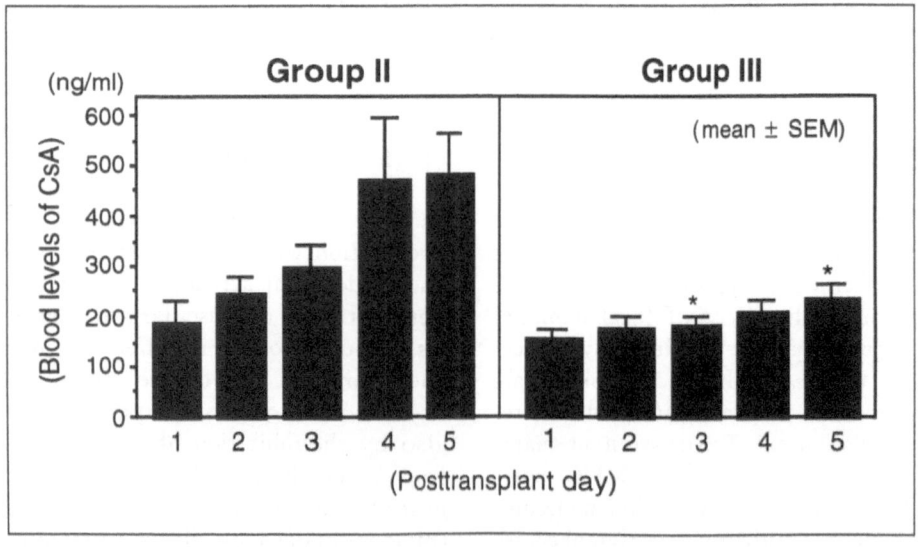

Fig. 10.5. Peripheral blood CsA levels in canine liver transplant recipients. Values are whole blood concentrations of CsA as measured by radioimmunoassay. Recipients in group II received 3 mg/kg/day CsA intravenously, and those in group III received the same dose intraportally. CsA levels in group III were significantly lower than those in group II on days 3 and 5 (*: P < 0.05 versus group II).

Table 10.2. Histological findings of the grafted liver in canine transplant recipients

Group*	Grade of acute rejection [#]				
	A-0	A-0-1	A-1	A-2	A-3
I				3	4
II		1		2	2
III	4	1	1	1	1

* Group I, no immunosuppression; group II, 3 mg/kg/day intravenous CsA; group III, 3 mg/kg/day intraportal CsA .
# Grade of rejection was determined according to Kemnitz's criteria as follows (ref. 12). A-0, no rejection; A-0-1, nondiagnostic; A-1, mild rejection; A-2, moderate rejection; A-3, severe rejection.

Table 10.3. CsA levels in the liver, kidney, pancreas, and spleen of canine liver transplant recipients

Dog No.	Group*	Day of autopsy	Tissue concentration (ng /g tissue)			
			Liver	Pancreas	Kidney	Spleen
1	II	7	2800	3500	3500	4100
2	II	10	1600	1100	730	1200
3	II	6	2800	4900	1900	3700
4	II	7	5300	6200	5500	6000
5	II	8	3100	6900	5300	4600
mean			3120	4520	3386	3920
6	III	13	4900	800	2600	580
7	III	10	6100	5500	5700	5800
mean			5500	3150	4300	3190

* Group II, 3 mg/kg/day intravenous CsA ; group III, 3 mg/kg/day intraportal CsA .

CONSIDERATION OF CLINICAL APPLICATION OF INTRAPORTAL CsA

One problem in local immunosuppression for liver transplantation is whether the portal vein or hepatic artery is a more beneficial route for drug administration. Both portal venous and hepatic arterial blood enter into the hepatic sinusoid. Comparable local graft concentration of the drug is obtained from both routes.[29,30] However, anomalous branches are frequently seen in the hepatic arterial system, and a catheter near the anastomotic portion of the hepatic artery in liver transplant recipients represents a hazard predisposing to hepatic arterial thrombosis. On the contrary, intraportal administration could be performed from a catheter placed in a peripheral branch of the mesenteric vein, and represents little hazard of thrombosis. In our study, intraportal administration of CsA was performed for 2 weeks without any complications such as thrombosis and infection.

CsA administered orally can be absorbed from the intestine and enter the portal blood. In the clinical liver transplant recipient, however, external drainage of the bile and decreased gastrointestinal function in the early postoperative period make it difficult to maintain stable CsA concentrations with oral administration.[1,13] Therefore, CsA is generally administered intravenously during this period. In many liver transplantation centers, CsA administration is begun only after adequate urinary output to monitor nephrotoxicity.[13] Local immunosuppression may be safely done even in this early posttransplant period because systemic adverse effects can be alleviated.

The result of our study on intraportal CsA suggests that local immunosuppression can enhance immunosuppressive effects and alleviate systemic side effects simultaneously in liver transplantation. This method would be useful in the early postoperative period, and could be applied to clinical use with significant benefits.

SUMMARY

Local immunosuppression with intraportal CsA effectively prevented hepatic allograft rejection in comparison with conventional same-dose systemic intravenous administration in a canine model. Despite the effective prevention of allograft rejection, peripheral blood levels of CsA in the recipient treated with intraportal CsA were significantly lower than in those receiving intravenous CsA, which might contribute to the alleviation of adverse effects such as nephrotoxicity and opportunistic infection due to systemic suppression of immune function. The results of this study indicate that local immunosuppression with intraportal CsA in liver transplantation could enhance the drug's immunosuppressive effects and alleviate systemic adverse effects simultaneously.

REFERENCES

1. Starzl TE, Demetris AJ. Prevention of rejection. In: Liver Transplantation. Chicago: Year Book Medical Publishers, 1990:71.
2. Kirby RM, McMaster P, Clements D et al. Orthotopic liver transplantation: postoperative complications and their management. Br J Surg 1987; 74:3.
3. Gruber SA. The case for local immunosuppression. Transplantation 1992; 54:1.
4. Gruber SA, Canafax DM, Cipolle RJ et al. Local immunosuppression of the vascularized allograft. Surgery 1991; 107:209.
5. Ruers TJM, Daemen JAP, Thijssen HHW et al. Sensitivity of graft rejection in rats to local immunosuppressive therapy. Transplantation 1988; 46:820.
6. Stepkowski SM, Goto S, Ito S et al. Prolongation of heterotopic heart allograft survival by local delivery of continuous low-dose cyclosporine therapy. Transplantation 1989; 47:17.
7. Gruber SA, Hrushesky WJ, Cipolle RJ et al. Local immunosupression with reduced systemic toxicity in a canine renal allograft model. Transplantation 1989; 48:936.
8. Gruber SA, Erdmann GR, Burke BA et al. Mizoribine pharmacokinetics and pharmacodynamics in a canine renal allograft model of local immunosuppression. Transplantation 1992; 53:12.
9. Ruers TJM, Buurman WA, Smits JFM et al. Local treatment of renal allografts, a promising way to reduce the dosage of immunosuppressive drugs. Transplantation 1986; 41:156.
10. Ko S, Nakajima Y, Kanehiro H et al. The significance of local immunosuppression in canine liver transplantation. Transplantation 1994; 57:1818.
11. Ko S, Nakajima Y, Kanehiro H et al. Immunologic aspect of local immunosuppression in canine liver transplantation. Transplant Proc 1994; 26:849.
12. Kemnitz J, Gubernatis H, Bunzendahl H et al. Criteria for histopathological classification of liver allograft rejection and their clinical relevance. Transplant Proc 1989; 21;2208.

13. Knobach T, Fischer V, Meyer UA. Cyclosporine metabolism in human liver: Identification of a cytochrome P-450III gene family as the major cyclosporine-metabolizing enzyme explains interactions of cyclosporine with other drugs. Clin Pharmacol Ther 1988; 43:630.

14. Takada K, Furuya Y, Yoshikawa H et al. Increased systemic availability of cyclosporin A by formulation design: pharmacokinetic consideration on its transport. Int J Pharmaceutics 1988; 44:107.

15. Maddrey WC, Van Thiel DH. Liver transplantation: An overview. Hepatology 1988; 8:948.

16. Ascher NL, Chen S, Hoffman RA et al. Maturation of cytotoxic T cells within sponge matrix allografts. J Immunol 1983;131:617.

17. Orosz CG, Zinn NF, Sirinek LP et al. In vivo mechanisms of alloreactivity: I. Frequency of donor reactive cytotoxic T lymphocytes in sponge matrix allografts. Transplantation, 1986; 41:75.

18. Orosz CG, Zinn NF, Sirinek LP et al. In vivo mechanisms of alloreactivity: II. Allospecificity of cytotoxic T lymphocytes in sponge matrix allografts as determined by limiting dilution analysis. Transplantation 1986; 41:84.

19. Orosz, CG, Zinn, NF, Sirinek, LP et al. In vivo mechanisms of alloreactivity: IV. Cyclosporine differentially impairs accumulation of donor-reactive CTL but not donor-reactive alloantibody in murine sponge matrix allografts. Int J Immunopharmacol 1988; 10:305.

20. Martinez OM, Krams SM, Sterneck M et al. Intragraft cytokine profile during human liver allograft rejection. Transplantation 1992; 53:449.

21. Hoffmann MW, Wonigeit K, Steinhoff G et al. Production of cytokines (TNF-alpha, IL-1-beta) and endothelial cell activation in human liver allograft rejection. Transplantation 1993; 55:329.

22. Adams DH, Shaw J, Hubscher SG et al. Intercellular adhesion molecule 1 on liver allografts during rejection. Lancet 1989; 2:1122.

23. Steinhoff G, Beherend M, Wonigeit K. Expression of adhesion molecules on lymphocytes/monocytes and hepatocytes in human liver grafts. Hum Immunol 1990; 28:123.

24. Palreoyo M, Makgoba MW. Leukocyte adhesion to cells in immune and inflammatory responses. Lancet 1989; 2:1139.

25. Palacios R. Mechanism of T cell activation: Role and functional relationship of HLA-DR antigens and interleukins. Immunol Rev 1982; 63:73.

26. Shevach EM, Dorsch SE. The effects of cyclosporine A on the immune system. Ann Rev Immunol 1985; 3:397.

27. Benson A, Ziegler HK. Macrophages as targets for inhibition by cyclosporine. Transplantation 1989; 47:696.

28. Nguyen DG, Eskandari MK, DeForge LE et al. Cyclosporine A modulation of tumor necrosis factor gene expression and effects in vitro and in vivo. J Immunol 1990; 144:3822.

29. Dedrick RL. Arterial drug infusion: pharmacokinetic problems and pitfalls. J Natl Cancer Inst 1988; 80:84.

30. Ziegler K, Polzin G, Frimmer M. Hepatocellular uptake of cyclosporine A by simple diffusion. Biochemica Biophysica Acta 1988; 938:44.

SECTION D:
OTHER DRUG TARGETING SYSTEMS FOR ACHIEVING LOCAL IMMUNOSUPPRESSION

CHAPTER 11

LIPOSOMAL CYCLOSPORINE A

Chris E. Freise, Nancy L. Ascher and John P. Roberts

BACKGROUND

Complications related to systemic immunosuppression continue to be a major cause of morbidity and mortality following solid organ transplantation. These complications result from the inability to reproducibly balance the toxicities of immunosuppressive agents (end organ toxicity and immunologic toxicity) and their benefits (prevention of allograft rejection). Targeting immunosuppressive agents to the allograft could alleviate systemic toxicities and still prevent rejection via local immunosuppressive effects. The ideal method to deliver agents locally to a vascularized allograft has not yet been elucidated. An obvious approach is to use a catheter delivering the agent directly to the blood supply of the allograft. This method has several potential problems including thrombotic and infectious complications.[1] A second method is to design an agent that is preferentially taken up by the allograft when given systemically. In the setting of liver transplantation, a potential approach to deliver the immunosuppressive agents locally could utilize liposomal technology. Liposomes are phospholipid vesicles with specific physical and biologic properties determined by the composition of the phospholipids, that can be loaded with many different pharmacologic agents.[2] These compounds are preferentially cleared from the systemic circulation by the reticuloendothelial system (RES). Since the liver is an important component of the RES, immunosuppressive agents incorporated into liposomes would potentially target the liver, with local delivery of the drug in adequate concentrations to inhibit the rejection response. The delivery of high concentrations of drug at the site of the allograft would also result in decreased systemic toxicity of the delivered agent. Our laboratory in a collaborative effort has developed a liposome containing cyclosporine (CsA). This prototypic agent has been examined with regard to its pharmacokinetic profile, the in vitro effects on mixed lymphocyte cultures, in vivo nephrotoxic side effects and immunosuppressive efficacy in a rat liver transplant model.

Local Immunosuppression of Organ Transplants, edited by Scott A. Gruber.
© 1996 R.G. Landes Company.

DEVELOPMENT AND CHARACTERIZATION OF A CsA LIPOSOME

The use of liposome technology for the delivery of pharmaceuticals has progressed over the last decade. Several agents are in use commercially, and the safety profile of systemically administered liposomes has been proven.[3-6] Design of a liposome for targeted delivery must take into consideration several physical properties of the planned compound including size, surface charge, fluidity, final lipid composition, in vitro and in vivo stability and characteristics of the loaded drug.[7] These various physical properties will influence the therapeutic performance of the final liposome.

There are several well described techniques for preparation of liposomes.[8] The technique used for the compound discussed in this chapter is reverse-phase evaporation and is outlined in Figure 11.1. Liposomes containing CsA were produced by dispersion of a homogeneous dry mixture obtained from a chloroform-ethanol solution of powdered CsA, phospholipids and cholesterol sulfate. The prototype compound consisted of CsA, phosphatidylserine/phosphatidylcholine, cholesterol sulfate and lysophosphatidylcholine in a ratio of 1:3:4:2. CsA content of the mixture was determined by high pressure liquid chromatography (HPLC). Efficiency of incorporation of CsA was typically 70%. The compound was stored at 4°C and thoroughly mixed before use. The size of the particles is relatively uniform, with the majority of particles measuring 450 nm as determined by laser light scattering measurements (Fig. 11.2). The particle size of 450 nm is

Fig. 11.1. Flow diagram depicting the process of liposomal manufacturing for the compound used in the following studies.

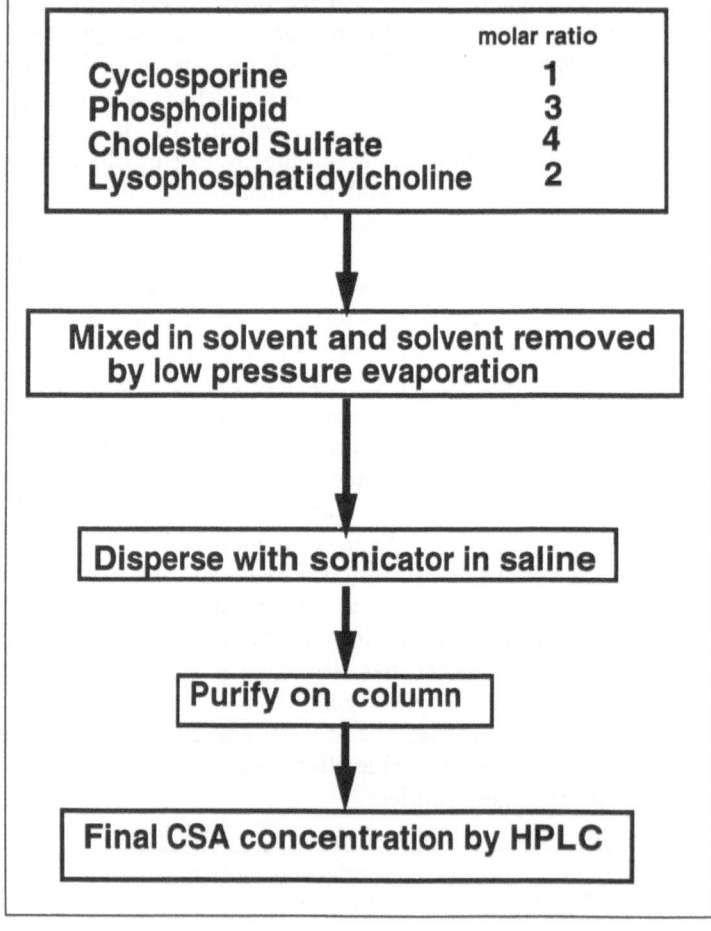

	molar ratio
Cyclosporine	1
Phospholipid	3
Cholesterol Sulfate	4
Lysophosphatidylcholine	2

Mixed in solvent and solvent removed by low pressure evaporation

Disperse with sonicator in saline

Purify on column

Final CSA concentration by HPLC

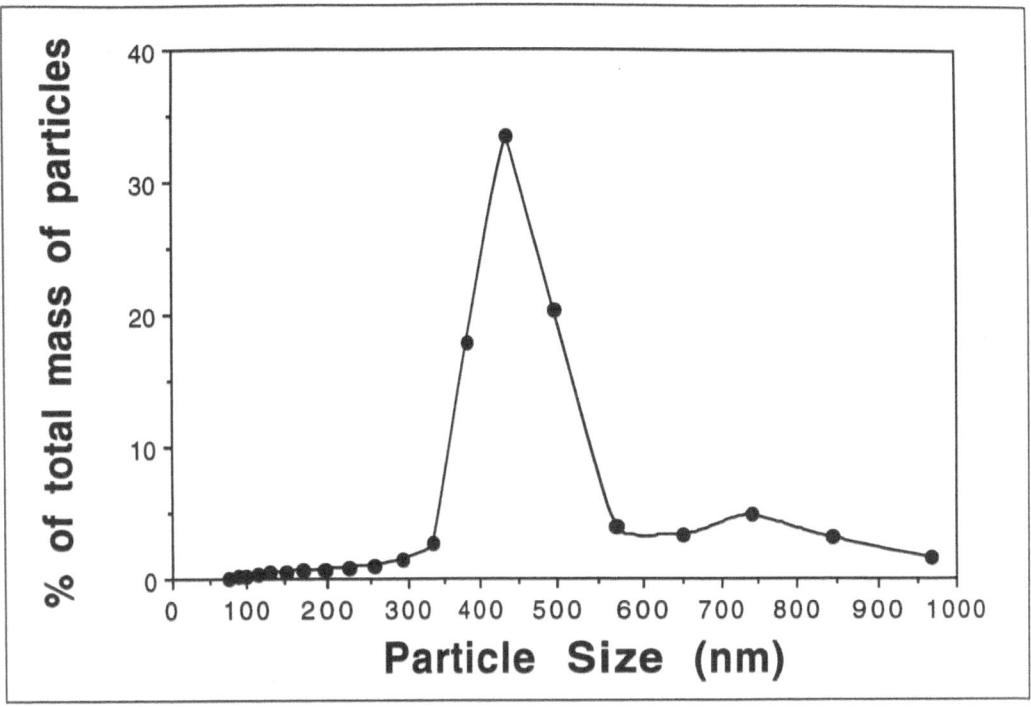

Fig. 11.2. Size of liposomal CSA particles measured using laser light scattering. Graph depicts the mass of particles distributed by size. The greatest mass of particles is in the range of 450 nm.

small enough to avoid trapping in the lung.[9] In addition, these liposomes are "well sealed" as demonstrated by the exclusion of gold particles in scanning electron microscopy studies. These microscopic studies also indicated that this compound most resembles a multilammellar liposome.

Initial work with this liposome was designed to demonstrate increased uptake in the liver compared with standard intravenous (i.v.) CsA when both drugs were administered systemically. Pharmacokinetic studies were performed in adult female Lewis rats weighing 300-350 grams. The drug (i.v. CsA or liposomal CsA) was administered as a bolus at a dose of 2 mg/kg at time 0. Samples of blood (200 μL) were collected at 5, 10, 15, 20, 30, 60, 90 and 120 minutes, with replacement of sampled volume with saline. Animals were sacrificed at 120 minutes with Nembutal injection and the liver, right kidney, spleen and a portion of intraabdominal fat were removed, weighed and later processed for tissue CsA measurements via the TDx fluo-

rescent polarization immunoassay system (Abbott Laboratories, Chicago, IL). This assay measures parent CsA as well as metabolites. In addition, blood samples collected at 120 minutes were also measured for parent CsA with HPLC. At the 2 hour time point, tissue to blood ratios of CsA were calculated for each of the sampled tissues.

Whole blood CsA levels for the prototype CsA liposome and standard i.v. CsA are shown in Figure 11.3. Differences in whole blood levels occur early (less than 10 minutes) and persist over the 2 hour sampling period. These curves suggest a faster clearance of the liposome compound from the systemic circulation compared with commercially-available CsA. Earlier clearance relative to standard i.v. CsA is suggestive of a preparation that may potentially be targeting the RES, and more specifically, liver tissue.

In an effort to determine which tissues were targeted by the liposome compound, liver tissue, splenic tissue, fat and kidney

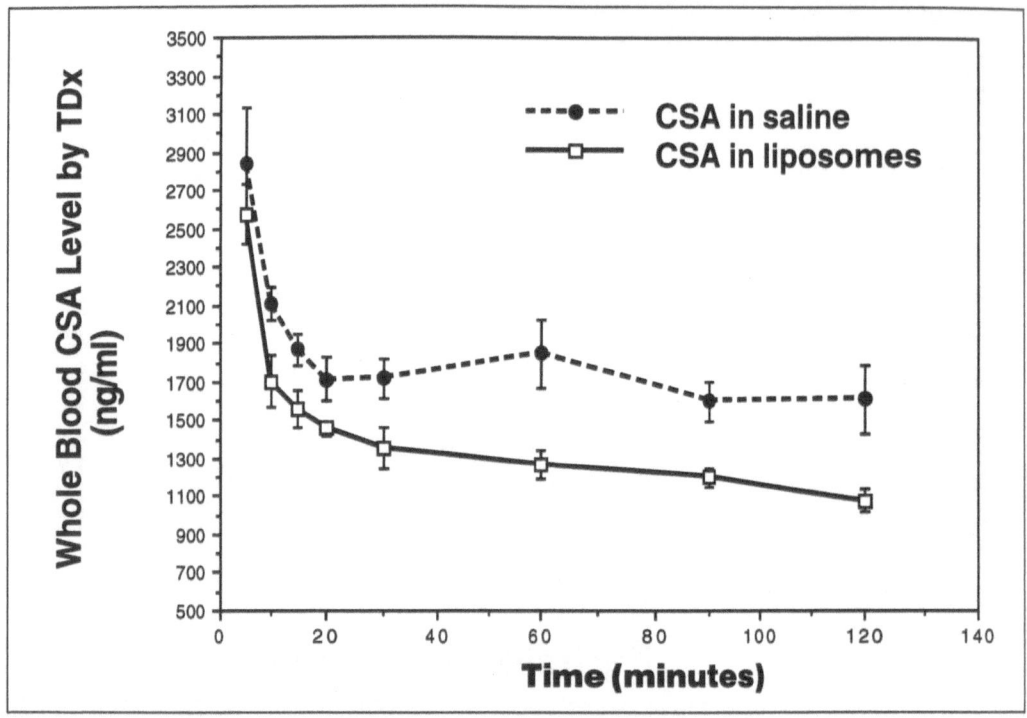

Fig. 11.3. Serial measurements of whole blood CSA levels using the TDx method were performed after injecting animals with 2 mg/kg of CSA in saline (n = 3) or CSA in liposomes (n = 4). Error bars represent standard error of the mean. Reproduced with permission from Freise CE et al, Transplantation 1994; 57:928.

were assayed for CsA parent compound and metabolites following tissue processing and extraction of CsA.[10] The ratio at 2 hours postinfusion of tissue CsA levels (ng/gm tissue) and whole blood CsA levels (ng/ml blood) were then determined for each tissue. CsA in liposome resulted in nearly a 2-fold increase in this ratio for liver tissue compared with CsA in saline (Fig. 11.4). This difference was statistically significant. The ratio in splenic tissue also increased in the liposome group, but this difference did not reach statistical significance. This compound, which exhibited liver-specific uptake and could be reproducibly manufactured, was used in all subsequent experiments.

IN VITRO CHARACTERISTICS OF CsA LIPOSOMES

In an effort to determine the effect of CsA liposomes on cellular responses in vitro and to assure no toxicity of this com-

pound to cells, the following experiments were undertaken. Murine mixed lymphocyte cultures containing responder cells that had been preincubated with various concentrations of CsA in saline, CsA in liposomes, blank liposome or plain saline for 2 hours were established. Splenocytes from 8-12 week old C3H/HeJ ($H2^k$) mice served as responders, and irradiated (3000 rads) splenocytes from 8-12 week old DBA/2 ($H2^d$) mice served as stimulators. Bulk cultures of responders at 4×10^6 cells/ml were preincubated in glass vials with the appropriate drug at 1, 10, 50 and 100 µg/ml for 2 hours. Cultures in nickel wells with 4×10^6 stimulators and 4×10^6 pretreated and subsequently washed responders were plated and harvested after 5 days for direct cytotoxicity using a chromium release assay and P815 tumor targets. For proliferation assays, 4×10^5 pretreated responders and 8×10^5 irradiated stimulators were plated in micro wells. Each day, new

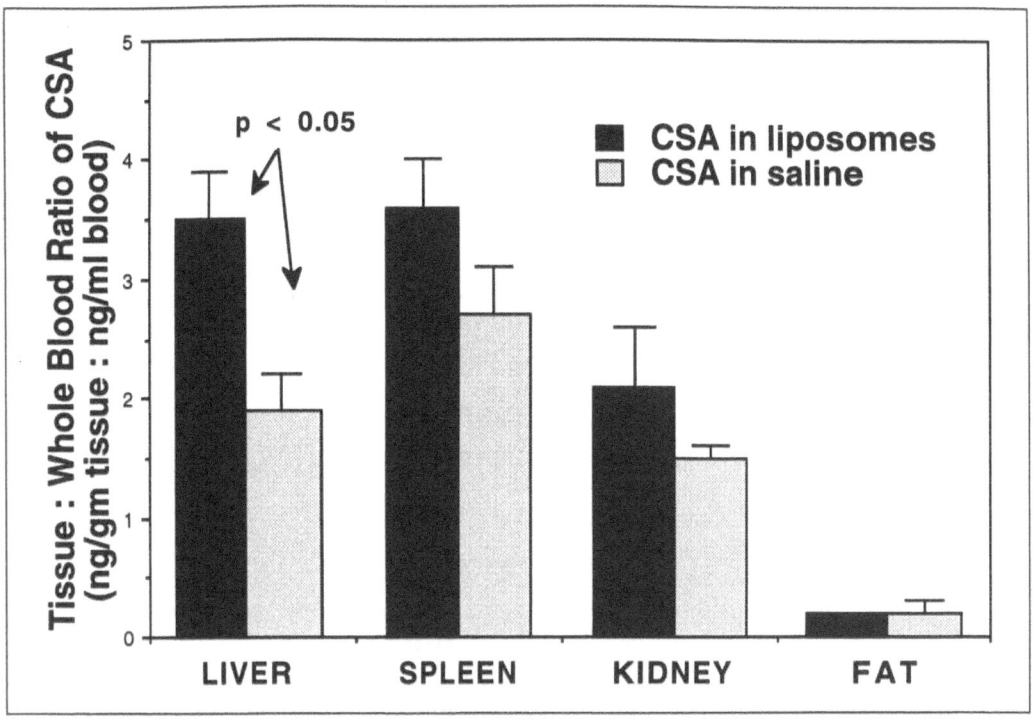

Fig. 11.4. Tissue to blood ratios of CSA (ng/gm tissue: ng/ml blood) were calculated 2 hours after a bolus injection of CSA in saline or CSA in liposomes. There was a significantly higher uptake in liver with the CSA in liposomes. Reproduced with permission from Freise CE et al, Transplantation 1994; 57:928.

wells were pulsed with tritiated thymidine for 24 hours and then frozen at 0°C. Plates were later harvested and thymidine incorporation quantitated with a Betaplate counter.

CsA contained in liposomes retained its immunosuppressive effects in vitro. Day 5 allospecific direct cytotoxicity was nearly abrogated after 2 hours pretreatment of responders at a dose of 50 µg/ml with CsA in liposomes. CsA in saline had little effect on direct cytotoxicity at this dose under these culture conditions (Plain saline 66.5% cell lysis, CsA in saline 61.0% cell lysis, CsA in liposome 1.7% cell lysis at effector to target ratio 30:1). This suggests that CsA in liposomes more readily affects cells important in the immune response. The mechanism and specific target cells responsible for this finding are unknown. CsA in liposomes was able to decrease proliferation at 6 days in a mixed lymphocyte culture (Fig. 11.5). This preparation again

appeared more effective than CsA in saline. Blank liposomes had no effect relative to the saline control indicating a lack of toxicity of this particular liposome preparation in these culture conditions.

Similar results were reported by Vadiei et al[11] utilizing CsA liposomes composed of dimyristoylphosphatidylcholine (DPMC) and stearylamine at a 7:1 ratio. A second liposome consisting of DPMC and dimyristoylphosphatidylglycerol at a ratio of 4:1 was also evaluated. These formulations had greater in vitro potency compared with commercially available i.v. CsA in a T-lymphocyte proliferation assay.[11] No in vivo data was reported for these liposomes.

EFFECT OF CsA LIPOSOMES ON NEPHROTOXICITY

One of the primary goals of targeted delivery of immunosuppressive agents is to avoid toxic side effects to other organs. In the case of CsA, neurotoxicity and nephro-

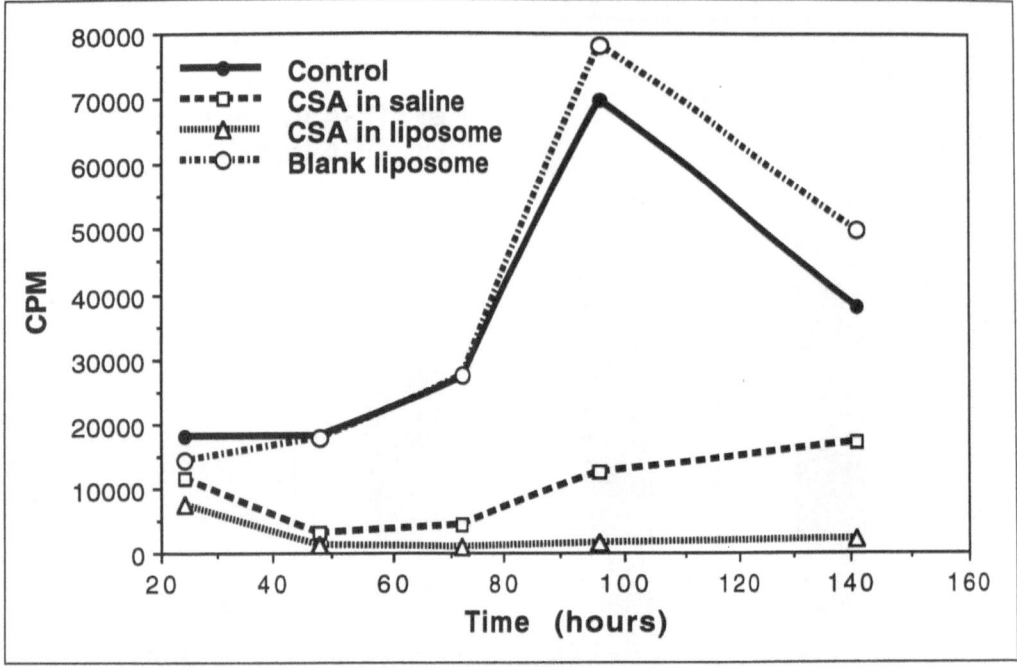

Fig. 11.5. Effect of in vitro administration of CSA liposomes, standard i.v. CSA, blank liposomes or saline on the proliferation of lymphocytes in a mixed lymphocyte culture. Liposomal CSA had the greatest effect at low concentration on inhibiting the proliferative response.

toxicity are the best-described complications of systemically-administered drug. To examine the potential decreased nephrotoxicity of liposomal CsA, a rat model of ischemic renal injury was used.[12,13]

Adult male Lewis rats were anesthetized with Nembutal and kept warm with a heating pad and warming light. The right kidney was completely mobilized down to the renal pedicle and the right renal artery was clamped for thirty minutes, followed by removal of the left kidney after clamp removal. Saline, CsA in saline or CsA in liposomes was then administered intravenously at a CsA dose of 10 mg/kg. Animals were allowed to recover and serum creatinine was measured on postoperative day 1, 2 and 4 via tail vein puncture.

There was a slight increase in serum creatinine on day 1 following this ischemic challenge and saline administration. This increase is more pronounced in animals receiving either CsA in saline or CsA in liposomes with nearly a doubling of serum creatinine from baseline. Animals receiving CsA in liposomes had a return of serum creatinine to control levels by 96 hours, suggesting a less severe toxic insult to the kidneys (Fig. 11.6).

In subsequent survival studies involving longer term administration of CsA liposomes in liver transplanted rats, no adverse effects on serum creatinine or urine production were noted. These studies utilized immunosuppressive doses far below the 10 mg/kg one-time dose used in these nephrotoxicity experiments.

The effect of a different CsA liposome on renal function was reported by Hsieh et al.[14] Lipids (specific composition undefined) or lipids plus cholesterol were used to encapsulate CsA in a 5:1 molar ratio. Drug was then administered to rats for 14 days at various doses. Glomerular filtration rates as measured by inulin clearance were significantly better in animals receiving the drug as a liposome, demonstrating decreased nephrotoxicity in a chronic delivery model. A similar benefit

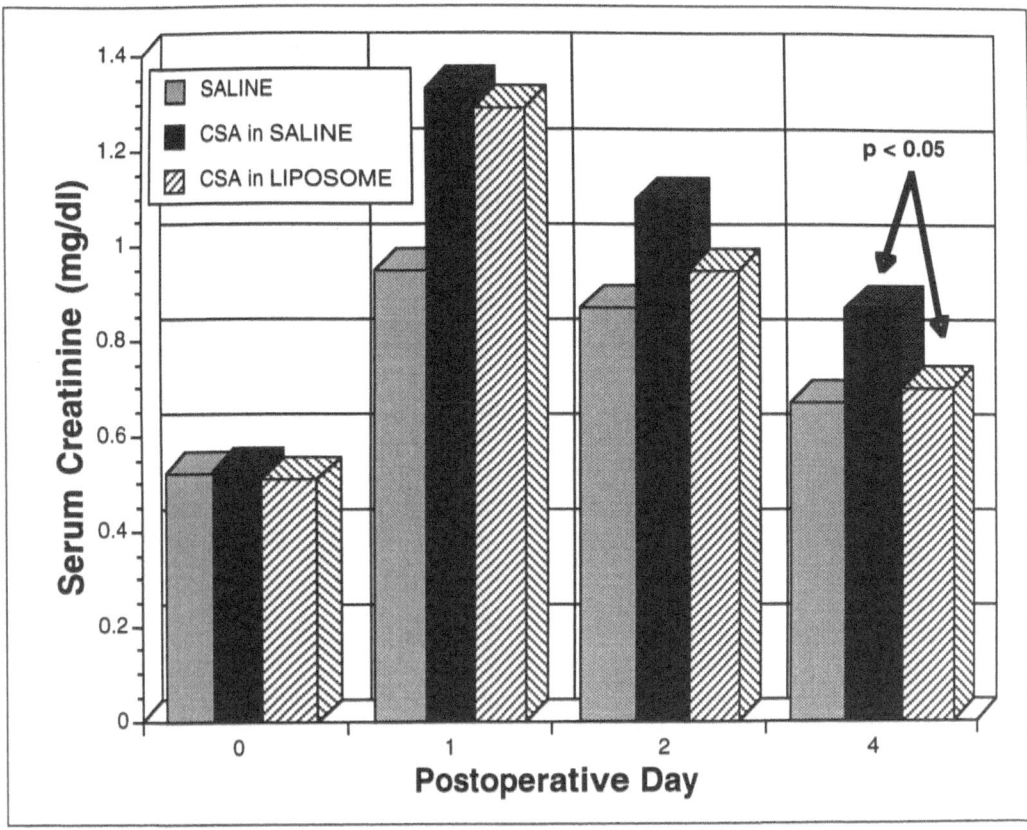

Fig. 11.6. Serial measurements of creatinine following 30 minutes of renal ischemia, contralateral nephrectomy and CsA administration at 10 mg/kg in saline or liposomes are shown. Animals receiving CsA in the liposome preparation returned to control levels of creatinine at 96 hours, a significant improvement compared with animals receiving standard i.v. CsA (P < 0.05).

of liposomal CsA on nephrotoxicity was also reported by Smeesters et al.[15]

INCREASED EFFICACY OF CsA LIPOSOME IN A RAT LIVER TRANSPLANT MODEL

The ultimate goal of this preliminary work was to demonstrate increased efficacy of CsA liposome in a rat liver transplant model. Improved efficacy translates into decreased systemic toxicity, since less drug is administered to achieve the same immunologic effect.

Orthotopic liver transplantation was performed in adult male rats in the high rejector strain combination D-Agouti (RT-1a) to Lewis (RT-1l). The standard technique of cuffed anastomosis as described by Kamada and Calne[16] with no

rearterialization was performed using an operating microscope. All animals received an indwelling subcutaneous port located in the right internal jugular vein for i.v. drug administration. Animals were randomized to three treatment groups, saline (n = 6), CsA in saline (n = 6) and CsA in liposomes (n = 6). Treated groups received CsA at a dose of 1.75 mg/kg/day for seven days postoperatively. Long term survivors were sacrificed at day 100 and the liver was sampled for histology. Rejection was graded by a blinded pathologist on hematoxylin and eosin sections.[17]

As shown in Figure 11.7, a dose of 1.75 mg/kg/day of commercially-available i.v. CsA results in some prolongation of survival compared with saline-treated animals (mean survival 51.8 days versus

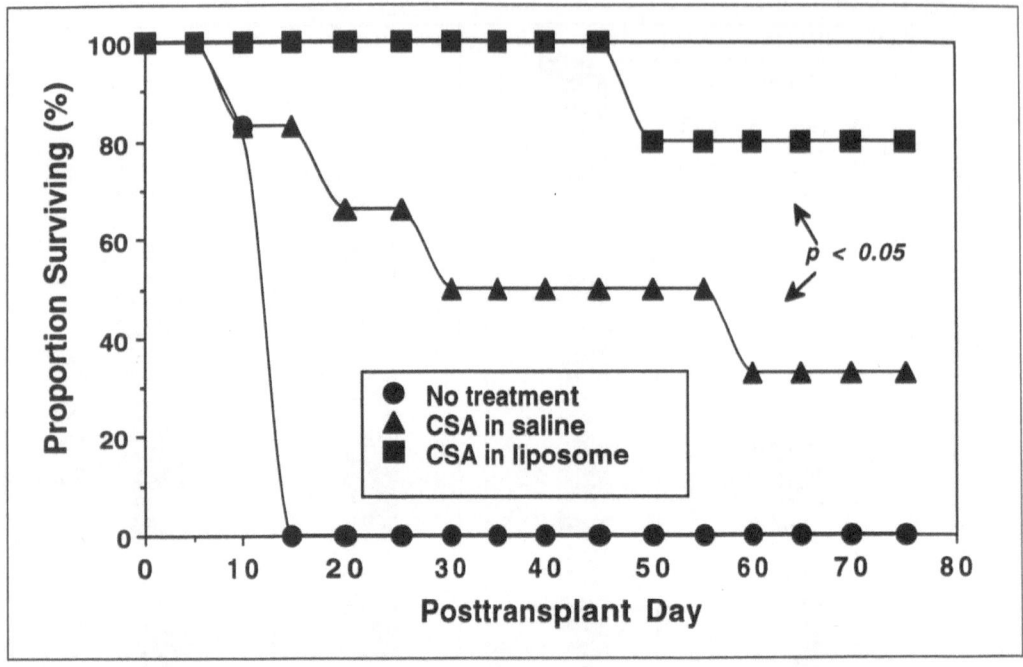

Fig. 11.7. Actuarial survival curves for the three treatment groups following liver transplantation. The CsA\ liposome group had a significantly prolonged survival with five of six animals surviving to 100 days posttransplant. Reproduced with permission from Freise CE et al, Transplantation 1994; 57:928.

11.33 days). However, animals receiving CsA liposome at this dose had a significantly prolonged survival (mean 92.6 days, $P < 0.05$ versus saline control or CsA in saline), with five of six animals surviving to day 100 at which time the study was terminated. The sixth animal actually died of biliary complications at day 48 and had no evidence of rejection on liver histology. Three of six animals in the CsA liposome group had no evidence of rejection and the other three animals had mild rejection at day 100. Four of six livers of animals receiving CsA in saline had mild rejection, one had moderate rejection and one died of severe rejection.

There was no evidence of adverse effects of the administered liposome. No infectious complications were seen in either the CsA in saline group or the CsA liposome group. Long-term survivors in both groups had eventual return to near baseline weight by day 30.

The mechanisms responsible for the increased efficacy are unknown. The im-

proved liver uptake of CsA liposome demonstrated in our pharmacokinetic experiments may allow for a higher local concentration of drug in liver parenchymal and nonparenchymal cells. The liposomes may be more effective at inhibiting T cell responses or may have some beneficial effect on Kupffer cells. This increased efficacy and decreased nephrotoxicity broadens the therapeutic index of CsA.

Other investigators working with a CsA liposome in a heart transplant model have also demonstrated increased efficacy and hypothesized that alteration of splenic function may play a role, since the spleen is the other major organ in the RES.[18] Local immunosuppression was probably not a factor in the heart transplant model, and the mechanism in our model may involve immunosuppressive effects in the spleen. Experiments to determine the role of the spleen are planned.

Future directions for the use of liposomal technology for local immunosuppression could involve several strategies. Other immunosuppressive agents or combinations of agents need to be evaluated in a large-animal model. Early work with tacrolimus in a canine liver transplant model has been reported and seems promising (see chapter 12).[19,20] The use of liposomes tagged with antibodies could also potentially improve targeting to immune effector cells within the liver allograft, further improving efficacy.[21] Antibodies to adhesion molecules or specific cytokines could likewise be incorporated in liposomes creating not only local immunosuppression but immune specificity.

The use of liposomes as a method of targeted drug delivery also opens up the opportunity to evaluate a stable model of local immunosuppression. The alterations in the immune response that occur at the local level (i.e., within the allograft) as well as the systemic level can be measured and compared. The ability to alter the host's immune responses differently at the allograft level and at the systemic level could potentially lead to new methods of tolerance induction, the ultimate method to decrease side effects of immunosuppressive agents.

REFERENCES

1. Gruber SA. The case for local immunosuppression. Transplantation 1992; 54:1.
2. Yatvin MB, Lelkes PI. Clinical prospects for liposomes. Medical Physics 1982; 9:149.
3. Lopez-Berestein G, Fainstain V, Hopfer R et al. Liposomal Amphotericin B for the treatment of systemic fungal infections in patients with cancer: a preliminary study. Journal of Infectious Dis 1985; 151:704.
4. Storm G, Regts J, Beijnen JH et al. Processing of Doxorubicin-containing liposomes by liver macrophages in vitro. Journal of Liposome Research 1989; 1:195.
5. Mayhew E, Ito M, Lazo R. Toxicity of non-drug containing liposomes for cultured human cells. Exp Cell Res 1987; 171:195.
6. Wasan K, Vadiei K, Lopez-Bernstein G et al. Pharmacokinetics, tissue distribution, and toxicity of free and liposomal amphotericin B in diabetic rats. Journal of Infectious Disease 1990; 161:562.
7. Fielding RM. Liposomal drug delivery. Clin Pharmacokinet 1991; 21:155.
8. Yatvin MB, Lelkes PI. Clinical prospects for liposomes. Med Phys 1982; 9:149.
9. Ascher NL, Stock PG, Bumgardner GL et al. Infection and rejection of primary hepatic transplants in 93 consecutive patients treated with triple immunosuppression therapy. Surg Gyn Obst 1988; 167:474.
10. Freise CE, Hong K, Clemens LE et al. Characterization of a cyclosporine containing liposome. Trans Proc 1991; 23:473.
11. Vadiei K, Lopez-Berestein G, Perez-Soler R et al. In vitro evaluation of liposomal cyclosporine. International Journal of Pharmaceutics 1989; 57:133.
12. Nalesnik MA, Lai HS, Murase N et al. The effect of FK 506 and CyA on the Lewis rat renal ischemia model. Trans Proc 1990; 22:87.
13. Jablonski P, Harrison C, Howden B et al. Cyclosporine and the ischemic rat kidney. Transplantation 1986; 41:147.
14. Hsieh H, Schreiber M, Stowe N et al. Preliminary report: the use of liposome-encapsulated cyclosporine in a rat model. Trans Proc 1985; 17:1397.
15. Smeesters C, Giroux L, Vinet B et al. Efficacy of incorporating cyclosporine into liposomes to reduce its nephrotoxicity. Canadian Journal of Surgery 1988; 31:34.
16. Kamada N, Calne R. A surgical experience with five hundred thirty-five transplants in the rat. Surgery 1983; 93:64.
17. Freise CE, Liu T, Hong K et al. The increased efficacy and decreased nephrotoxicity of a cyclosporine liposome. Transplantation 1994; 57:928.
18. Gorecki DC, Jakobisiak M, Kruszewski A et al. Evidence that liposome incorporation of cyclosporine reduces its toxicity and potentiates its ability to prolong survival of cardiac allografts in mice. Transplantation 1991; 52:766.
19. Ko S, Nakajima Y, Kanehiro H et al. Significance of newly developed liposomal FK 506 in canine liver transplantation. Trans Proc 1995; 27:351.

20. Ko S, Nakajima Y, Kanehiro H et al. The
enhanced immunosuppressive efficacy of
newly developed liposomal FK506 in canine liver transplantation. Transplantation
1995; 59:1384.

21. Debs RJ, Heath TD, Papahadjopoulos D.
Targeting of anti-Thy 1.1 monoclonal antibody conjugated liposomes in Thy 1.1 mice
after intravenous administration. Biochimica
Biophysica Acta 1987; 901:183.

CHAPTER 12

LIPOSOMAL FK506 IN A CANINE HEPATIC ALLOGRAFT MODEL

Saiho Ko, Yoshiyuki Nakajima and Hiroshige Nakano

INTRODUCTION

FK506 is a potent immunosuppressant in clinical use, and has improved the results of organ transplantation.[1,2] However, adverse effects of FK506, including nephrotoxicity and neurotoxicity, restrict the permissible dosage.[2,3] Local immunosuppression is a potential approach to reduce the adverse effects of systemic immunosuppression. This attractive option in immunosuppressive therapy has been demonstrated to enhance efficacy while simultaneously alleviating systemic adverse effects.[4,5] In order to take advantage of this concept, we developed a liposome-incorporated formulation of FK506. Liposomes are artificially constructed phospholipid vesicles which can be formulated to incorporate a variety of agents, and are preferentially taken up by the reticuloendothelial system (RES) following intravenous administration.[6] Since the liver and spleen are primary components of the RES, liposome-incorporated FK506 would target the liver and spleen. Because the liver is the site of the allograft in hepatic transplantation and the spleen is a major lymphoid depot, we hypothesized that local delivery of FK506 to these organs via the liposomal formulation would increase immunosuppressive efficacy. On the other hand, liposomal FK506 would unlikely distribute to the brain and kidney, alleviating the nephrotoxicity and neurotoxicity of FK506. In this chapter, we introduce the pharmacokinetic characteristics and immunosuppressive effects of liposomal FK506.

Local Immunosuppression of Organ Transplants, edited by Scott A. Gruber.
© 1996 R.G. Landes Company.

GENERAL CHARACTERISTICS OF THE LIPOSOMES

Liposomes which we used for incorporating FK506 are multilayered phospholipid vesicles. Figure 12.1 shows the electron microscopic appearance of liposomes. Autoradiography after intravenous injection of C^{14}-radiolabeled liposomes revealed intense accumulation in the liver, spleen and bone marrow.[6]

LIPOSOMAL INCORPORATION OF FK506

Liposomal FK506 was prepared by incorporating FK506 in multilamellar phospholipid vesicles using the solvent evaporation method.[7] A solution of phosphatidylcholine and cholesterol in chloroform was mixed with FK506 crystalline powder. The molecular ratio of phosphatidylcholine, cholesterol and FK506 was 7:7:0.8. This

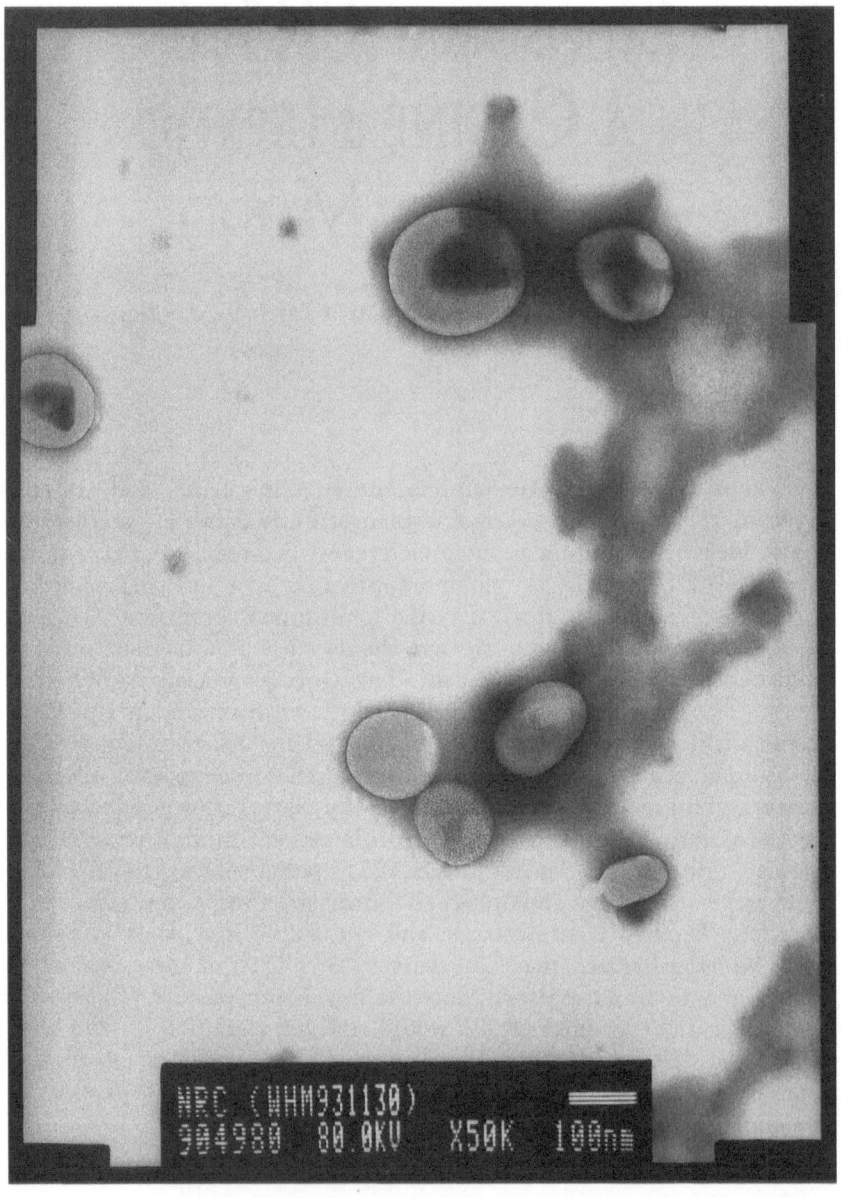

Fig. 12.1. Electron microscopic appearance of liposomes. Mean diameter of the liposomes is 145 nm.

solution was dried by an evaporator (Ohtake Works Co., Ltd., Tokyo, Japan). After evaporation, the mixture was hydrated with saline, then vigorously shaken in the Frenchpress. The suspension of liposomes was extruded under high pressure through a 0.45-micron membrane filter to control the diameter of the particles. The surface of the liposomes was treated with HSPE-PEG5K (hydrogenated soy phosphatidyl ethanolamine bounded with polyethylene glycol) to stabilize the structure in vivo.[8] The suspension of liposome-incorporated FK506 was used for administration. The mean diameter of the liposomes was 145 nm, and the FK506 concentration of the suspension was 0.56 mg/ml.

PHARMACOKINETICS OF LIPOSOMAL FK506

The pharmacokinetics of liposomal FK506 were compared with that of the conventional intravenous formulation in a rat model.[7] Male Wistar rats weighing 180-220 g were used. FK506 was administered intravenously into the tail vein at a dose of 0.5 mg/kg as the liposome-incorporated formulation (liposome group, n = 12) and as the standard formulation (i.v. formula group, n = 12).

Ten minutes (n = 3), 1 hour (n = 3), 6 hours (n = 3) and 24 hours (n = 3) after injection of FK506, the rats in each group were anesthetized with ethyl ether inhalation. After laparotomy, blood samples were taken from the inferior vena cava, and the abdominal aorta was cut to flush out the blood. Subsequently, spleen, liver, kidney, pancreas, intestine (jejunum), cerebrum and cerebellum tissue samples were excised.

FK506 levels were measured by an enzyme immunoassay method using anti-FK506 monoclonal antibody as previously described.[9] For the determination of tissue levels of FK506, samples were homogenized in saline and centrifuged. FK506 levels in the supernatant were measured, and tissue FK506 levels were calculated as the amount of FK506 in 1 g of tissue.

Ten minutes after injection of FK506, whole blood levels of FK506 in the liposome group were higher than in the i.v. formula group (Fig. 12.2). However, FK506 levels in the liposome group rapidly decreased and the values at 1 hour were significantly lower than those in the i.v. formula group. These data suggested that liposomal FK506 was distributed from the blood more rapidly than the i.v. solution of FK506 within 10 minutes of administration.

FK506 levels in the kidney and cerebrum were significantly lower in the liposome group than in the i.v. formula group (Figs. 12.3, 12.4). On the contrary, FK506 levels in the spleen were significantly higher in the liposome group than in the i.v. formula group at 10 minutes and 1 hour (Fig. 12.5). FK506 levels in the liver at 10 minutes were also significantly higher in the liposome group than in the i.v. formula group (Fig. 12.6). Preferential accumulation of liposomal FK506 in the liver suggested that it might have enhanced effects in preventing hepatic allograft rejection with less systemic side effects.

IMMUNOSUPPRESSIVE EFFECTS OF LIPOSOMAL FK506

Immunosuppressive effects of liposomal FK506 in liver transplantation were evaluated in a canine allograft model.[10] Outbred young adult beagle dogs of both sexes, weighing 8-14 kg, were used. Orthotopic canine allotransplantation of the liver was performed, and the recipients were divided into the following groups: Group I, controls, no immunosuppression (n = 5); group II, 0.05 mg/kg/day FK506 was administered intravenously as the commercially-available i.v. formulation for 14 days postoperatively (n = 5); group III, 0.05 mg/kg/day of FK506 was administered intravenously as the liposomal formulation for 14 days postoperatively (n = 5). Open biopsies of the liver and spleen were performed on the 14th day in the recipients that survived for more than 14 days. Autopsies were routinely performed and the cause of death was confirmed by gross and microscopic examination. Microscopic findings of

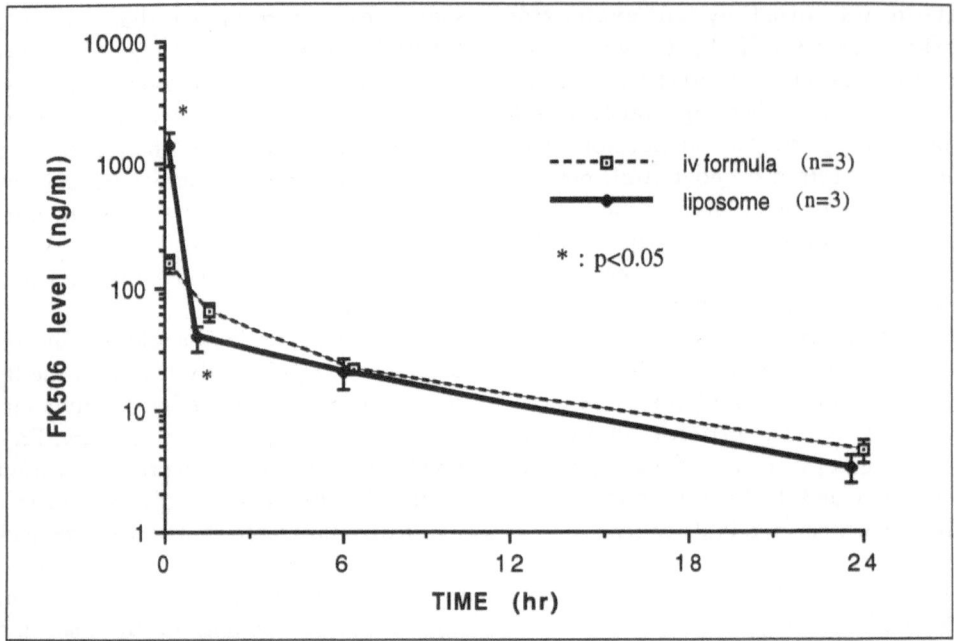

Fig. 12.2. *Whole-blood FK506 levels after an injection of 0.5 mg/kg FK506 as the conventional i.v. and liposomal formulations in a rat model.*

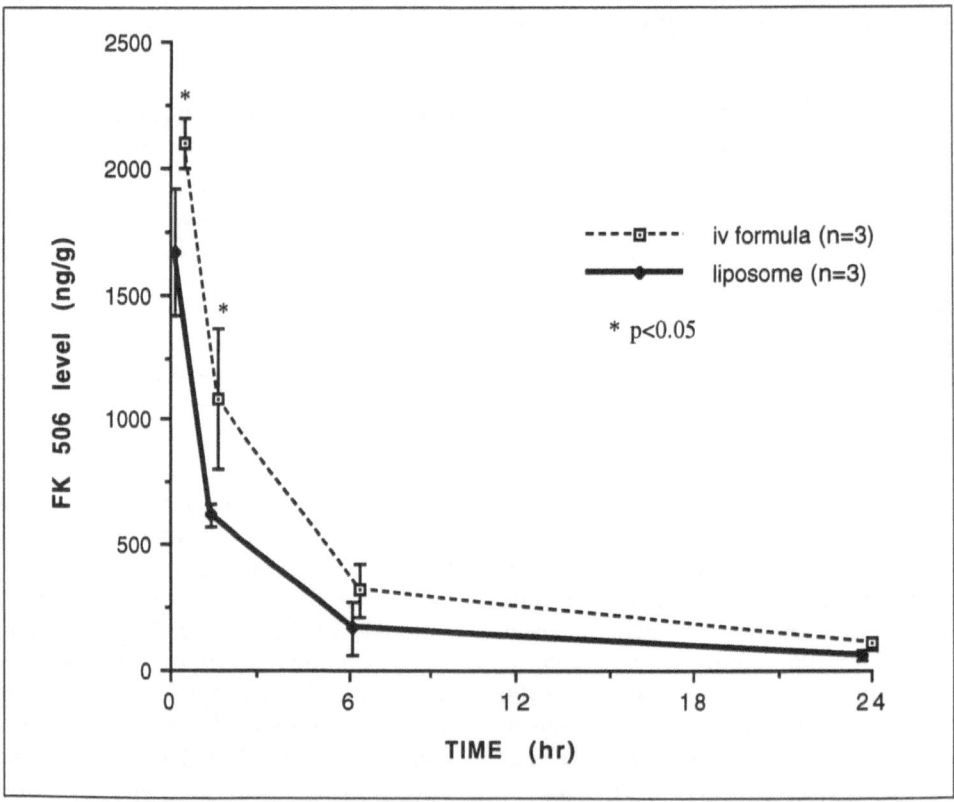

Fig. 12.3. *FK506 levels in the kidney after an injection of 0.5 mg/kg FK506 as the conventional i.v. and liposomal formulations in a rat model.*

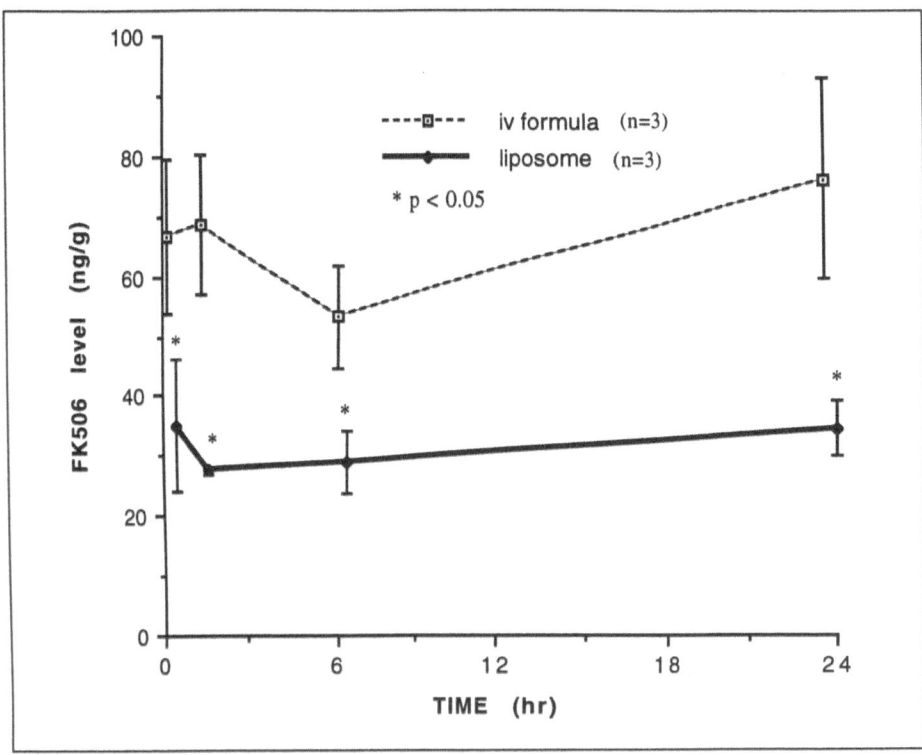

Fig. 12.4. FK506 levels in the cerebrum after an injection of 0.5 mg/kg FK506 as the conventional i.v. and liposomal formulations in a rat model.

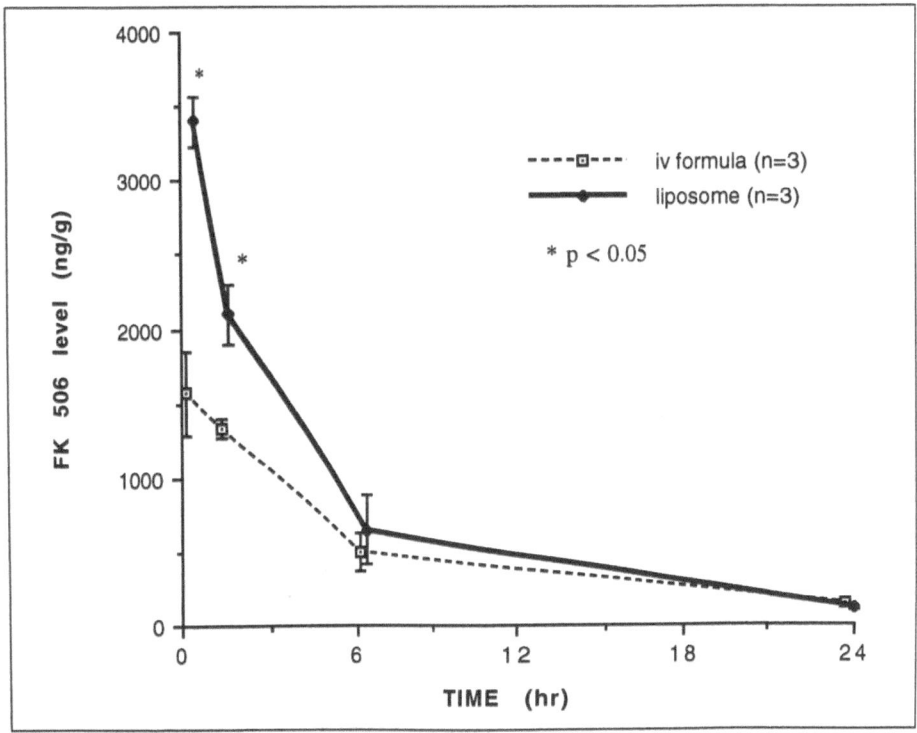

Fig. 12.5. FK506 levels in the spleen after an injection of 0.5 mg/kg FK506 as the conventional i.v. and liposomal formulations in a rat model.

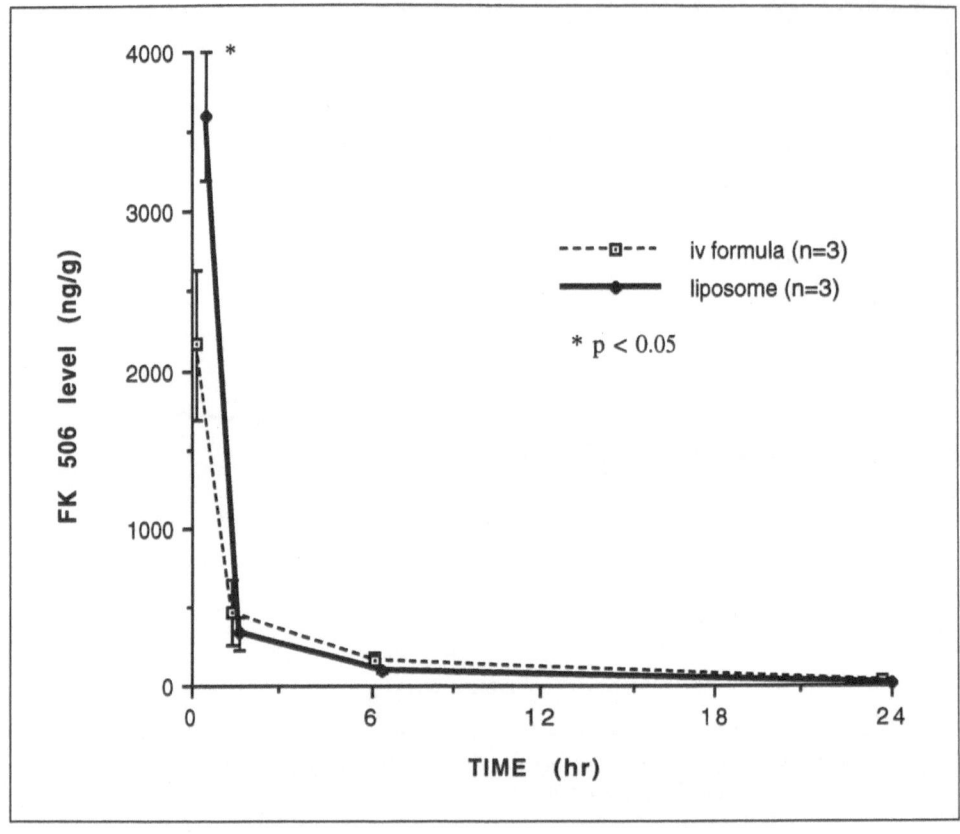

Fig. 12.6. FK506 levels in the liver after an injection of 0.5 mg/kg FK506 as the conventional i.v. and liposomal formulations in a rat model.

rejection in the grafted liver were assessed by H&E staining according to Kemnitz's criteria.[11] The following evaluations were performed in each group: (a) survival time after transplantation; (b) peripheral blood trough levels of FK506 on days 4, 7 and 14 (groups II and III); (c) tissue trough levels of FK506 in the spleen on day 14 (groups II and III); (d) histological evaluation of graft rejection in the biopsy specimen on day 14 and the autopsy specimen and (e) DNA analysis of peripheral blood mononuclear cells (PBMC) and splenic mononuclear cells (SMC) on day 14. For DNA analysis, the sum of S and G2M phase populations, designated SG2M%, is an indicator of proliferative activity of mononuclear cells related to the rejection reaction.[12]

As shown in Figure 12.7, recipients in group III had a significantly prolonged survival when compared with those in groups I and II. All recipients in group I died of severe acute rejection within 2 weeks (median survival 10 days). In group II, two out of five recipients also died within 2 weeks, and the remaining three recipients died of rejection on days 24, 27 and 33 (median survival 24 days). In group III, three out of five recipients survived for more than 200 days despite discontinuation of immunosuppressive therapy on day 14 (median survival 202 days, P < 0.05 versus group I or group II). In the three recipients in group II that survived for more than 2 weeks, the histological grade of rejection on day 14 was mild or moderate, but was severe at au-

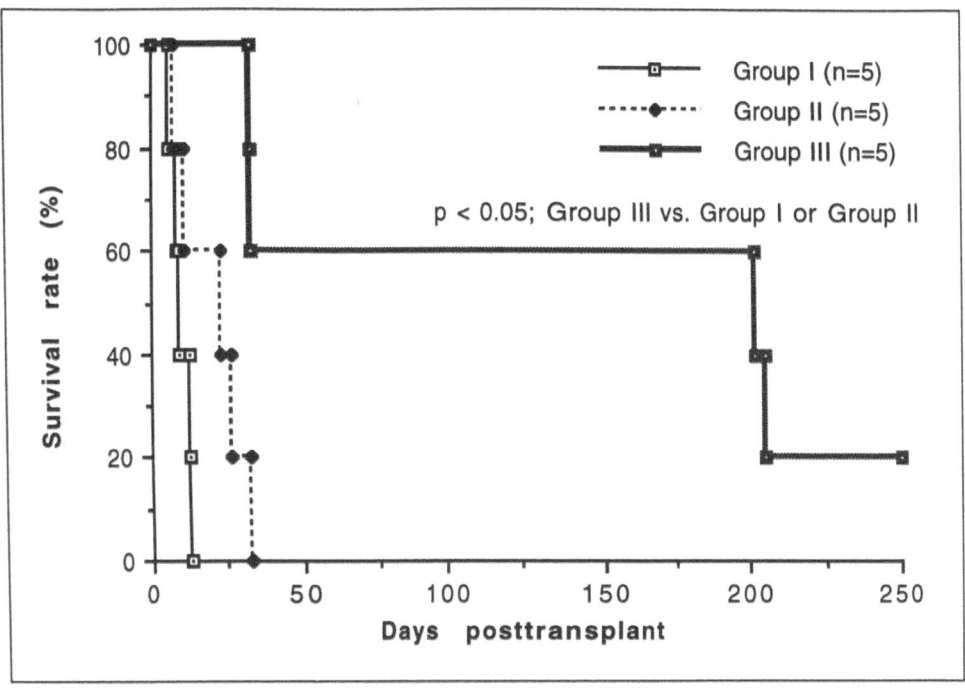

Fig. 12.7. Actual survival after canine liver transplantation.[10] Group III (liposomal formulation) had a significantly prolonged survival when compared with group I (control) or group II (i.v. formulation). Reproduced with permission from Transplantation 1995; 59:1384-1388.

topsy. In group III, day 14 histology revealed no or mild rejection. Two out of the three long-term survivors in group III had typical chronic rejection at autopsy (Table 12.1).

Peripheral whole-blood trough levels of FK506 in group III were as low as those in group II (Fig. 12.8). On the other hand, mean ± SD FK506 levels in the spleen on day 14 in group III were 64 ± 13 ng/g, significantly higher than those in group II (18 ± 5 ng/g; $P < 0.01$).

The present study demonstrated that low-dose liposomal FK506 treatment for 14 days significantly prolonged canine liver allograft survival compared with the commercially-available standard i.v. formulation. This result suggests that liposomal incorporation is a useful method for increasing the immunosuppressive efficacy of FK506 in liver transplantation. Since liposomal incorporation did not delay clearance of FK506 from the systemic circulation and

tissues, the altered tissue distribution of liposomal FK506 appears to play an important role in enhancing its immunosuppressive efficacy. Recently, we reported the significance of local immunosuppression in preventing allograft rejection in a liver transplantation model using intraportal administration of cyclosporine A.[5] Other investigators also have reported the efficacy of local immunosuppressive therapy in sponge matrix, kidney, heart and pancreatic islet transplantation models.[4,13,14] In the present study, increased FK506 levels in the liver, which was the site of the allograft, might have resulted in increased immunosuppressive efficacy.

In addition, increased FK506 levels in the spleen might also play a role in the immunosuppressive efficacy of liposomal FK506. FK506 inhibits the release of interleukin-2 from allosensitized T-lymphocytes, and this immunological reaction is believed to progress in the spleen and

Table 12.1. *Histology of the graft in a canine liver transplantation model*

Group	FK506 Dose (mg/kg/day)	Survival (days)	Rejection Grade POD 14	Autopsy
I (n = 5)	none	6	–	severe
		9	–	severe
		10	–	severe
		13	–	severe
		13	–	severe
II (n = 5)	0.05	8	–	severe
	in iv formula	11	–	severe
	for 14 days	24	moderate	severe
		27	mild	severe
		33	mild	severe
III (n = 5)	0.05	32	none	moderate
	in liposome	33	none	undiagnosed
	for 14 days	202	mild	chronic
		205	none	chronic
		>250	none	–

Reproduced with permission from Transplantation 1995; 59:1384-1388.

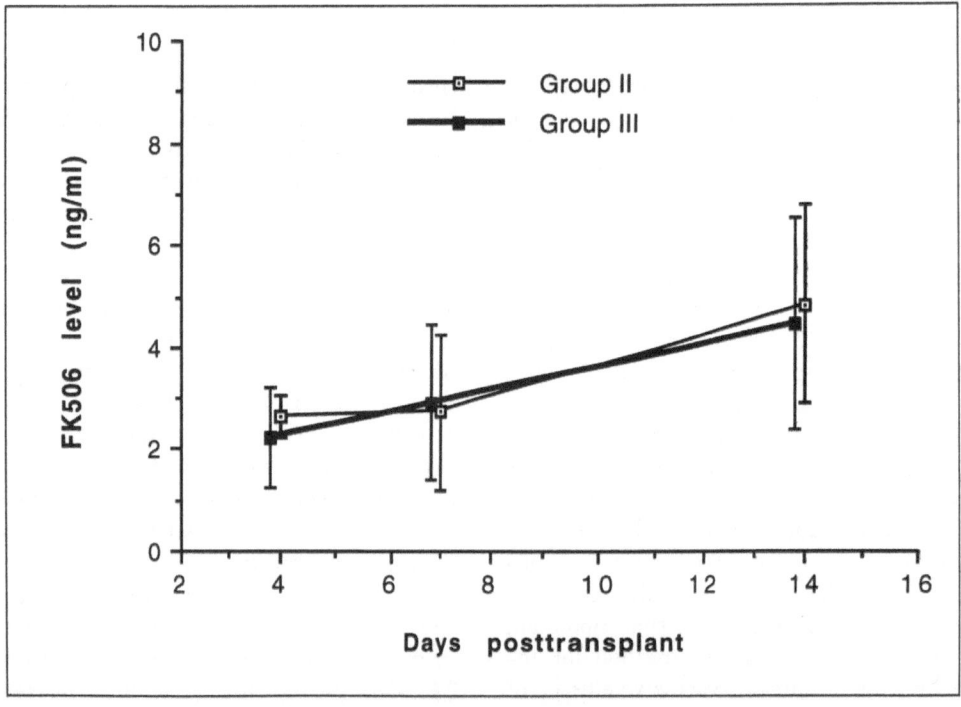

Fig. 12.8. *Peripheral whole- blood FK 506 trough levels in canine liver transplant recipients in group II and group III.*[10] *Levels in group III (liposomal formulation) were as low as those in group II (i.v. formulation). Reproduced with permission from Transplantation 1995; 59:1384-1388.*

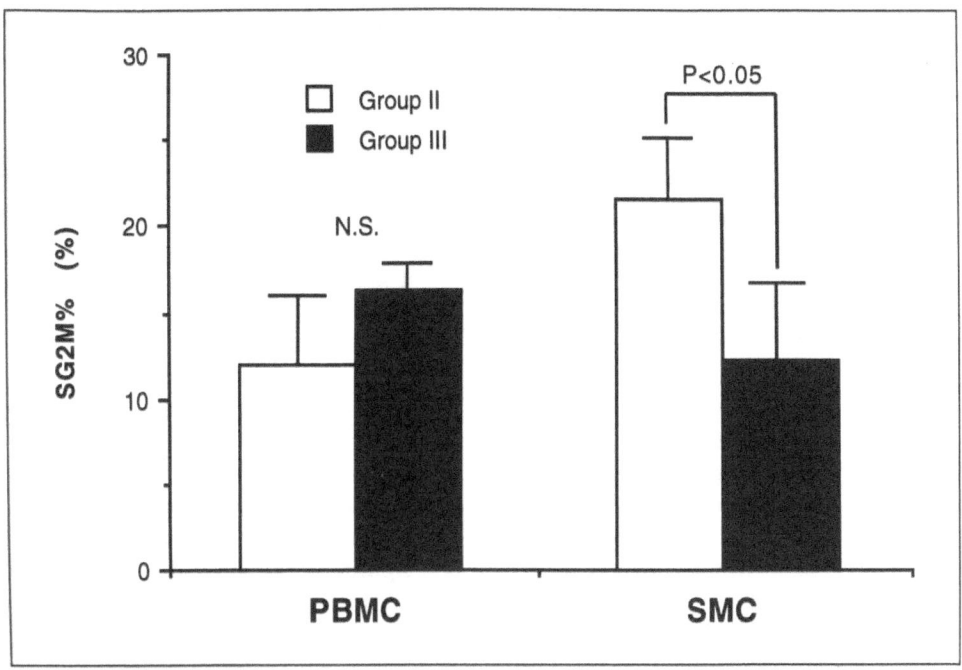

Fig. 12.9. DNA SG2M% of peripheral blood and splenic mononuclear cells on day 14 in canine liver allograft recipients.[10] SG2M% of PBMC on day 14 in group III (liposomal formulation) was as much as that in group II (i.v. formulation). On the contrary, SG2M% of SMC in group III was more effectively suppressed than that in group II (P < 0.05). Reproduced with permission from Transplantation 1995; 59:1384-1388.

regional lymph nodes.[4,6] Therefore, the spleen may be one of the main target organs of FK506. Moreover, as shown in Figure 12.9, SG2M% of SMC in group III was significantly lower than that in group II, which suggested that liposomal FK506 more effectively suppressed splenocyte proliferation activity than the i.v. formulation of FK506.[10] This significant suppression of splenocyte proliferation might contribute to enhancement of immunosuppressive efficacy of liposomal FK506. It remains to be elucidated whether a local immunosuppressive effect in the liver or suppression of splenocyte proliferation played the dominant role in enhancing overall immunosuppressive efficacy.

Our results in this model suggest that a kind of tolerance was induced by liposomal FK506 because some recipients survived for a long time even after discontinuation of immunosuppressive therapy. Meiser et al[15] demonstrated that alteration of splenic immune function was essential to cyclosporine-induced allograft tolerance in a rat model. Since the mechanism of action of FK506 is similar to that of cyclosporine,[16] significant suppression of splenocyte proliferation by liposomal FK506 might contribute to long-term graft acceptance. However, the precise mechanism of long-term graft acceptance after discontinuation of liposomal FK506 needs to be explored.

BENEFITS OF LIPOSOMAL INCORPORATION WITH RESPECT TO THE ADVERSE EFFECTS OF FK506

As mentioned above, altered tissue distribution of FK506 by liposomal incorporation provided increased efficacy in preventing hepatic allograft rejection. From the viewpoint of adverse effects, decreased FK506 levels in the kidney and brain with the liposomal preparation would be expected to alleviate the nephrotoxic and neurotoxic side effects of the drug. In our canine liver transplantation model, blood chemical analysis did not demonstrate any evidence of nephrotoxicity with either formulation of FK506, presumably due to the low doses utilized. There were no demonstrable toxic effects related to administration of the liposomes observed with follow-up of more than 200 days in our canine model.

CONCLUSION

The results of our study suggest that liposomal incorporation would be an attractive method to increase the therapeutic index of FK506 in liver transplantation. Optimal doses and adequate treatment after discontinuation of liposomal FK506 should be evaluated in further investigation. There were no demonstrable toxic effects observed with follow-up of more than 200 days in our canine model. It is expected that liposomal FK506 may be applied in clinical liver transplantation with significant therapeutic benefits.

SUMMARY

The pharmacokinetics and immunosuppressive effects of liposomal FK506 were studied. Increased FK506 levels in the liver and spleen, and decreased FK506 levels in the kidney and brain were noted in comparison with the commercially-available i.v. formulation. In a canine liver allograft model using beagle dogs, 0.05 mg/kg/day of FK506 administered i.v. in a liposomal formulation for 14 days significantly prolonged survival when compared with the same dose of the commercially-available i.v. formulation.

These results suggest that liposomal incorporation markedly increases the immunosuppressive efficacy of FK506 in liver transplantation. Both local immunosuppressive effects in the grafted liver and significant suppression of splenocyte proliferation might contribute to the overall enhancement of immunosuppressive efficacy observed. In addition, decreased FK506 levels in the kidney and brain with liposomal incorporation would alleviate the nephrotoxicity and neurotoxicity of FK506.

REFERENCES

1. Starzl TE, Todo S, Fung J et al. FK506 for human liver, kidney, and pancreas transplantation. Lancet 1989; 8670:1000.
2. European FK506 Multicentre Liver Study Group. Randomised trial comparing tacrolimus (FK506) and cyclosporin in prevention of liver allograft rejection. Lancet 1994; 344:423.
3. Platz KP, Mueller AR, Blumhardt G et al. Nephrotoxicity following orthotopic liver transplantation. A comparison between cyclosporine and FK506. Transplantation 1994; 58:170.
4. Gruber SA. The case for local immunosuppression. Transplantation 1992; 54:1.
5. Ko S, Nakajima Y, Kanehiro H et al. The significance of local immunosuppression in canine liver transplantation. Transplantation 1994; 57:1818.
6. Sakaguchi K, Suzuki M, Ogata Y et al. Biodistribution of the neo red cell and effect on the phagocytic activity of the reticuloendothelial system. Jpn J Artif Organs 1993; 22:560.
7. Ko S, Nakajima Y, Kanehiro H et al. The pharmacokinetic benefits of newly developed liposome-incorporated FK506. Transplantation 1995; 58:1142.
8. Yoshioka H, Suzuki K, Miyauchi Y et al. Characteristics of Neo Red Cells and their in vivo oxygen transport capacity. Artificial Organs 1990; 14:211.
9. Tamura K, Kobayashi M, Hashimoto K. A highly sensitive method to assay FK506 levels in plasma. Transplant Proc 1987; 19:23.
10. Ko S, Nakajima Y, Kanehiro H et al. The enhanced immunosuppressive efficacy of newly developed liposomal FK506 in canine liver transplantation. Transplantation 1995; 59:1384.
11. Kemnitz J, Gubernatis H, Bunzendahl H et al. Criteria for histopathological classification of liver allograft rejection and their clinical relevance. Transplant Proc 1989; 21:2208.
12. Nakajima Y, Hisanaga M, Taki J et al. Cytoimmunologic monitoring using DNA analysis in canine liver transplantation. Transplantation 1993; 55:480.

13. Ruers TJM, Daemen MJAP, Thijssen HHW et al. Sensitivity of graft rejection in rats to local immunosuppressive therapy. Transplantation 1988;46:850.

14. Todo S, Ueda Y, Demetris JA et al. Immunosuppression of canine, monkey, and baboon allografts by FK506: with special reference to synergism with other drugs and to tolerance induction. Surgery 1988; 104:239.

15. Meiser BM, Morris RE. The importance of the spleen for the immunosuppressive action of cyclosporine in transplantation. Transplantation 1991; 51:690.

16. Metcalfe SM, Richards FM. Cyclosporine, FK506, rapamycin. Transplantation 1990; 49:798.

CYCLOSPORINE AEROSOL IN LUNG TRANSPLANTATION

Gilbert J. Burckart, Robert J. Keenan,
Aldo T. Iacono and Bartley P. Griffith

In solid organ transplantation, the graft is generally inaccessible to localized pharmacologic therapy. Lung transplantation represents the exception, however, in that aerosolized pharmacologic agents have direct access to the donor graft, and the technology for delivering medication by the inhalational route is well developed for other pulmonary disorders. In 1988, a team of investigators at the University of Pittsburgh made the decision to pursue aerosolized immunosuppression for lung transplant recipients based upon the success of other experimental models of localized immunosuppression.

The driving force for pursuing new approaches to immunosuppression in lung transplantation was the significant incidence of chronic rejection in the recipients. Chronic rejection most frequently manifests histologically as obliterative bronchiolitis, a progressive inflammatory process leading to scarring and occlusion of small airways.[1,2] Early in the disease, no demonstrable change in pulmonary function may be observed, but the usual course of chronic rejection is progressive deterioration with worsening pulmonary function and increasing symptoms of dyspnea and fatigue.[3-5] Obliterative bronchiolitis is traditionally treated with short-term enhancement of immunosuppression consisting of pulse corticosteroids and antilymphocyte globulin, after which maintenance immunosuppression is increased to tolerance.[6-8] These treatments are associated with significant morbidity and mortality, as evidenced by the fact that 49% of the 65 patients at our center with this diagnosis have experienced serious infectious complications following therapy, with three deaths resulting. In over 30% of lung transplant patients treated for obliterative bronchiolitis, persistent histological evidence of scarring of small airways and progressive loss of lung function is observed.[3,6-9] These patients have a dismal prognosis with a life expectancy of less than two years.

Local Immunosuppression of Organ Transplants, edited by Scott A. Gruber.
© 1996 R.G. Landes Company.

Hepatic and renal toxicity often limit the dosing of cyclosporine (CsA, Sandimmune, Sandoz, East Hanover, NJ) in patients with graft rejection.[10] If CsA could be delivered directly into the transplanted lung by aerosol inhalation, higher concentrations of CsA in the graft may be achieved which could result in improvement of rejection with acceptable systemic toxicity. The concept of using CsA as an aerosol was originally proposed by Dr. Rene Duquesnoy, but the task of turning this concept into a clinical reality was larger than anyone in the investigative team imagined at the time.

The clinical use of CsA as an immunosuppressive aerosol in lung transplantation was encouraged by a diverse group of studies that had been previously conducted by other investigators. Work in the sponge matrix allograft model first demonstrated the local development of cells within the graft that are responsive against the donor.[11] Local radiation therapy had been used in canine renal and heterotopic heart allografts with some success.[12,13] Human kidney allografts also have been reported to benefit from local radiation therapy.[14] Regional delivery of steroids by intra-arterial infusion results in down-regulation of class II MHC antigen and interleukin-2 (IL-2) receptor expression,[15] and prolongation of heterotopic cardiac allograft survival in rats.[16] Intraarterial CsA administration prolonged rat heterotopic heart allograft survival beyond that observed with similar intravenous or oral dosing,[17] and produced the highest CsA tissue concentrations in recipient lungs. Therefore, the stage was set for the development of a therapeutic regimen that could directly deliver CsA to the transplanted lung in our patient population.

ANIMAL STUDIES

Our first attempts to deliver aerosolized CsA were in normal anesthetized and intubated dogs.[18] The CsA was dissolved in ethanol, since this appeared to be the only reasonable vehicle for administration to animals or human subjects that could solubilize CsA to the extent necessary. In this initial protocol, 200 mg of CsA powder was dissolved in 5 ml of 95% USP ethanol and nebulized via a small particle aerosol generator (SPAG-2, ICN Pharmaceuticals, Cosa Mesa, CA). Nebulization was complicated by the precipitation of CsA within the nebulization chamber as the ethanol was volatilized off, which clogged the SPAG-2 generator. Future protocols used 100% absolute ethanol in an attempt to overcome this problem.

Five dogs received the 200 mg nebulized CsA daily for eight doses via endotracheal tube, and blood and tissue concentrations were measured. Sufficient tissue was available to distinguish proximal airway, distal airway and lung parenchymal concentrations of CsA. Trough blood levels (by high-performance liquid chromatography [HPLC]) before the final nebulized dose of CsA were less than 50 ng/ml in all cases, while lung parenchymal levels were greater than 700 ng/gm. Whole-blood levels did increase following CsA dosing, and peaked at 100-250 ng/ml 60 minutes postdose. The CsA concentrations observed in proximal and distal airway (up to 25,000 ng/gm) were 10 to 100 times the concentrations observed in kidney and heart tissue. The aerosolized administration of CsA did not appear to cause any damage to lung tissue, as assessed by blood gases in the animals or by histologic examination. Therefore, we concluded that while the daily intubation of the dogs was labor-intensive and time-consuming, this model of aerosolized CsA delivery was adequate for an initial trial in canine lung transplantation.

The study of aerosolized CsA in a canine single lung transplant model that followed was reported by Dowling et al in 1990.[19] Two-hundred mg CsA was aerosolized daily for eight doses to each of eight animals as in the previous study in nontransplanted animals. Six dogs were transplanted but received no immunosuppressive therapy as the control group. Table 13.1 gives the grade of rejection present in an open lung biopsy specimen taken on postoperative day 7 in the control and CsA-treated groups.

Over 75% of the whole-blood trough drug concentrations obtained in the CsA-aerosol treatment group were less than 100 ng/ml. The average blood concentrations at 20 and 60 minutes after the CsA dose rose to 165 and 185 ng/ml, respectively. Mean trough and 60 minutes postaerosol lung parenchymal levels were 2424 and 25,550 ng/gm respectively, but considerable variation existed between animals. Grade 0 histologic rejection was observed in the animals with the highest measured concentrations of CsA in lung tissue. This initial lung transplant study demonstrated that aerosolized CsA was effective in suppressing the rejection process even when very low concentrations of drug could be measured systemically.

The evolution of this therapy required that a greater number of animals be studied to both investigate the toxicologic properties of aerosolized CsA and further validate its therapeutic effect. The procedures used in the initial dog studies were too difficult to carry out in large numbers of animals. Therefore, the next studies were performed in a rat model of lung transplantation.

The rodent studies were conducted with the collaboration of Drs. Michelle Schaper and Andrew Duncan using the Pitt generator for the production of CsA aerosol. The first study in nontransplanted rats involved administering 50 mg/m³ aerosolized CsA to 15 Lewis rats for 45 minutes.[5] Five rats were sacrificed at 90 minutes, five were sacrificed at 6 hours, and the remaining five were sacrificed at 24 hours. Table 13.2 presents the CsA tissue and blood concentrations observed in these animals. This study provided the basis for dosage selection in a 30 day toxicology trial and in a rat lung transplant trial that followed.

The toxicology study was conducted in 10 nontransplanted Lewis rats exposed to 50 mg/m³ CsA aerosol for 90 minutes per day.[5] Five animals were exposed for 15 days and sacrificed, and five animals were exposed for 30 consecutive days. Histopathological and microbiologic examination of the lungs, kidneys, livers and hearts of the ten exposed rats revealed no lesions or

Table 13.1. Grade of rejection in the CsA-aerosol treated and control groups following canine single lung transplantation

Histologic Grade of Rejection	Control Group (n = 6)	CsA Aerosol Group (n = 7)
0	0	1
1+	0	1
2+	0	3
3+	0	2
4+	6	0

Table 13.2. Tissue and blood CsA levels after a single exposure to aerosolized CsA in rats (50 mg/m³)

	90 Min Post (n = 5)	6 Hr Post (n = 5)	24 Hr Post (n = 5)
Lung	7102 ± 756	1670 ± 285	208 ± 35
Liver	1668 ± 368	1045 ± 68	ND
Kidney	639 ± 56	647 ± 71	ND
Heart	248 ± 23	88 ± 11	ND
Blood	93 ± 22.5	71 ± 13	ND

Concentrations by HPLC expressed as ng/mL in whole blood and ng/gm in tissues (mean ± SD)
ND = not detectable (< 50 ng/gm or mL)
Reprinted with permission from Zenati M et al, Eur J Cardiothorac Surg 1991; 5:266.

infections. All whole-blood CsA concentrations were less than 50 ng/ml in all animals.

The rat lung transplant experiment compared an untreated control group with animals given a one-time or daily (x 4 days) 25 mg/kg dose of intramuscular (i.m.) CsA, and with rats receiving aerosolized CsA, 180 mg/m^3 for 3 hours daily for 7 days.[5] Microbiologic and histologic studies were performed in all groups, and the results on postoperative day 6 are presented in Table 13.3.

A question that remained was whether there was a definite dose-response relationship with aerosolized CsA. This question was addressed in an extension of the previous study, in which low-, intermediate- and high-dose aerosolized CsA groups were added.[20] As can be seen in Table 13.4, a clear relationship was apparent between the dose of aerosolized CsA administered to the transplanted rat, the concentrations of CsA that were achieved in blood and lung tissue, and the histologic grade of rejection after 7 days of aerosolized therapy. This observation may be critically important as we attempt to develop dosing regimens in patients with differing needs for immunosuppressive therapy.

A concurrent avenue of investigation was to develop a different method of administration of the CsA aerosol to dogs. More sophisticated studies of the administration of aerosolized CsA to beagle dogs were conducted in collaboration with Drs. Bruce Muggenberg and Mark Hoover of the Lovelace Inhalation Toxicology Research Institute.[21] These studies included the use of radiolabeled CsA aerosol by adding ^{99m}Tc as a sulfur colloid to the CsA, and making an assessment of whole-body and lung deposition with a gamma camera. The Lovelace nebulizer was used to administer the aerosol to the dogs via an oral mouthpiece. However, while 20 to 78% of the aerosolized dose was deposited in the body of the dog, only 5 to 24% was deposited in the lungs. Therefore, significant amounts of CsA given by this method were deposited in the mouth and swallowed, or were cleared from large airways by mucociliary action and swallowed. Bronchoalveolar lavage (BAL) was performed 24 hours after the aerosol dose and identified only one biochemical abnormality, an increase in lactate dehydrogenase in the BAL fluid when compared with that in animals given CsA by other routes.

Table 13.3. Rejection grade and incidence of pneumonia in rat lung transplant recipients treated with aerosolized or intramuscular CsA

	CsA Dose/Route	Mean Rejection Grade	Pneumonia
Group 1	None	4	–
Group 2	25 mg/kg IM x 1	2.2	3/10
Group 3	25 mg/kg IM x 4	1.8	5/10
Group 4	3.6 mg/kg aerosol x 7	1.2	0/6

Table 13.4. Correlation of aerosolized CsA dose in a rat left lung transplant model with blood/tissue drug concentrations and grade of histologic rejection

CsA Aerosol (mg/kg/day)	CsA Blood (ng/mL)	CsA Lung (ng/gm)		Grade of Rejection
		Left	Right	
0.98	198	1580	2853	3.25
1.94	390	3423	5253	2.3
3.6	1057	7838	10,516	1.3

In 1991, collaborative studies were initiated with Drs. Gerald Smaldone and Thomas O'Riordan which expanded the ^{99m}Tc studies initiated at Lovelace, and eventually allowed for depositional studies of CsA aerosol to be performed in lung transplant patients. An in vitro study using an AeroTech II jet nebulizer (CIS-US, Bedford, MA) demonstrated that a CsA aerosol could be generated whose aerodynamic dimensions were not altered by the addition of the radiolabel to the nebulizer solution.[22]

HUMAN STUDIES

The initial human trials were designed to include lung transplant patients with chronic rejection and end-stage obliterative bronchiolitis. Although aerosolized CsA was used as the primary immunosuppressant in the animal studies described above, it was added concomitantly to a background of either oral CsA or tacrolimus maintenance immunosuppression in the human subjects. The clinical trial was begun in December, 1991, and nine patients have been enrolled in the refractory chronic rejection study.[23] The success of the chronic refractory rejection program has led to expansion of the protocol to lung transplant patients with refractory acute rejection.

REFRACTORY CHRONIC REJECTION

From December, 1991 to September, 1994, we studied nine lung transplant patients with biopsy-proven active obliterative bronchiolitis and rapidly deteriorating pulmonary function.[23] Patients were eligible to enter the study if they had persistent histologic rejection despite having received at least five cycles of enhanced immunosuppression, and were predicted to have a limited life expectancy.

Aerosolized CsA treatments were given in the pulmonary function laboratory or at bedside using the AeroTech II jet nebulizer. Inhalation was performed through a mouthpiece during spontaneous respiration while patients were monitored with continuous pulse oximetry. Treatments were given in a special facility room to ensure

the absence of environmental contamination or in the patient's room using a commercially available high efficiency particulate air filter (AeroStar, BioSafety Systems, San Diego, CA).

Patients were premedicated by inhalation of 2% lidocaine (5 ml) via a conventional nebulizer, since the CsA preparation was found to cause pharyngeal irritation during inhalation. After receiving aerosolized lidocaine, patients were given one test dose of the vehicle used in solubilizing CsA (5 ml ethanol or 4.8 ml propylene glycol). Absolute 100% ethanol was used as the vehicle for the original subjects, but poor tolerance of the ethanol stimulated the change to 100% propylene glycol as the current vehicle for aerosolized CsA. Subjects received aerosolized CsA in the following sequence: 100 mg was given the first day, 200 mg the 2nd day, 300 mg on the 3rd and subsequent days for ten consecutive days and then 300 mg thrice weekly. CsA was ideally administered until consecutive transbronchial biopsies performed at 4-6 week intervals showed no evidence of obliterative bronchiolitis or acute rejection.

In seven of the nine patients (Table 13.5), transbronchial biopsies showed reduction in the active mononuclear cell infiltrate as manifested by transition from an active obliterative bronchiolitis to a less active or inactive form (e.g., C1a to C1b), or by downgrading of acute cellular rejection (e.g., A2 to A1). These histologic responses were seen within the first 86 days of therapy.

Stabilization of lung function correlated with histologic improvement in the seven patients after initiating aerosolized CsA. The average FVC and FEV_1 prior to aerosolized CsA were 2.64 ± 0.7 L and 1.49 ± 0.6 L respectively, and after a mean of 200 days of treatment, the FVC and FEV_1 stabilized (2.70 ± 0.7 L and 1.48 ± 0.6 L, respectively).

Adverse effects related to CsA inhalation consisted of cough (9/9), pharyngeal soreness (5/9) and acute breathlessness (4/9). Symptoms following inhalation gen-

Table 13.5. Histology prior to and within 86 days of aerosol CsA treatment and radiolabeled CsA deposition in lung transplant recipients[a]

Patient	Histology		Radiolabeled CsA deposition (mg)	
	Pre (Grade)	Rx CsA (Grade/Day)	Right Lung	Left Lung
#1	Active OB (C1a) Mild AR (A2a)	Inactive OB (C1b/43) No AR (43)	25.4 (allograft)	9.5 (allograft)
#2	Active OB (C1a)	Active OB (C1a/21) Mild AR (A2a/21)	15.8 (native)	6.9 (allograft)
#3	Active OB (C1a) Mild AR (A2c)	Minimal AR (A1c/14)[b]	12.3 (native)	20.5 (allograft)
#4	Active OB (C1a)	No OB (86) Moderate AR (A3a/86)	11.0 (allograft)	9.4 (allograft)
#5	Active OB (C1a) Moderate AR (A3a,c)	No OB (14) Minimal AR (A1b/14)	NA	–
#6	Active OB (C1a) Moderate AR (A3)	Inactive OB (C1b/47) Minimal AR (A1b/47)	NA	–
#7	Active OB (C1a)	Active OB (C1a/24)[c]	NA	–
#8	Active OB (C1a)	Lymphocytic bronchitis (B1/65)	NA	–
#9	Active OB (C1a)	Inactive OB (C1b/26)	NA	–

[a] *Definition of abbreviations:* Rx CsA = during aerosol CsA treatment; C = chronic rejection, with 1 = total, a = active, b = inactive; OB = obliterative bronchiolitis; AR = acute rejection, with A1 = minimal, A2 = mild, A3 = moderate, a = with small airways, b = without small airways, c = large airways; NA = not available.
[b] No small airways to assess OB
[c] The degree of active airways inflammation during aerosol CsA is diminished when compared with the pre-therapy biopsy.

Reprinted with permission from Iacono A et al, Am J Resp Crit Care Med (in press).

erally lasted for less than 30 minutes and improved following β-agonist therapy.

Three patients who received CsA in ethanol experienced airway irritation which improved with a change in vehicle to propylene glycol. In the three other patients who received CsA in ethanol, propylene glycol was not used and treatments were discontinued.

Significant changes in serum creatinine, urea nitrogen or liver function tests did not occur during aerosolized CsA administration. Bone marrow suppression, lymphoproliferative disease, neurological symptoms and cardiovascular adverse effects were also not observed. Periodic endoscopic examinations of the trachea, bronchi and upper airways were unremarkable.

These studies demonstrated that aerosolized CsA can be safely administered even in the patient with refractory chronic rejection and obliterative bronchiolitis. In this patient population, aerosolized CsA may help to stabilize pulmonary function for a period of time.

Pulmonary deposition studies of aerosolized CsA have been reported in five patients.[24] Regional deposition of the ^{99m}Tc tagged CsA was measured using a gamma camera, and the lung dose delivered ranged from 20 to 53 mg. Three patients were single-lung recipients and two patients received a double-lung transplant, and additional studies were conducted on regional volume and perfusion using intravenous ^{99m}Tc macroaggregates. A significant relationship was observed between regional drug deposition and regional perfusion to the allograft (r = 0.891, P < 0.0001).

REFRACTORY ACUTE REJECTION

The positive experience with aerosolized CsA in patients with chronic rejection encouraged us to expand the protocol to include patients with refractory acute rejection. Consequently, eight consecutive lung transplant recipients with refractory acute rejection were treated with aerosolized CsA.[25] Seven of the eight patients sustained improvement in the histologic grade of rejection (grade 2 to 0, four patients; grade 3 to 0, one patient; grade 3 to 1, one patient; and grade 2 to 1, one patient). BAL cell IL-6 expression decreased 4- to 6-fold in five patients. In addition, pulmonary function improved significantly from baseline during a 6-month interval.

The incidence of pulmonary bacterial, viral or fungal infection has not increased in this patient population on aerosolized CsA. The most common adverse effects were cough and pharyngeal soreness. None of these subjects required premature discontinuation of the drug. Overall, aerosolized CsA appears to be more effective than conventional therapy in suppressing rejection in patients with persistent acute rejection.

Pulmonary deposition studies were conducted in six of these patients.[25] The lung dose delivered ranged from 6.8 to 24.8 mg. In five patients, a significant relationship existed between the amount of CsA deposited in the allograft after aerosolized drug delivery and the improvement in FEV_1 as a percentage of the baseline established at the beginning of aerosol therapy (r = 0.981, P = 0.019).

PHARMACOKINETIC STUDIES

Initial pharmacokinetic studies were difficult to interpret since the patients were also receiving oral CsA, but this situation was remedied when tacrolimus was used as the primary immunosuppressant. The trough blood concentrations of CsA did not change significantly in patients receiving concomitant oral maintenance CsA therapy, but acute changes in concentration following inhalation were easily recognized in subjects on oral tacrolimus therapy. A rapid increase in CsA blood concentration was observed immediately after inhalation of the aerosol dose, and then a prolonged return to the preinhalation concentration is apparent (Fig. 13.1). This pattern of change in blood concentration indicates that a small portion of the drug is immediately solubilized in lung tissue and, with its lipid solubility characteristics, readily passes into the bloodstream. The remaining portion of the deposited drug may be present in an insoluble form which is slowly absorbed over time, producing a decline in blood concentration which is slower than that normally observed following an intravenous dose. In one patient in whom we have sufficient information from both the ^{99m}Tc and pharmacokinetic studies, a 20 mg drug deposition was predicted by both.

SUMMARY

The modulation of immune responses within the lungs is of value for transplant rejection and for other pathophysiologic processes such as asthma. Investigational work with oral CsA has already been initiated in both animal models of asthma and in limited clinical trials. The ability to administer CsA by inhalation will not only benefit lung transplant patients, but will also benefit other patients with inflammatory pulmonary disease.

Our studies have demonstrated that aerosolized CsA can modify the course of acute rejection in an animal model and the course of both refractory acute and chronic rejection in lung transplant patients. Considerable refinement of our techniques is necessary to properly adjust patient doses and to make this therapy easier for the patient to administer. Newer anti-cytokine agents may be more amenable to inhalational administration due to their increased potency or due to their solubility characteristics in the propellants used in metered dose inhalers. Animal work with agents

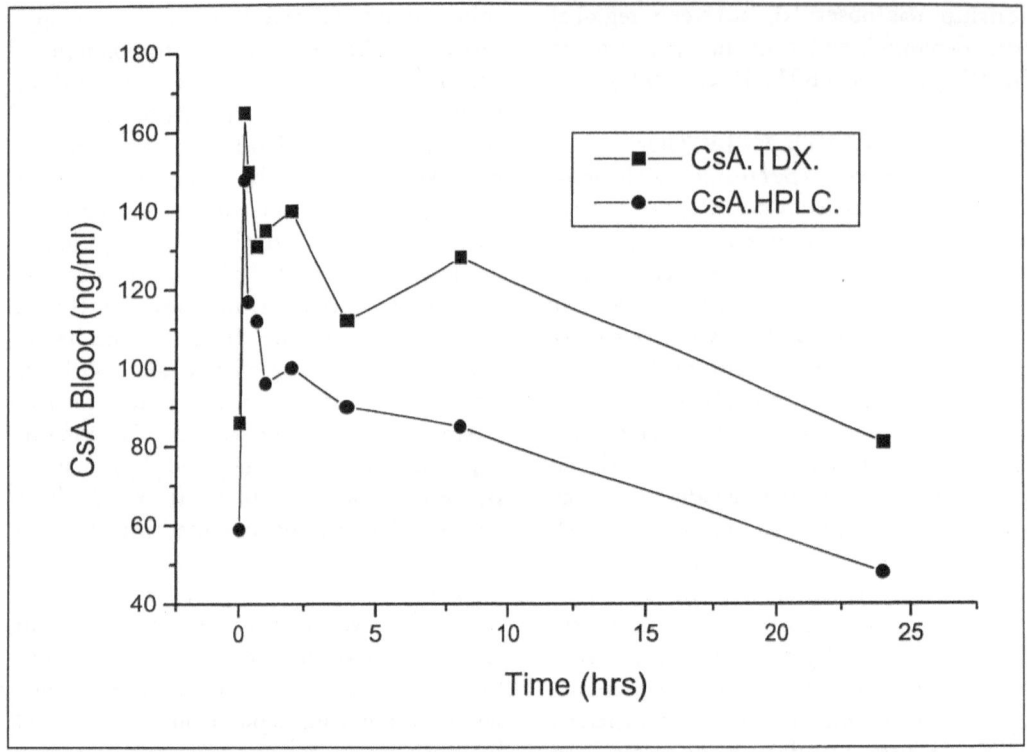

Fig. 13.1. CsA blood concentrations in a lung transplant patient receiving oral tacrolimus maintenance immunosuppression following an aerosolized dose. Concentrations were measured by both HPLC and a nonspecific immunoassay (TDX, Abbott Laboratories).

such as tacrolimus has demonstrated that this approach is possible.[26] Local immunosuppression in pulmonary transplant patients is a very realistic goal, and the aforementioned studies with aerosolized CsA have taken a major step toward achieving that goal.

REFERENCES

1. Griffith BP, Paradis IL, Zeevi A et al. Immunologically mediated disease of the airways after lung transplantation. Ann Surg 1988; 208:371.

2. Yousem SA, Berry GJ, Brunt EM et al. A working formulation for the standardization of nomenclature in the diagnosis of heart and lung rejection: Lung rejection study group. J Heart Lung Transplant 1990; 9:593.

3. Paradis I, Yousem S, Griffith BP. Airway obstruction and bronchiolitis obliterans after lung transplantation. Clin Chest Med 1993; 14:751.

4. Cooper JD, Billingham M, Egan T et al. A working formulation for nomenclature and for clinical staging of chronic dysfunction in lung allografts. J Heart Lung Transplant 1993; 12:713.

5. Zenati M, Duncan AJ, Burckart GJ et al. Immunosuppression with aerosolized cyclosporin for prevention of lung rejection in a rat model. Eur J Cardiothorac Surg 1991; 5:266.

6. Trulock EP. Management of lung transplant rejection. Chest 1993; 103:1566.

7. Bando K, Paradis IL, Konishi H et al. Obliterative bronchiolitis after lung and heart-lung transplantation: an analysis of risk factors and management. J Thoracic Cardiovas Surg 1995;110:4.

8. Glanville GR, Baldwin JC, Burke CM et al. Obliterative bronchiolitis after heart-lung transplantation: apparent arrest by augmented immunosuppression. Ann Int Med 1987; 107:300.

9. Theodure J, Starnes VA, Lewiston NJ. Obliterative bronchiolitis. Clin Chest Med 1990; 11:309.

10. Kahan BD. Cyclosporine. N Engl J Med 1989; 321:1725.

11. Ascher NL, Chen S, Hoffman RA et al. Maturation of cytotoxic T cells within sponge matrix allografts. J Immunol 1983; 131:617.

12. Wolf JS, McGavic JD, Hume DM. Inhibition of the effector mechanism of transplant immunity by local graft irradiation. Surg Gynecol Obstet 1969; 128:584.

13. Gergely NF, Coles JC. Prolongation of heterotopic cardiac allografts in dogs by topical irradiation. Transplantation 1970; 9:193.

14. Fidler JP, Alexander JW, Smith EJ et al. Radiation reversal of acute rejection in patients with life threatening infection. Arch Surg 1973; 107:256.

15. Ruers TJM, Buurman WA, van der Linden CJ et al. Local inhibition of major histocompatibility complex class II induction within the graft: an effective way to induce immunosuppression. Transplant Proc 1987; 19:246.

16. Ruers T, Daemen M, Thijssen H et al. Sensitivity of graft rejection in rats to local immunosuppressive therapy. Transplantation 1988; 46:820.

17. Stepkowski SM, Goto S, Ito T et al. Prolongation of heterotopic heart allograft survival by local delivery of continuous low-dose cyclosporine therapy. Transplantation 1989; 47:17.

18. Burckart GJ, Dowling R, Zenati M et al. Cyclosporine administration by aerosol. J Clin Pharmacol 1989; 29:860.

19. Dowling RD, Zenati M, Burckart GJ et al. Aerosolized cyclosporine as single agent immunotherapy in canine lung allografts. Surgery 1990; 108:198.

20. Keenan RJ, Duncan AJ, Yousem SA et al. Improved immunosuppression with aerosolized cyclosporine in experimental pulmonary transplantation. Transplantation 1992; 53:20.

21. Muggenburg BA, Hoover MD, Griffith BP et al. Administration of cyclosporine by aerosol: A feasibility study in beagle dogs. J Aerosol Med 1990; 3:1.

22. O'Riordan TG, Duncan SR, Burckart GJ et al. Production of an aerosol of cyclosporine as a prelude to clinical studies. J Aerosol Med 1992; 5:171.

23. Iacono A, Keenan RJ, Duncan SR et al. Aerosolized cyclosporine in lung recipients with refractory chronic rejection. Am J Resp Crit Care Med (in press).

24. O'Riordan TG, Iacono A, Keenan RJ et al. Delivery and distribution of aerosolized cyclosporine in lung allograft recipients. Am J Resp Crit Care Med 1995; 151:516.

25. Iacono A, Keenan R, Zeevi A et al. Improvement of acute allograft rejection refractory to conventional immunosuppressive therapy with aerosolized cyclosporine in lung transplant recipients. Am J Resp Crit Care Med 1995; 151:A85.

26. Akutsu I, Fukuda T, Majima K et al. Inhibitory effect of inhaled FK-506 on increased bronchial responsiveness and eosinophil infiltration in the airway mucosa. Arerugi 1992; 41:543.

CHAPTER 14

SITE-SPECIFIC IMMUNOSUPPRESSION WITH TOPICAL AGENTS

Kirby S. Black and Charles W. Hewitt

SIGNIFICANCE OF TOPICAL IMMUNOSUPPRESSANTS

Novel immunosuppressive compounds derived from fungi have unique properties compared to conventional immunosuppressants: they are selective in their mechanism of action, and are potent anti-inflammatory compounds. Cyclosporin (CsA), FK506 and rapamycin (Fig. 14.1) derivatives are well recognized for their powerful ability to permanently alter immune responsiveness, in comparison to conventional agents, so that some degree of selective immunologic nonreactivity can be achieved. Therefore, it would be extremely advantageous to develop topical formulations of novel immunosuppressants for localized site-specific action.[1]

One of the newest and most exciting areas in the pharmaceutical industry is development of novel techniques for drug delivery. New methods of drug delivery are being investigated to produce compounds that will target active agents to specific tissue sites for superior results and reduced side effects. One of the primary choices for application of this technology is in local delivery of drugs to diseased skin, or through the skin (transcutaneous delivery) to underlying target tissues. Several of the chemical principles necessary for directing immunosuppressive molecules to specific tissue sites are currently being established in the authors' laboratories using in vivo skin graft and contact hypersensitivity models. Several formulations of these topical immunosuppressive and anti-inflammatory compounds have been successfully developed and tested in animal studies.[2-6] A lead product now needs to be devised and tested clinically. A great deal of research concerning other site-specific, and tissue-directed anti-inflammatory compounds is ongoing including topical

Local Immunosuppression of Organ Transplants, edited by Scott A. Gruber.
© 1996 R.G. Landes Company.

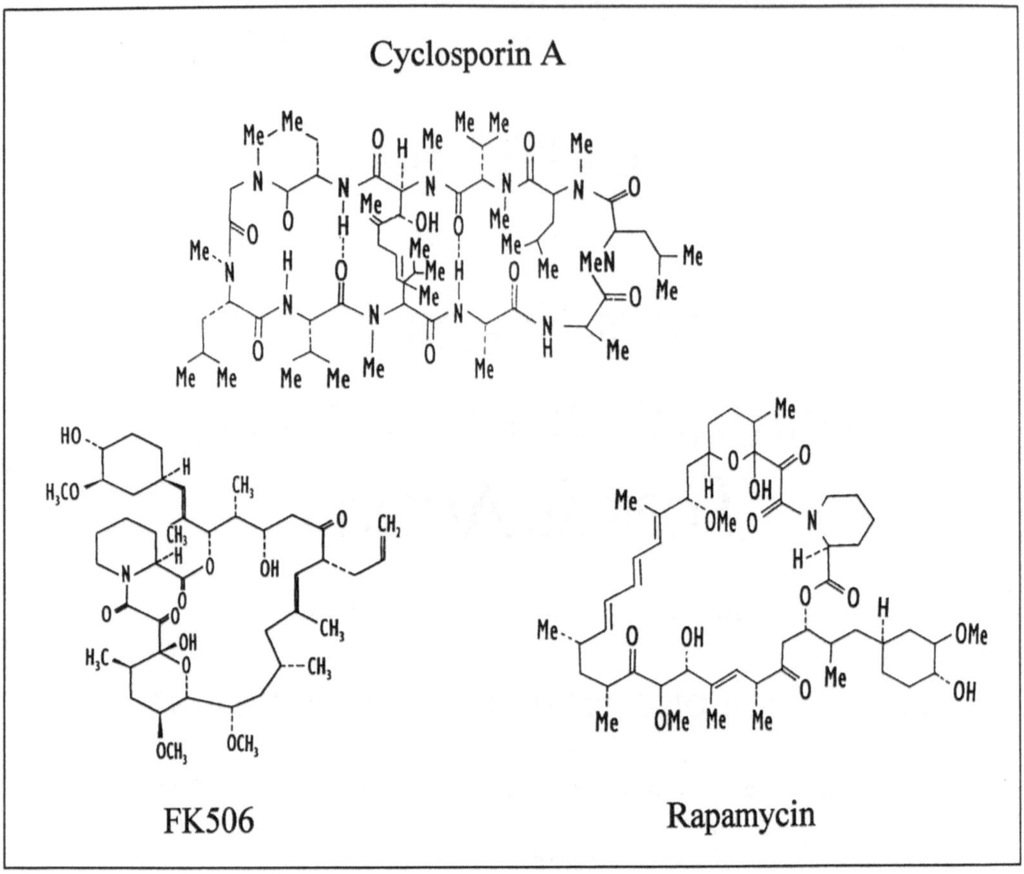

Fig. 14.1. Structure of CsA, FK506, and rapamycin. Adapted from reference 55.

rapamycin and combinational immunosuppressive and anti-inflammatory agents.[6] Lead topical drugs now need to be tested in long-term animal studies and, clinically, in patients suffering from inflammatory skin diseases. These diseases include psoriasis, contact hypersensitivity, alopecia areata and others, but the primary focus by most investigators is on psoriasis at this time. Certain formulations that provide very effective transdermal drug delivery in animal studies also need to be examined clinically, and for potential transmuscular delivery into joint spaces for treatment of arthritis (i.e., rheumatoid arthritis). In additional applications, CsA and other immunosuppressants can also be formulated for local delivery to donor tissues to protect organ transplants from rejection. It may also be possible to treat massive burn victims with cadaver skin grafts and topical immunosuppressants to inhibit their rejection.[7]

BACKGROUND

Systemic CsA has provided a means of attenuating T cell mediated events including rejection of allografted tissues and autoimmune disorders of the skin in both animal and human studies.[8-15] One method to achieve immunosuppression with CsA and other immunosuppressants and reduce their potential toxic systemic side effects involves targeting the drug to a specific tissue site and local responding immunocytes. This would have obvious and important clinical relevance: localized CsA delivery would be possible in such varied indications as suppressing autoimmune inflammatory skin diseases;[8-13,16,17] or even inhibiting skin allograft rejection for immediate wound coverage following massive thermal injury.

Induction of localized site-specific immunosuppression (SITE) is not a new concept. In 1951, Billingham et al[18] successfully prolonged the survival of skin allografts with topical steroids. Their evidence for the local inhibition of the rejection response was acquired from a rabbit skin allograft model using several allografts and autografts on the same animal. Half of the allografts were treated with the active compound and half were treated with vehicle control. In this model, concomitant systemic alloactivation occurred via the untreated contralateral grafts. The presence of the untreated grafts in the system effectively eliminated the prolongation of survival of the skin allografts normally observed upon topical application. Steroids, however, have a detrimental effect on other cellular processes including wound healing and nonspecific immunity against bacterial infection.[19] It was postulated that autoimmune disorders of the skin could benefit from transdermal (localized) treatment with CsA.[16]

Previous studies have shown that topically-applied CsA in dimethyl sulfoxide (DMSO) was effective in prolonging skin allograft survival.[20-22] It was demonstrated that a topical CsA formulation which does not contain DMSO is also effective in inhibiting skin graft rejection.[2] In addition, CsA has been used topically to eliminate contact hypersensitivity in guinea-pigs.[23] Topical CsA has also been shown to be effective in treating alopecia areata and contact hypersensitivity in humans, yet was not found effective in psoriasis.[24-29] Additionally, neither topical rapamycin nor CsA was found to be effective in inhibiting contact hypersensitivity to dinitrofluorobenzene in pigs.[30] Yet, in the same test system, topical FK506 was shown to be efficacious.[30] Thomson et al[29] commented that further laboratory experiments to determine the efficacy of topical CsA formulations were needed. Corneal grafts were treated with topical CsA in rabbits and rats

and demonstrated decreased histopathological evidence of rejection.[31-33] However, the results seemed to be dependent on the vehicle used to carry CsA. Foets et al[31] felt that increased survival of corneal allografts by topical CsA was primarily due to a local immunosuppressive effect.

Duncan and colleagues[34] demonstrated that enhanced percutaneous absorption of topical CsA could be obtained with the penetration enhancers, azone and propylene glycol. With this formulation, there was a reduction in infiltrating lymphocytes in areas undergoing delayed-type hypersensitivity reactions with dinitrofluorobenzene using the guinea pig model. However, these investigators could not demonstrate a site-specific effect with this formulation in psoriatic patients, grossly.[35] Yet, there was a reduction in CD3$^+$ and CD25$^+$ cells in the epidermis along with decreased CD25$^+$ and MHC class II expressing cells in the dermis, microscopically. In agreement with these findings, Surber et al[36] could not demonstrate a beneficial effect with topical CsA in allergic contact dermatitis in man. However, CsA has shown excellent therapeutic effects in psoriasis, pyoderma gangrenosum, lichen planus and other autoimmune diseases of the skin when used systemically.[17] Topically-applied CsA was shown to have excellent site-specific efficacy when used on oral tissues of patients with lichen planus[37] and graft versus host disease (GVHD).[38] Additionally, SITE of psoriasis using intralesional injections has been shown to be very effective.[39]

Studies have been undertaken using a dual rat skin allograft model with various oil-based and amphipathic topical CsA formulations.[2-6] The dual skin allograft model contains internal controls to monitor the immune responses both locally and systemically. These experiments showed that a critical requirement for inducing efficacious local immune suppression with topical CsA involved modulating both systemic and local immune mechanisms.[2-6] Therefore, topical CsA when used in conjunction with a short-term limited systemic CsA schedule (8 mg/kg/day x 10 days) effectively abrogated skin allograft rejection, without toxicity to the tissues. In fact, skin allograft survival was significantly prolonged with this regimen when compared with matched vehicle control treatment. As long as topical CsA was applied, the skin grafts survived, grew hair and appeared relatively normal. Other investigators have also shown a site-specific effect with topical CsA used on rat skin allografts.[20-22,40] These findings should be directly transferable clinically to localized inflammatory skin reactions including contact hypersensitivity, alopecia areata, psoriasis, cutaneous GVHD, skin graft rejection and other autoimmune diseases of the skin. In general, topical CsA should inhibit all types of T cell mediated immune inflammatory reactions at a localized level.

The basic technology of SITE involves the physicochemical properties of the active agent as it relates to drug delivery and targeting to specific tissue sites and immune principles discovered that are necessary for inhibiting activated immune responses during a disease state. Anti-inflammatory efficacy has been proven grossly, histopathologically and immunologically on a local level.[2-6] Systemic T cell mediated immunity was unaffected by local treatment. Drug levels were low systemically, and showed relative site-specificity in terms of tissue concentration.

Conclusions concerning these investigations to date include:

1. Inhibition of an activated immune response in a site-specific manner is possible. A critical mechanism involves attenuating the systemic phase of immune responsiveness in conjunction with local intervention. Additionally, CsA formulations that penetrate the skin barrier and localize in dermal tissue, or other formulations that cross the transdermal barrier to provide systemic therapeutic levels have been successfully developed and tested in animal models.

2. The skin allograft model is excellent for studying cutaneous inflammatory/immune disease and SITE. The dual skin allograft model is comparable grossly and histopathologically to bilateral paired comparisons utilized in clinical topical drug trials for autoimmune conditions.

3. Further study of the mechanism(s) of action of SITE is needed.

4. Dose and timing requirements should be studied and varied for both systemic and topical phases of treatment.

MECHANISMS OF SITE

Many scientific efforts are currently focused on developing novel selective immunosuppressive agents for the treatment of inflammatory/immune diseases. These compounds include cyclosporines, rapamycin, rapamycin analogs, FK506 and FK506 analogs (Fig. 14.1). CsA is well established, while FK506 has recently been developed, and rapamycin is in the research and development pipeline. The mechanism of action of each of these novel immunosuppressants is not completely known. However, such compounds derived from fungi, including the cyclosporines and macrolides (FK506 and rapamycin), possess similar properties. They are lipophilic antifungal antibiotics that inhibit the transcription of T cell activation genes (CsA and FK506), or transduction of T cell activation gene products involved in T cell activation (rapamycin).[41] A prominent mechanism of action for novel immunosuppressants is inhibition at the level of the CD4⁺ MHC class II responsive helper T cell (Th). In particular, these agents can inhibit the release of cytokine cellular growth factors such as interleukin-2 (IL-2), IL-3, IL-4, granulocyte/macrophage colony-stimulating factor, interferon-gamma (IFN-γ) and tumor necrosis factor-alpha in the case of CsA and FK506, or cellular responsiveness to such cytokines in the case of rapamycin. Systemic administration is well known to block the inflammatory immune cascade and facilitate permanent allograft acceptance (actively acquired immunological tolerance) in various experimental animal models by inhibitory effects upon Th cells with sparing of immunoregulatory cell expression. Intracellular targets of these immunosuppressive compounds are a class of receptor proteins known as immunophilins, which are important in signaling pathways for T cell activation.[41] The immunophilin-immunosuppressant complex then inhibits calcineurin, a calcium/calmodulin dependent phosphatase required for dephosphorylation and activation of the IL-2 transcription factor, nuclear factor of activated T cells (NF-AT).[41]

The mechanisms of SITE are currently under investigation. Experiments confirm that certain novel immunosuppressants can indeed have potent modulatory effects on preactivated and activated immune cells when successfully delivered locally at relatively high concentrations. Other novel compounds show surprising efficacy even

on activated immune cells at relatively moderate-to-low local concentrations. Certain cells of the immune system (Th cells) were found to be inhibited at a local level. Moreover, once treated, immunocytes were preferentially responsive to further site-specific treatment. It was found that site-specific immune modulation down-regulates the local expression of MHC class I and class II cell surface molecules.[5] Digital image analysis of immunostained grafts showed that MHC class I expression was dramatically increased for the rejecting vehicle grafts versus CsA treated grafts (Fig. 14.2; P < 0.0001). MHC class I expression was increased due to greater numbers of positive cells and increased cell size in the

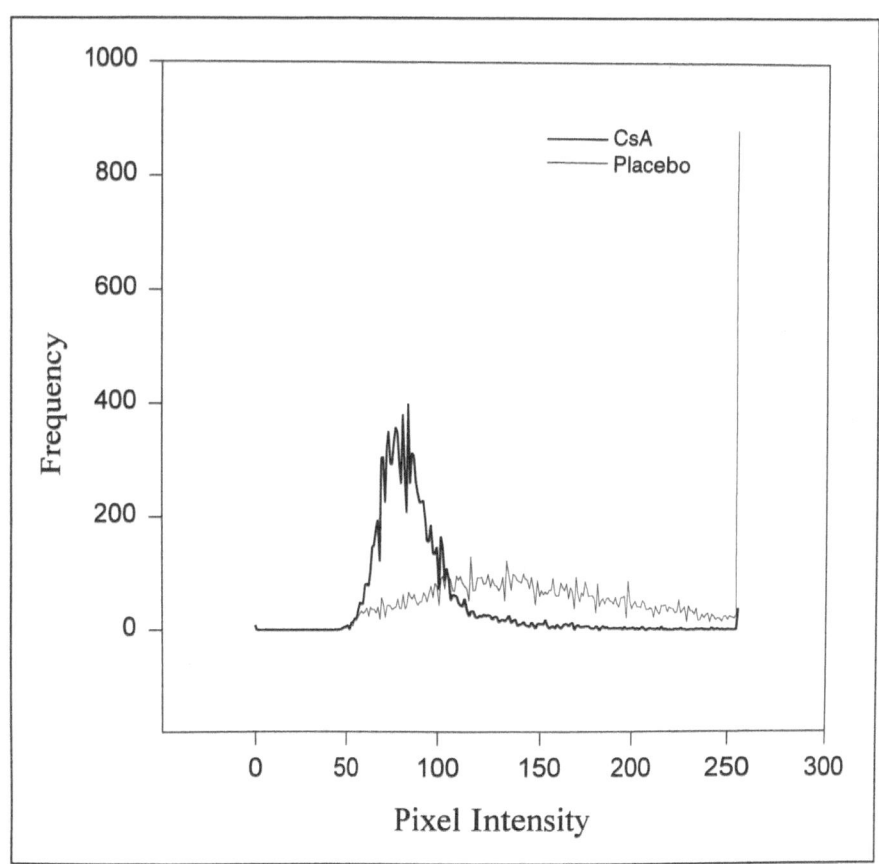

Fig. 14.2. MHC class I (OX-18) expression during SITE was dramatically increased for the rejecting placebo-treated versus topically CsA-treated grafts. Fluorescent images of immunostained skin graft sections were digitally processed and analyzed. Increasing pixel intensity (Black = 0, White = 255) correlates with a "whiter", and therefore more intensely stained, cell population and greater class I expression.

dermis. Similar results were obtained for MHC class II expression (Fig. 14.3). Expression of MHC class II determinants was increased in the vehicle-treated grafts due primarily to a dramatic increase in cell surface area.[5] In addition, it was demonstrated that site-specific therapy could even modulate systemic disease mechanisms possibly via local induction of antigen-specific T-suppressor cells and/or clonal inactivation.

It has been demonstrated that CsA will locally inhibit the immune response in a dual graft system with concurrently activated cells provided by the untreated contralateral graft.[2-6] The mechanism of action must involve one or more steps of the lymphocyte activation cascade (i.e., initial recognition of antigen, lymphocyte differentiation and activation, migration to the site of inflammation and/or target recognition and killing), specifically local immunocyte inhibition and/or alteration of the target tissue in response to inflammatory challenge. Although CsA does not appear to inhibit the initial recognition of antigen, there is evidence for inhibition of target tissue antigen expression (target tissue adaptation).[42,43] Inhibition of the maturation of Th1, Th2 and cytotoxic T cells (CTLs) via transcribed cytokines (IL-2, IFN-γ and IL-4) appears to be the primary target of CsA.[41] However, in the present proposed studies, treatment is localized and the po-

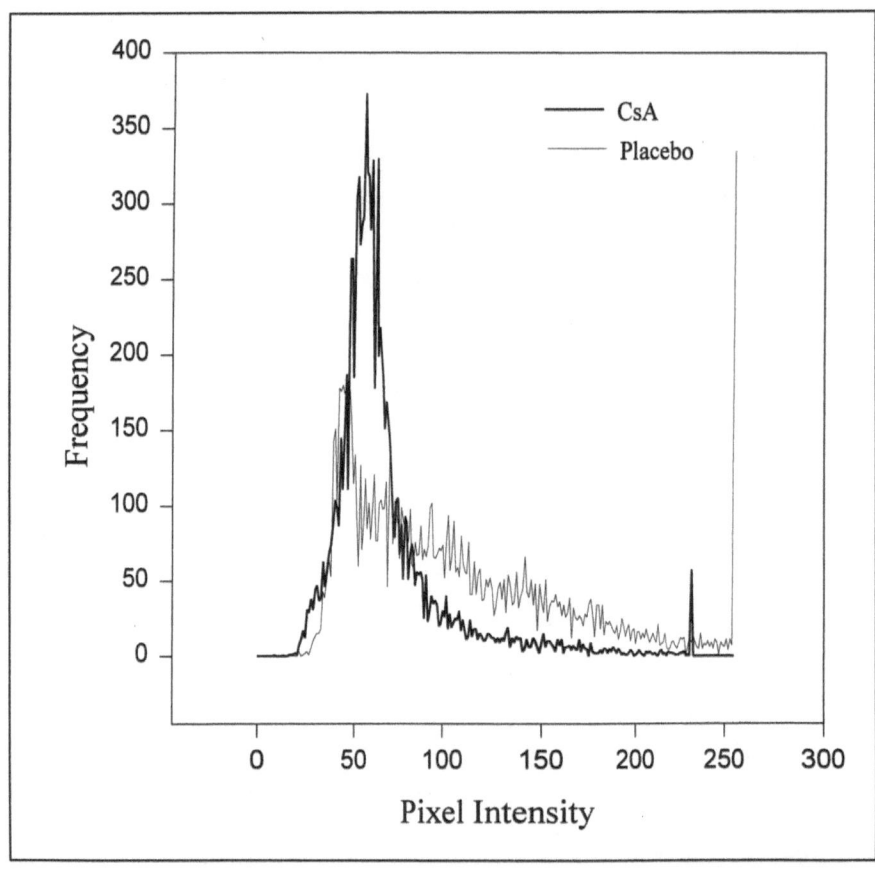

Fig. 14.3. MHC class II (OX-3) expression during SITE was also dramatically increased for the rejecting placebo-treated grafts versus topically CsA-treated grafts. Fluorescent images of immunostained skin graft sections were digitally processed and analyzed. Increasing pixel intensity (Black = 0, White = 255) correlates with a "whiter", and therefore more intensely stained, cell population and greater class II expression.

tential for maturation of Th1, Th2 and CTLs distal to the site of treatment exists. If there were distal maturation of these cell lines, then they could migrate to the site of CsA treatment. Although CsA is not thought to directly impair lymphocyte trafficking, the local tissue concentration of CsA after topical treatment can be much greater than therapeutic levels developed through systemic administration.

Wilkinson and Higgins[44] have shown that CsA can inhibit mitogen activated, but not phorbol ester activated, locomotion of human lymphocytes in vitro. It has been speculated that local inflammatory responses may be in part due to the local proliferation of antigen-reactive cells,[45] as well as to lymphocyte influx into the area of inflammation. Norin et al[46] determined that CsA cessation resulted in an increase in con A-dependent cell mediated cytotoxicity of lymphocytes isolated from lung allografts. This may have resulted from an inhibition of the cells' ability to migrate to the allograft, or a lack of chemotactic factors produced by cells in the allograft. However, the results of Hanto et al[47] indicate that intragraft amplification of both CD4[+] and CD8[+] cells may be an important initial phase of allograft rejection. Therefore, supplying the immunosuppressive agent to the site of activation may provide certain advantages over systemic administration.

Mayer et al[48] found that the tempo of rejection of skin allografts did not directly correlate with the number of infiltrating T cells. Studies by Orosz et al[49,50] using an infiltrating sponge matrix allograft model demonstrated that, at the peak of infiltration, only 0.2% of the cells were antigen-specific CTLs. Thus, the other 99.8% of the infiltrate is apparently comprised of nonspecific inflammatory cells responding to production of cytokines by small numbers of immune cells possessing epitope-specific T cell receptors. Therefore, the local inhibition of these relatively few antigen-specific cells may prevent the expansion and infiltration of the overwhelming majority of nonspecific immune cells.

However, one question remains: if immunocytes have initially recognized antigen, become activated, differentiate and migrate to the site of target antigen while under topical CsA treatment, can they then recognize and effectively kill the target antigen? Havele et al[51] demonstrated that antigen-dependent CTLs can be blocked by physiological levels of CsA parent compound as a result of an IL-2-independent mechanism. Therefore, the possibility exists that CsA and/or other novel immunosuppressants could block preactivated epitope-specific immunocytes that migrate to the site of treatment, if the immunosuppressant tissue levels were maintained at high concentrations. Another important consideration is that in vitro experiments generally utilize CsA parent compound. This may not be relevant to in vivo studies in which CsA is metabolized in the tissues following systemic treatment. Topical or local treatment could potentially provide greater levels of parent compound concentrated locally.

COMMERCIAL APPLICATION

Psoriasis affects 2%-4% of the population, representing greater than 5 to 10 million prospective patients in the U.S. However, only 2 to 3 million patients per year are actually treated for psoriasis, with approximately 70% of psoriatic patients requiring topical therapy alone. One-third of all patients visiting dermatology clinics suffer from eczematous dermatitis, which includes the subclassifications contact dermatitis, atopic dermatitis and drug-related dermatitis. Topical corticosteroid preparations represent the most frequently prescribed therapy for psoriasis, although their effectiveness and side effects have raised concern. In contrast, topical cyclosporines and other novel immunosuppressants represent a potential new class of potent anti-inflammatory drugs. They possess superior properties compared with conventional anti-inflammatories due to their tissue-specific and selective actions upon the immune response with reduced side effects.

The lead candidate products developed from the technology outlined in this chapter include topical immunosuppressant/anti-inflammatory drugs. They are projected for use in autoimmune and inflammatory diseases of the skin, such as psoriasis, contact dermatitis, skin allografts for burn treatment and others. Additional indications being explored for site-specific immunosuppressive therapeutic systems include rheumatoid arthritis, joint and soft tissue injury and inflammatory reactions of the lung and ear. The technology involves targeting immunosuppressive agents to specific tissue sites. Certain biologic and chemical principles have been defined, with respect to the vehicle, as important and necessary to achieve the desired effects. Various topical drug formulations have been studied for both transdermal penetration (penetration through the skin) in order to achieve effects on the whole system (systemic effects), and their ability to act locally at specific sites within target tissues. The technology has been tested successfully in the laboratory, but, more extensive tests are required clinically, particularly in the dermatology realm.

In addition to cyclosporines, rapamycins and FK analogs, off-patent chemical entities and unique combinational products are currently being explored for new topical and site-specific drug development. Multiple classes of active agents can be successfully combined to produce extremely potent topical immunosuppressive drugs. New compounds that combine more than one active principle can be designed to attenuate multiple immune mechanisms. This affords the opportunity for developing new drugs for topical application by utilizing and combining off-patent active principles.

Since CsA is primarily known to work by affecting early phase T cell activation gene products, localized corticosteroids (CS) would theoretically synergize with topical CsA because they act as potent nonselective immunosuppressive agents that may inhibit late-phase antigen-independent inflammatory reactions.[52-54] Thus, it was hypothesized that site-specific immune modulation of early immune/inflammatory events would be achieved with topical CsA during the induction phase, followed by topical CS during the maintenance phase.[6] The dual skin allograft model was utilized to evaluate this hypothesis. Three groups of animals were tested: (1) topical CsA (2.5%) was used continuously throughout rejection; (2) concomitant CsA/CS was used until full rejection and (3) topical CsA was utilized during the induction phase and, subsequently, CsA/CS was used during the maintenance phase. Topical CsA provided significant graft prolongation and disparity ($P < 0.04$). SITE with topical CsA/CS was equivalent and did not provide an additive or synergistic effect. However, topical CsA administered during the antigen-dependent induction phase with subsequent suppression of antigen-independent inflammation by topical CsA/CS provided significant ($P < 0.001$) and dramatic synergism with optimal efficacy (Figs. 14.4 and 14.5) Therefore, we concluded that a beneficial local immunoregulatory mechanism was induced by topical CsA during the early induction phase that was steroid-sensitive.

SUMMARY

It is proposed that local CsA delivery to skin via topical application is efficacious for inhibiting site-specific T cell-mediated inflammatory immune processes. Important clinical relevance is obvious: localized CsA delivery would be possible in such varied indications as suppressing autoimmune inflammatory skin diseases; or even inhibiting skin allograft rejection for immediate wound coverage following massive thermal injury. The objective of these continuing studies is to define the most efficacious dose and formulation of topical CsA and other novel immunosuppressants for clinical trials. The elucidation of the mechanisms underlying local immunosuppression achieved with topical CsA will provide a basis to proceed with other locally-applied immunosuppressive compounds.

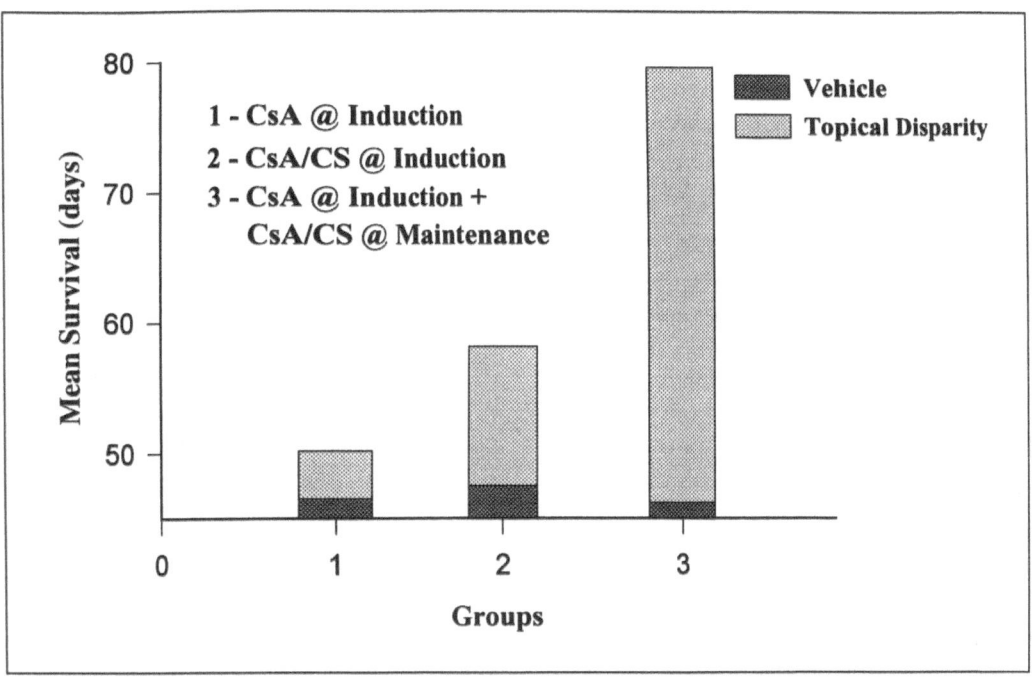

Fig. 14.4. Mean disparity in dual skin allograft survival (difference in survival time between matched experimental and vehicle-treated grafts) with topical CsA/CS immunosuppression (group 1, n = 4; group 2, n = 5; group 3, n = 6). Adapted from reference 6.

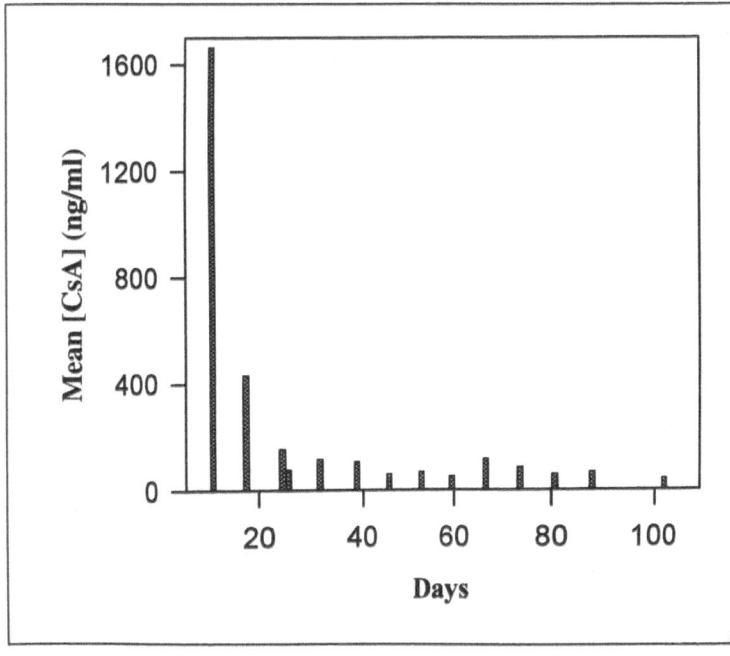

Fig. 14.5. Systemic serum CsA profile over time in the experimental animals in Figure 14.4. Mean values from all three groups combined are shown (n = 15). CsA levels were determined by radioimmunoassay (Sandoz Pharmaceuticals Corp., East Hanover, NJ). Subtherapeutic concentrations were achieved by day 25. Adapted from reference 6.

Specifically, the following has been accomplished:

1. A definitive dual skin allograft model has been developed for purposes which include but are not limited to defining the concept, analyzing modulators and elucidating mechanisms of SITE. The skin allograft model has served as an excellent representation of many varied inflammatory immune processes such as rejection and autoimmune skin diseases. In studying the model, the strength of the inflammatory component can be dictated by the tissue transplant barrier and via the genetically defined donor-recipient combination.

2. CsA, when applied to a local area of tissue in the model, will inhibit a T cell mediated inflammatory immune reaction (rejection) in a site-specific fashion.

3. Depending upon the formulation developed and its transdermal carrier properties, pharmacokinetic studies have demonstrated minimal systemic CsA concentrations, relative site-specificity and absence of systemic toxicity in animals undergoing topical drug application with excipients designed for localized delivery. Other formulations developed have been shown capable of delivering transdermal drug levels at systemic therapeutic doses using in vivo animal models. Long-term animal efficacy and toxicity studies on lead topical drugs now need be instituted with both transdermal and localized carriers.

4. Contributing mechanisms to site-specific nonresponsiveness have been shown to involve important local and systemic immune events. Further investigations are needed to better characterize and understand these local and systemic immunosuppressive mechanisms.

ACKNOWLEDGMENTS

Supported in part by grants from Robert Wood Johnson Medical School, Camden; International Association of Fire Fighters Burn Foundation; Orthopaedic Research and Education Foundation; and Plastic Surgery Education Foundation.

REFERENCES

1. Gruber SA. The case for local immunosuppression. Transplantation 1992; 54(1):1.
2. Black KS, Hewitt CW, Chau CLC et al. Transdermal application of cyclosporine prolongs skin allograft survival. Transplant Proc 1988; 20(2 Suppl 2):660.
3. Black KS, Nguyen DK, Proctor CM et al. Site-specific suppression of cell-mediated immunity by cyclosporine. J Invest Dermatol 1990; 94(5):644.
4. Black KS, Patel MP, Patel AP et al. Mechanisms of site-specific immunosuppression. Transplant Proc 1991; 23(1):120.
5. Tatem L, Hou A, Black KS et al. Digital image analysis of major histocompatibility complex class I and class II expression during site-specific immune suppression with topical cyclosporine. Transplant Proc 1995; 27(1):344.
6. Llull R, Lee TP, Vu AN et al. Site-specific immune suppression with topical cyclosporine. Synergism with combined topical corticosteroid added during the maintenance phase. Transplantation 1995; 59:1483.
7. Achauer BM, Hewitt CW, Black KS et al. Long-term skin allograft survival after short-term cyclosporine treatment in a patient with massive burns. Lancet 1986; 1:14.
8. Mueller W, Herrmann B. Cyclosporin A for psoriasis. N Engl J Med 1979; 301:555.
9. Thomson AW, Moon DK, Inoue Y et al. Modification of delayed-type hypersensitivity reactions to ovalbumin in cyclosporine A-treated guinea-pigs. Immunology 1983; 48:301.
10. Harper JI, Keat ACS, Staughton RCD. Cyclosporin for psoriasis. Lancet 1984; 2:981.
11. Thivolet J, Barthelemy H, Rigot-Muller G et al. Effects of cyclosporin on bullous pemphigoid and pemphigus. Lancet 1985; 1:334.
12. van Hooff JP, Leunissem KM, v.d. Staak W. Cyclosporin and psoriasis. Lancet 1985; 1:335.
13. Velthuis PJ, Jesserun RF. Improvement of ichthyosis by cyclosporin. Lancet 1985; 1:335.
14. Borel JF. Cyclosporine: historical perspectives. Transplant Proc 1983; 15(4):2219.

15. Hess AD, Esa AH, Colombani PM. Mechanisms of action of cyclosporine: effect on cells of the immune system and on subcellular events in T cell activation. Transplant Proc 1988; 20(2):29.

16. Valdimarsson H, Baker BS, Jonsdottir I et al. Psoriasis: a disease of abnormal keratinocyte proliferation induced by T lymphocytes. Immunol Today 1986; 7(9):256.

17. Aldridge RD, Simpson JG, Whiting PH et al. Cyclosporin and skin disease. Lancet 1985; 1:160.

18. Billingham RE, Krohn PL, Medawar PB. Effect of locally applied cortisone acetate on survival of skin homografts in rabbits. Br Med J 1951;2:1049.

19. Boss P, Jolley W, Ainsworth E. Mechanisms of action of topically applied triamcinolone acetonide in prolonging skin allograft survival time. Transplantation 1973; 15:17.

20. Lai CS, Wesseler TA, Alexander W et al. Long-term survival of skin allografts in rats treated with topical cyclosporine. Transplantation 1987; 44(1):83.

21. Zhao XF, Schroeder TJ, Alexander JW et al. The prolongation of skin allograft survival by topical use of cyclosporine A. Transplant Proc 1988; 20(2 Suppl 2):670.

22. Zhao XF, Alexander JW, Schroeder T et al. The synergistic effect of low-dose cyclosporine and fluocinolone acetonide on the survival of rat allogeneic skin grafts. Transplantation 1988; 46:490.

23. Aldridge RD, Thomson AW, Rankin R et al. Inhibition of contact sensitivity reactions to DNFB by topical cyclosporin application in the guinea-pig. Clin Exp Immunol 1985; 59(1):23.

24. De Prost Y, Teillac D, Paquez F et al. Placebo-controlled trial of topical cyclosporin in severe alopecia areata. Lancet 1986; 2:803.

25. Parodi A, Rebora A. Topical cyclosporine in alopecia areata. Arch Dermatol 1987; 123(2):165.

26. Thompson AW, Aldridge RD, Sewell HF. Topical cyclosporin in alopecia areata and nickel contact dermatitis. Lancet 1986; 2:971.

27. Aldridge RD, Sewell HF, King G et al. Topical cyclosporin A in nickel contact hypersensitivity: results of a preliminary clinical and immunohistochemical investigation. Clin Exp Immunol 1986; 66(3):582.

28. Griffiths CE, Powles AV, Baker BS et al. Topical cyclosporine and psoriasis. Lancet 1987; 1:806.

29. Thomson AW, Sewell HF, Aldridge RD. Topical cyclosporin and immunologically-mediated skin disorders. Lancet 1987; 1:1212.

30. Meingassner JG, Stutz A. Immunosuppressive macrolides of the type FK 506: a novel class of topical agents for treatment of skin diseases? J Invest Dermatol 1992; 98(6):851.

31. Foets B, Missotten L, Vanderveeren P et al. Prolonged survival of allogeneic corneal grafts in rabbits treated with topically applied cyclosporin A: systemic absorption and local immunosuppressive effect. Br J Ophthalmol 1985; 69(8):600.

32. Behrens-Baumann W, Theuring S, Brewitt H. The effect of topical cyclosporin A on the rabbit cornea. A clinical and electron microscopic study. Graefes Arch Clin Exp Ophthalmol 1986; 224(6):520.

33. Williams KA, Erickson SA, Coster DJ. Topical steroid, cyclosporin A, and the outcome of rat corneal allografts. Br J Ophthalmol 1987; 71(3):239.

34. Duncan JI, Payne SN, Winfield AJ et al. Enhanced percutaneous absorption of a novel topical cyclosporin A formulation and assessment of its immunosuppressive activity. Br J of Dermatol 1990; 123(5):631.

35. Duncan JI, Wakeel RA, Winfield AJ et al. Immunomodulation of psoriasis with a topical cyclosporine A formulation. Acta Dermato-Venereologica 1993; 73(2):84.

36. Surber C, Itin P, Muchner S et al. Effects of new topical cyclosporin formulation on human allergic contact dermatitis. Contact Dermatitis 1992; 26(2):116.

37. Eisen D, Ellis CN, Duell EA et al. Effect of topical cyclosporine rinse on oral lichen planus. A double-blind analysis. N Engl J Med 1990; 323(5):290.

38. Epstein JB, Reece DE. Topical cyclosporine A for treatment of oral chronic graft-versus-host disease. Bone Marrow Transplantation 1994; 13(1):81.

39. Ho VC, Griffiths CE, Ellis CN et al. Intralesional cyclosporine in the treatment

of psoriasis. A clinical, immunologic, and pharmacokinetic study. J Am Acad Dermatol 1990; 22(1):94.

40. Sonmez YE, Ercan E, Savci N et al. Long-term survival of skin allograft in rats by topical use of cyclosporine A. Turk J Med Biol Res 1991; 2(2):143.

41. Bierer BE. Cyclosporin A, FK506, and rapamycin: Binding to immunophilins and biological action. Chem Immunol 1994; 59:128.

42. Schleuning M, Duggan A, Reem GH. Cyclosporine does not inhibit the early transducing signals generated by the activation of human thymocytes. Transplant Proc 1988; 20(2):63.

43. Hewitt CW, Black KS, Gonzalez GA et al. Decreased reactivity of allosera against target lymphocytes obtained following thermal injury or long-term cyclosporine treatment. Clin Immunol Immunopathol 1987; 45:395.

44. Wilkinson PC, Higgins A. Cyclosporin A inhibits mitogen-activated but not phorbol ester-activated locomotion of human lymphocytes. Immunology 1987; 61:311.

45. Hopt UT, Erath F, Schareck W et al. Effect of cyclosporin A on local inflammation in rejecting allografts. Transplant Proc 1988; 20(2):163.

46. Norin AJ, Kamholz SL, Pinsker KL et al. Concavalin A-dependent cell-mediated cytotoxicity in bronchoaleolar lavage fluid. Transplantation 1986; 42(5):466.

47. Hanto DW, Ulrich HT, Hoffman R et al. Recruitment of unsensitized circulating lymphocytes to sites of allogeneic cellular interactions. Transplantation 1982; 33(5):541.

48. Mayer TG, Bhan AK, Winn HJ. Immunohistochemical analysis of skin graft rejection in mice. Transplantation 1988; 46(6):890.

49. Orosz CG, Zinn NE, Sirinek L et al. In vivo mechanisms of alloreactivity 1. Frequency of donor-reactive cytotoxic T lymphocytes in sponge matrix allografts. Transplantation 1986; 41:75.

50. Orosz CG, Zinn NE, Sirinek LP et al. In vivo mechanisms of alloreactivity. II. Allospecificity of cytotoxic T lymphocytes in sponge matrix allografts as determined by limiting dilution analysis. Transplantation 1986; 41(1):84.

51. Havele C, Paetkau V. Cyclosporine blocks the activation of antigen dependent cytotoxic T lymphocytes directly by an IL-2 independent mechanism. J Immunol 1988; 140(10):3303.

52. Mellert J, Hopt UT, Erath F et al. Differential effects of azathioprine (Aza), cyclosporine A (CsA) and dexamethaxone (Dexa) on lymphokine mediated inflammation in rejecting allografts. Transplant Proc 1989; 21:98.

53. Erjefalt I, Greiff L, Alkner U et al. Allergen-induced biphasic plasma exudation responses in guinea pig large airways. Am Rev Respir Dis 1993; 148(3):695.

54. Holgate ST, Djukanovic R, Wilson J et al. Allergic inflammation and its pharmacological modulation in asthma. Int Arch Allergy Appl Immunol 1991; 94:210.

55. Bierer BE. Immunosuppressive agents targeting T-cell activation pathways. In: Przepiorka D, Sollinger H, eds. Recent Developments in Transplantation Medicine. Physicians & Scientists Publishing Co., Inc. 1994:9.

LOCAL IMMUNOSUPPRESSION IN CORNEAL TRANSPLANTATION

Ali R. Djalilian and Edward J. Holland

INTRODUCTION

Corneal transplantation (penetrating keratoplasty) is currently the most common and successful type of tissue transplant performed in the U.S. The remarkable survival of corneal allografts can be largely attributed to their unique avascular structure. This feature allows the graft to remain hidden from the host's immune system, and effectively renders it immunologically-privileged status. Nonetheless, immune-mediated rejection remains the leading cause of graft failure.[1] Up to 30% of penetrating keratoplasty patients will have at least one episode of rejection.[2] These usually occur between 4 and 18 months postoperatively, but may occur up to years after successful transplantation. The incidence of rejection is further increased in corneal grafts that develop neovascularization (e.g., due to previous rejection).[1,2] In these vascular corneas, the recipient's immune system can recognize and attack the donor tissue much more readily, thus leading to a higher failure rate. Other factors that can increase the risk of immune-mediated rejection include repeat grafts, bilateral grafts, history of inflammatory eye disease and presence of adhesions.[2]

The highly accessible location of the cornea further contributes to the success of transplantation. This feature allows rejection episodes to be recognized early and treated locally under close monitoring. Traditionally, topical as opposed to systemic pharmacologic therapy has been the mainstay of preventing corneal graft rejection, in part because the morbidity and mortality associated with systemic immunosuppression cannot be justified for this non-life-threatening condition. Typically, more than half of all rejection episodes can be reversed with appropriate topical immunosuppressive therapy,[1,2] although occasionally systemic therapy becomes necessary as well. In addition to topical administration,

Local Immunosuppression of Organ Transplants, edited by Scott A. Gruber.
© 1996 R.G. Landes Company.

subconjunctival, intracameral (into the anterior chamber) and periocular injections are also effective means of local drug delivery to the eye.

The local immunosuppressive therapy of corneal transplants provides a useful model for the study of target-directed drug delivery systems. It allows graft immunosuppression to be achieved with far less systemic side effects. Currently, corticosteroids are the gold-standard for achieving ocular immunosuppression in corneal transplantation. However, promising newer agents may soon provide a safe and effective adjunct for the local immunosuppressive therapy of corneal allografts.

CORTICOSTEROIDS

Corticosteroids are the drugs of choice for both the prevention and treatment of acute corneal graft rejection. They are currently the most effective ocular immunosuppressants available. Local drug delivery is most commonly via topical administration, though sometimes subconjunctival injections are used as well.

Steroids exert their regional immunosuppressive effects by inhibiting many aspects of the local inflammatory response. They have been shown to block the synthesis of prostaglandins through inhibition of phospholipase A2, decrease cellular and fibrinous exudation, inhibit fibroblastic and collagen-forming activity, restore capillary permeability, stabilize the lysosomal membranes of polymorphonuclear leukocytes and inhibit graft vascularization.[3]

Currently, three different synthetic corticosteroid bases are available for topical administration in the eye: prednisolone, dexamethasone and fluorometholone. Ophthalmic absorption of these agents depends heavily on the type of preparation. In particular, the alcohol and acetate derivatives, which are soluble in hydrophobic media, easily traverse the epithelial and endothelial layers of the cornea, while the phosphate salt derivatives do not readily pass through the intact epithelium. Therefore, in an uninflamed eye with intact corneal epithelium, the acetate and alcohol derivatives of prednisolone or dexamethasone produce significantly higher corneal and aqueous humor drug levels than the phosphate derivatives.[4]

Subconjunctival (or sub-Tenon's) injection of corticosteroids also appears to suppress the local immune response. This route of administration is less effective than, but seems to act synergisticly with, topically-delivered drug.[5] Since no preparations have been specifically manufactured for subconjunctival administration, frequently a preparation suitable for intravenous injection is used. This route also has the advantage of providing a local reservoir which could last up to days for some preparations.

Following corneal transplantation, a standard preventive regimen involves a corticosteroid drop such as 1% prednisolone acetate. Typically, this is applied four times a day for the first 3 months postoperatively, and is then gradually decreased over the next 3-12 months. The optimal preventive dose for each patient is determined by their clinical response. Some patients may be able to stop using steroids altogether, while high-risk patients with significant neovascularization or repeat grafts may require large preventive doses for prolonged periods.

Mild graft rejections are treated by reinstituting or increasing the dose of topical steroids. A subconjunctival injection of steroids may also be given as an adjunct. Severe rejections are treated immediately and more aggressively. Initially, methylprednisolone 125-250 mg is given by intravenous bolus, followed by intensive topical therapy (every hour) as well as oral prednisone 1 mg/kg/day. Treatment is continued until signs of waning inflammation become visible. Most cases begin to respond within the first few days, and subsequently, the doses can be gradually reduced. Approximately 50% to 70% of the rejection episodes can be reversed with local steroids, though sometimes a short course of systemic steroids may also be necessary.[1,2]

Overall, topical steroids are extremely beneficial and are considered to be the benchmark against which all other ocular immunosuppressive agents are tested.[6] While the complications of systemic steroid therapy are avoided, topical use is still associated with significant side effects. In particular, chronic use can lead to such complications as cataracts, steroid-induced glaucoma, delayed wound healing and surface immunosuppression which predisposes to infections or recurrence of herpes simplex virus.[7] Subconjunctival injections can additionally cause problems such as conjunctival scarring, ptosis and scleral thinning.[8] These complications become particularly important in patients whose grafts are significantly vascularized and require chronic therapy to maintain their graft. To effectively manage these high-risk patients, more specific and less toxic agents would be preferable. Nonetheless, topical corticosteroids will continue to be the primary immunosuppressive agents in routine keratoplasty, given their superior efficacy and ease of use.

CYCLOSPORINE A (CsA)

The use of CsA in corneal transplantation has yet to produce the same enthusiasm and excitement as it has in solid organ transplantation. The significant associated side effects have restricted its systemic use mainly to one-eyed high-risk patients that are dependent on their graft for vision,[9] while its topical use has been limited because of suboptimal absorption into the cornea.

CsA is a hydrophobic cyclic peptide that can easily cross the corneal epithelium; however, it cannot readily penetrate the hydrophilic stroma. Its ocular absorption has been enhanced using several vehicles, most commonly, olive oil.[10] Other substances with demonstrated benefit include arachis oil,[11] castor oil,[12] cremophor/ethanol,[13] Azone[14] and cyclodextrin.[15] More recently, liposomal encapsulation has been used to promote the penetration of CsA into the eye and was shown to be superior to oil formulations.[16] Using these vehicles, it appears that the delivery of topical CsA to the eye may no longer be a significant issue.

As a topical agent, CsA is thought to work by the same mechanisms as it does systemically, namely, by inhibiting IL-2, interferon-gamma and IL-2 receptor expression, as well as down-regulating class II antigen expression.[17] Several animal and clinical studies have demonstrated its efficacy as a topical immunosuppressant.[14,18-20] In a report of 11 high-risk keratoplasty patients treated with 2% CsA in sterile olive oil, 10 corneas remained clear at 16 month follow-up examination.[19] Zhao and associates[20] used 0.5% CsA to treat 16 patients with refractory corneal graft rejection and achieved a complete cure in nine eyes and marked improvement in another six eyes. Thus, topical CsA appears to be effective for both the prevention and treatment of corneal graft rejection.

Topically, CsA is well tolerated. Belin et al[19] reported a self-limiting transient epithelial keratitis in their patients following topical administration of CsA. In a review of 43 patients treated with topical CsA for a variety of anterior segment inflammatory conditions, only two patients experienced severe ocular discomfort.[10] The remaining patients tolerated the medication well, including several patients receiving hourly application.

There has been a concern regarding the systemic absorption of topical CsA, partly stimulated by a few reports noting significant systemic levels following topical administration.[18,19,21] However, other investigators have found whole-blood CsA levels to be undetectable by high-performance liquid chromatography after topical therapy.[10,20] Moreover, there have not been any reports of nephrotoxicity or other systemic side effects associated with the topical use of CsA. Foets and associates[18] studied eccentric corneal grafts in a rabbit model and applied CsA either to the ipsilateral (grafted) or the contralateral (nongrafted) eye. They found that all ipsilaterally-treated grafts remained clear, while contralaterally-treated grafts were rejected, even though systemic drug levels as determined by radioimmunoassay were similar in both groups. These results suggest that the suppression of allograft rejection by topical CsA is primarily a local effect and the systemic drug absorption is unlikely to play a clinically-significant role.

Overall, topical CsA is a well-tolerated and effective ocular immunosuppressant. Its main role currently is in the management of high-risk keratoplasty. While systemic absorption may no longer be a major concern, the long-term safety and efficacy of topical CsA has not yet been studied in a randomized prospective trial. With future studies, topical CsA has the potential for becoming an extremely valuable tool in preventing and treating corneal graft rejection, particularly in cases where steroids are ineffective or intolerable.

FK506

Although used clinically in solid organ transplantation, the application of FK506 to corneal transplantation has been limited to animal studies. Similar to CsA in action, the topical absorption of FK506 has likewise been hindered by its hydrophobic structure. Cyclodextrin,[22] olive oil,[23] and liposomes[23] have all been used effectively as vehicles to promote the ocular absorption of topical FK506. Pleyer and associates[23] have demonstrated superior efficacy with liposomal preparations when compared with oil formulations. Alternatively, subconjunctival[24] or periocular[25] injections have been used for local administration of FK506.

Kobayashi et al[24] was first to report the use of FK506 subconjunctivally in rabbits for prolonging corneal graft survival. Since then, numerous other studies have demonstrated its beneficial role in preventing corneal graft rejection following topical, subconjunctival, or periocular administration in both rats and rabbits.[22,23,25] So far, no significant side effects have been noted in these studies. Serum levels were undetectable following topical administration of FK506 using various vehicles.[23] Thus, as an inhibitor of T cell activation, the ocular immunosuppressive effects of topical FK506 are most likely mediated via local mechanisms.

Without clinical studies, the safety and efficacy of topical FK506 in humans is unknown. Based on animal studies, it appears to be an effective local agent for preventing corneal graft rejection. Future clinical trials may prove FK506 to be a safe and useful adjunct for the management of high-risk keratoplasty.

MONOCLONAL ANTIBODIES

Monoclonal antibodies directed against T cell antigens have been used extensively to reverse acute graft rejection in solid organ transplantation.[26,27] Both monoclonal antibodies and heterologous antilymphocyte serum have been shown to prolong corneal graft survival in animal models when given systemically.[28,29] Until now topical therapy with antibodies has not been effective due to their poor absorption across the cornea.[29] Recently, however, Pleyer et al[30] were able to suppress corneal graft rejection in rats using topically-administered, liposome-encapsulated anti-CD4 monoclonal antibodies.

Subconjunctival administration of monoclocal antibodies has also been used with variable success. Using the rabbit corneal graft model, Shirao et al[31] examined the effect of subconjunctivally-injected monoclonal antibodies, either unmodified or coupled to the immunotoxin ricin A, and failed to show any significant benefit. In contrast, Hoffman and associates[32] demonstrated that antibodies against the IL-2 receptor can prolong corneal allograft survival in rats following subconjunctival or intraperitoneal injection.

Alternatively, intracameral (into the anterior chamber) injections have been used in both animal and clinical studies. Williams et al[33] examined the phenotype of cells infiltrating rejecting corneal allografts in rabbits and demonstrated that injecting monoclonal antibodies directed against a peripheral T cell determinant and major histocompatibility complex class II antigen into the anterior chamber could reverse rejection in that model. Ippoliti and associates[34] clinically demonstrated that intracameral injection of anti-CD3 or anti-CD6 anti-T cell monoclonal antibodies can reverse acute corneal allograft rejection. Finally, monoclonal antibodies directed against intercellular adhesion molecule-1 (ICAM-1) and lymphocyte function-associated antigen-1 (LFA-1) have proven effective in preventing experimental corneal graft rejection.[35]

Despite its demonstrated clinical benefit, intracameral injection of monoclonal antibodies is unlikely to become a standard protocol for corneal transplantation in the near future. Intracameral injection is not a suitable mode of drug delivery for repeated use. It not only carries the risk of infection and mechanical damage to the anterior chamber structures, but also could potentially lead to an intraocular cytokine-mediated inflammatory reaction.[36] However, liposome encapsulation may provide a safe and effective alternative for local drug delivery, and future clinical studies are needed to evaluate the safety and efficacy of topical liposomal preparations of a variety of different monoclonal antibodies.

EXPERIMENTAL AGENTS AND TECHNIQUES

In addition to FK506, several other immunosuppressive drugs have been studied in animal models. Most studies have involved only systemic administration, demonstrating prolonged graft survival using agents such as rapamycin,[37] 15-deoxyspergualin,[38] and urocanic acid[39] in rats or rabbits. Systemic azathioprine, which has actually been used clinically in corneal transplantation, was found not to be effective topically.[40] Recently, Van der Veen and associates[41] were able to show that subconjunctival administration of liposomes containing dichloromethylene diphosphonate prevents corneal graft rejection in rats.

Other groups have focused on strategies for reducing the antigenicity of the donor tissue. Specifically, techniques such as pretreatment of corneal allografts with UV light,[42] or heterologous antibodies[43] have been employed to reduce the antigenic load of the donor graft. HLA matching has been advocated by some as a means of pro-

longing graft survival.[44] However, although one recent study found the risk of rejection to be directly proportional to the number of HLA-A and -B mismatches and inversely proportional to the number of HLA-DR mismatches,[45] another collaborative study did not find a significant association between HLA matching and the risk of rejection.[46]

SUMMARY

The location of the cornea makes it an ideal candidate for local immunosuppressive therapy following transplantation. Currently corticosteroids remain the most effective topical immunosuppressive agents available. More specific drugs such as CsA and FK506 are likely to gain wider acceptance since they help avoid the complications of chronic steroid therapy. Liposomal encapsulation is an exciting new technique which has been demonstrated to significantly enhance intraocular drug delivery following topical administration. It can potentially provide a safe and effective route for administering agents with poor ocular absorption such as monoclonal antibodies. In the meantime, other approaches, including HLA matching and reduction of donor antigenicity, may be used to further improve the results of corneal transplantation.

REFERENCES

1. Khodadoust AA. The allograft rejection reaction: the leading cause of late failure of corneal grafts. In: Porter R, Knight J, ed. Corneal Graft Failure, Ciba Found Symp 15. Amsterdam: Elsevier, 1973:151.

2. Alldredge OC, Krachmer JH. Clinical types of corneal rejection: their manifestations, frequency, preoperative correlates and treatment. Arch Ophthalmol 1981; 99:599.

3. Duke-Elder S, Ashton N. Action of cortisone on tissue reactions of inflammation and repair with special reference to the eye. Br J Ophthalmol 1951; 35:695.

4. Leibowitz HM, Kupferman A. Bioavailability and therapeutic effectiveness of topically administered corticosteroids. Trans Am Acad Ophthalmol Otolaryngol 1975; 79:78.

5. Leibowitz HM, Kupferman A. Periocular injection of corticosteroids. Arch Ophthalmol 1977; 95:1387.

6. Coster DJ, Williams KA. Immunosuppression for corneal transplantation and treatment of graft rejection. Transplant Proc 1989; 21:3125.

7. Frangie JP, Leibowitz HM. Steroids. Int Ophthalmol Clin 1993; 33(4):9.

8. O'Connor GR. Periocular corticosteroid injection: uses and abuses. Eye Ear Nose Throat Mon. 1976; 55(3):26.

9. Hill JC. Systemic cyclosporine in high-risk keratoplasty. Short- versus long-term therapy. Ophthalmology 1994; 101:128.

10. Holland EJ, Olsen TW, Ketcham JM et al. Topical cyclosporin A in the treatment of anterior segment inflammatory disease. Cornea 1993; 12:413.

11. Williams KA, Grutzmacher RD, Roussel TJ et al. A comparison of the effects of topical cyclosporine and topical steroid on rabbit corneal allograft rejection. Transplantation 1985; 39:242.

12. Weiderholt M, Kossendrup D, Schulz W et al. Pharmacokinetics of topical cyclosporin A in the rabbit eye. Invest Ophthalmol Vis Sci 1986; 27:519.

13. Williams KA, Erickson SA, Coster DJ. Topical steroid, cyclosporin A, and the outcome of rat corneal allografts. Br J Ophthalmol 1987; 71:239.

14. Newton C, Gebhardt BM, Kaufman HE. Topically applied cyclosporine in a zone prolongs corneal allograft survival. Invest Ophthalmol Vis Sci 1988; 29:208.

15. Cheeks L, Kawsan RL, Green K. Influence of vehicle and anterior chamber protein concentration on cyclosporine penetration through the isolated rabbit cornea. Curr Eye Res 1992; 11:641.

16. Pleyer U, Elkins B, Ruckert D et al. Ocular absorption of cyclosporin A from liposomes incorporated into collagen shields. Curr Eye Res 1994; 13:177.

17. Belin MW, Bouchard CS, Philips TM. Update on topical cyclosporin A: Background, immunology, and pharmacology. Cornea 1990; 9:184.

18. Foets B, Missoten L, Vanderveeren P et al. Prolonged survival of allogenic corneal grafts in rabbits treated with topically applied cyclosporin A: systemic absorption and local immunosuppressive effect. Br J Ophthalmol 1985; 69:600.

19. Belin MW, Bouchard CS, Frantz BS et al. Topical cyclosporine in high-risk corneal transplants. Ophthalmology 1989; 96:1144.

20. Zhao JC, Jin XY. Local therapy of corneal allograft rejection with cyclosporine. Am J Ophthalmol 1995; 119:189.

21. Gregory CR, Hietala SK, Pederson NC et al. Cyclosporine pharmacokinetics in cats following topical ocular administration. Transplantation 1989; 47:516.

22. Mills RA, Jones DB, Winkler CR et al. Topical FK-506 prevents experimental allograft rejection. Cornea 1995; 14:157.

23. Pleyer U, Lutz S, Jusko J et al. Ocular absorption of topically applied FK-506 from liposomal and oil formulations in the rabbit eye. Invest Ophthalmol Vis Sci 1993; 34:2737.

24. Kobayashi C, Kanai A, Nakajima A et al. Suppression of corneal graft rejection in rabbits by a new immunosuppressive agent, FK-506. Transplant Proc 1989; 21:3156.

25. Dickey JB, Cassidy EM, Bouchard CS. Periocular FK-506 delays allograft rejection in rat penetrating keratoplasty. Cornea 1993; 12:204.

26. Cosimi AB, Burton RC, Colvin RB et al. Treatment of acute renal graft rejection with OKT3 monoclonal antibody. Transplantation 1981; 32:525.

27. Cosimi AB, Cho SI, Delmonico FL et al. A randomized clinical trial comparing OKT3 and steroids for the treatment of hepatic allograft rejection. Transplantation 1987; 43:91.

28. Waltman SR, Faulkner WM, Burde RM. Modification of the ocular immune response. I. Use of antilymphocytic serum to prevent immune rejection of penetrating corneal homografts. Invest Ophthalmol 1972; 8:196.

29. Polack FM, Townsend WM, Waltman S. Antilymphocyte serum and corneal graft rejection. Am J Ophthalmol 1972; 72:52.

30. Pleyer U, Milani JK, Dukes A et al. Effects of topically applied anti-CD4 monoclonal antibodies on orthotopic corneal allografts

in a rat model. Invest Ophthalmol Vis Sci 1995; 36:52.

31. Shirao, Deschenes J, Char DH. Corneal allograft rejection in rabbits. Curr Eye Res 1986; 5:817.

32. Hoffman F, Kruse HA, Meinhold H et al. Interleukin-2 receptor—targeted therapy by monoclonal antibodies in the rat corneal graft. Cornea 1994; 13:440.

33. Williams KA, Standfield SD, Wing AJ et al. Patterns of corneal graft rejection in the rabbit and reversal of rejection with monoclonal antibodies. Transplantation 1992; 54:38.

34. Ippoliti G, Fronterrè A. Usefulness of CD3 or CD6 monoclonal antibodies in the treatment of acute corneal graft rejection. Transplant Proc 1989; 21:3133.

35. Yamagami S, Obata H, Tsuru T et al. Suppression of corneal allograft rejection after penetrating keratoplasty by antibodies to ICAM-1 and LFA-1 in mice. Transplant Proc 1995; 27:1899.

36. Williams KA, Coster DJ. Use of monoclonal antibodies in corneal transplantation. Clin Immunother 1994; 2:32.

37. Olsen TW, Benegas NM, Joplin AC et al. Rapamycin inhibits corneal allograft rejection and neovascularization. Arch Ophthalmol 1994; 112:1471.

38. Holland EJ, Olsen TW, Sterrer J et al. Suppression of graft rejection using 15-deoxyspergualin in the allogeneic rat penetrating keratoplasty model. Cornea 1994; 13:28.

39. Guymer RH, Mandel TE. Urocanic acid as an immunosuppressant in allotransplantation in mice. Transplantation 1993; 55:36.

40. Elliot JH, Leibowitz HM. Chemotherapeutic immunosuppression of corneal graft rejection. 3. Topical azathioprine. Arch Ophthalmol 1966; 76:709.

41. Van der Veen G, Broersma L, Dijkstra CD et al. Prevention of corneal allograft rejection in rats treated with subconjunctival injection of liposomes containing dichloromethylene diphosphonate. Invest Ophthalmol Vis Sci 1994; 35:3505.

42. Hill JC, Sarvan J, Maske R et al. Evidence that UV-B irradiation decreases corneal Langerhans cells and improves corneal graft survival in the rabbit. Transplantation 1994; 57:1281.

43. Binder PS, Gebhardt BM, Chandler JW et al. Immunologic protection of rabbit corneal allografts with heterologous blocking antibody. Am J Ophthalmol 1975; 79:949.

44. Boisjoly HM, Roy R, Dube I et al. HLA-A, B and DR matching in corneal transplantation. Ophthalmology 1975; 93:1290.

45. Vail A, Gore SM, Bradley BA et al. Influence of donor and histocompatibility factors on corneal graft outcome. Transplantation 1994; 58(11):1210.

46. Fink N, Stark WJ, Maguire MG et al. Effectiveness of histocompatibility matching in high-risk corneal transplantation: A summary of results from the Collaborative Corneal Transplantation Studies. Ceskoslobenska Oftalmologie 1994; 50(1):3.

CHAPTER 16

CONTROLLED-RELEASE DRUG MATRICES FOR LOCAL IMMUNOSUPPRESSION OF ORGAN TRANSPLANTS

Steven F. Bolling, Vinod Labhasetwar and Robert J. Levy

INTRODUCTION

The use of improved immunosuppression is responsible for the wide-spread application of organ transplantation. However, systemic immunosuppression frequently results in well-known, but unavoidable, side effects. Conversely, the phenomenon of transplant rejection has been recognized as a local cellular event, with extreme variability noted in rejection even between adjacent cells.[1] Effective local immunosuppression by controlled-release drug delivery systems, such as polymer or biodegradable matrices, might be able to minimize immunosuppressive problems by delivering agents directly to the affected target cells, and optimal drug activity could be achieved with less systemic side effects.

Controlled-release local drug delivery systems have been successfully used for preventing cardiovascular calcification,[2] ventricular arrhythmias,[3] pacer threshold elevation[4] and endocarditis.[5] These delivery systems have often utilized polymer matrices, configured to have both sustained-release properties (potentially years) and to serve functionally as valve prosthesis sewing rings (for preventing bioprosthetic calcification), cardiac pacing lead tips and epicardial patch implants (for preventing ventricular arrhythmias). Other types of more biodegradable controlled-release matrix materials have the advantage of a finite release duration without the residual presence of a foreign body implant, and are well suited for delivery of water insoluble, biologically-active agents, such as cyclosporine.

Additionally, long-term configurations of both release matrices have been possible by optimizing controlled-release parameters.[2] Presently, the use of long-term implantable pumps for drug delivery is a clinical reality in the realm of cancer and pain treatment, and this concept has been applied to local drug delivery for immunosuppression.

RATIONALE

The phenomenon of graft rejection has long been recognized as a local individual cellular event because of the extreme variability noted at transplant biopsy in terms of differential rejection and cellular destruction patterns between adjacent cells.[1] Investigators have attempted to inhibit rejection with local drug administration, since studies have shown that development and expression of T lymphocyte immunoeffector cells can occur within the transplanted organ,[6] with activation and maturation of lymphocytes at a remote site and subsequent migration to the transplant.[7,8] Furthermore, local immunoregulatory mechanisms involved with transplant organ rejection may be altered at the local cellular level, including production of important local chemokines and cytokines from T lymphocytes.[9,10] For example, tumor necrosis factor (TNF) plays an important role in T cell immune reactions. These immune reactions are typically characterized by the elicitation and activation of lymphocytes, macrophages and cytotoxic T cells.[11] Consequently, the local anti-TNF effect of steroids could have an important role in modulating the transplant rejection response. Conceptually therefore, very specific effective local immunosuppression could be achieved, if therapy could be targeted optimally.

REVIEW OF EXPERIMENTAL RESULTS

Local immunosuppressive steroid therapy has been utilized previously. Prednisolone (4 mg/kg/day) delayed rat kidney transplants from rejecting when delivered intraarterially by an osmotic pump[12] (chapter 4). In these transplanted rats, there was a significant increase in mean graft survival time (28 days) when compared with rats which received the identical dosage of steroid by intravenous injection (9 days). In that study, local delivery prolonged graft survival presumably by producing high intrarenal levels of prednisolone in comparison with the systemic group. In confirmation, it has been shown that elevated local and regional steroid levels inhibit the function of effector cells migrating to transplanted organs and can depress the recognition of grafted tissue. Kidneys treated with prednisolone locally show almost no staining for class II major histocompatibility complex (MHC) antigens, and do not express interleukin-2 receptors.[12] All of these findings suggest that the rejection process can be modulated locally. Recent studies[13] have demonstrated a decrease in immune-activated cytolytic cells present when local immunosuppression was produced with a matrix containing methylprednisolone topically applied to an experimental skin allograft (chapter 14). Mechanisms of action in that study were postulated to involve reduction in class I and II MHC expression and inhibition of local CD4+ lymphocytes, but the immunosuppressive effect may also in part be due to steroid inhibition of TNF-α synthesis by blocking its transcription at the cellular level.

Along the lines of the above findings, we demonstrated that local, controlled-release administration of dexamethasone significantly delayed rejection in a Brown-Norway to Lewis rat cervical heterotopic cardiac transplant model.[14,15] Local release matrices were formulated by dissolving dexamethasone in a high molecular weight polyanhydride consisting of repeating subunits of sebacic acid (60%) and carboxyphenoxypropane (40%). Dexamethasone and polyanhydride were formed by solvent casting in methylene chloride at 37°C and evaporation adjusted to yield polymers containing 2%, 0.2% or 0.02% dexamethasone. Heart transplant rejection as assessed by mean survival time to cessation of cardiac contraction is shown in Table 16.1. Administration of local high-dose dexamethasone significantly delayed time to allograft rejection (mean survival time = 10.8 days for 2.0% dexamethasone-treated rats versus 6.9 days in controls, P < 0.05). In addition, the controlled-release preparation with 0.2% dexamethasone delivery resulted in an equally significant prolongation of graft survival (10.2 days). However, the controlled-release preparation with 0.02% dexamethasone delivery resulted in no prolongation of graft survival (7.2 days) compared with controls, demonstrating a decreasing dose-dependent effect. No animals received any systemic immunotherapy. Daily wound examination revealed poor healing in 50% of the animals (3/6) in the highest steroid (2.0% Dex) group. All other animals had excellent primary wound healing.

In our next series of studies, cyclosporine A biodegradable local controlled-release matrices were formulated by adding rat tail collagen and acetic acid to cyclosporine dissolved in acetone.[16] Cyclosporine matrices were formulated at 2 and 10% (0.2 or 1 mg/kg/day released).

Formaldehyde cross-linking was employed to extend cyclosporine delivery (Fig. 16.1). Again, heart transplant rejection, as assessed by mean survival time to cessation of cardiac contraction, was evaluated using a rat cervical heterotopic transplant model (Table 16.1, Fig. 16.2). Local immunosuppression with high-dose cyclosporine A in a controlled-release matrix resulted in a significant survival advantage (mean survival time = 17.1 days; control = 6.9 days, P < 0.001). The lower dose of cyclosporine also demonstrated significant survival benefit (10.1 days) versus controls (Fig. 16.2). The cyclosporine-treated (0.2 mg/kg/day) animals had whole-blood cyclosporine levels (measured by high-performance liquid chromatography) monitored for 6 weeks following implantation. Mean cyclosporine levels peaked at 7-10 days after transplant at 119 ± 26 (SE) ng/ml and decayed to < 50 ng/ml by day 42 (Fig. 16.3). At no time did whole-blood cyclosporine concentrations reach clinically significant levels, and kidney tissue levels were also noted to be very low on day 6 posttransplant. However, both doses of local-release cyclosporine were well absorbed locally, resulting in

Table 16.1. The effect of cyclosporine A (Cy) and dexamethasone (Dex) controlled-release matrices implanted around rat heterotopic heart transplants

	n	Graft Survival (days)	Cyclosporine Levels at Day 6 Posttransplant		
			Blood (ng/ml)	Heart (ng/mg)	Kidney(ng/mg)
Control	10	6.9 ± 0.3	0	0	0
Cy 0.2 mg	8	$10.1 \pm 0.2^*$	100 ± 20	$9800 \pm 4300\#$	$460 \pm 257\#$
Cy 1 mg	6	$17.1 \pm 0.6^*$	$746 \pm 114\#$	$107,000 \pm 3300\#$	$5373 \pm 347\#$
Cy distal (0.2 mg)	6	8.2 ± 0.6	156 ± 29	725 ± 151	1214 ± 121
Dex distal (0.2%)	5	7.5 ± 0.4			
Dex 0.02%	5	7.2 ± 0.4			
Dex 0.2%	6	$10.2 \pm 0.6^*$			
Dex 2%	6	$10.8 \pm 0.4^*$			
Cy/Dex (0.2 mg/0.2%)	7	$10.6 \pm 0.6^*$			

Graft survival times (days) are given as mean ± SE; * = P < 0.05 versus untreated controls. Cyclosporine A levels are shown from whole blood, heart and kidneys obtained on postoperative day 6 following transplantation as mean ± SE; # = P < 0.05 vs controls.
Reproduced from Polymers for Advanced Technology 1992; 3:45-50 by permission of John Wiley & Sons, Ltd.

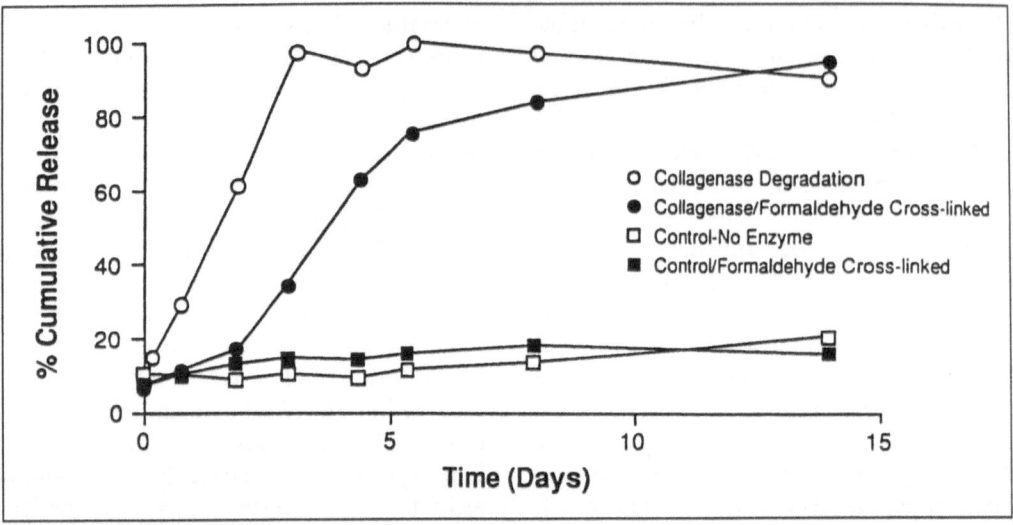

Fig. 16.1. *In vitro release curve at pH 7.4 of cyclosporine from rat tail collagen matrices showing the effect of formaldehyde cross-linking and collagenase degradation. Reproduced with permission from J Heart Lung Transplant 1991; 10:577-83.*

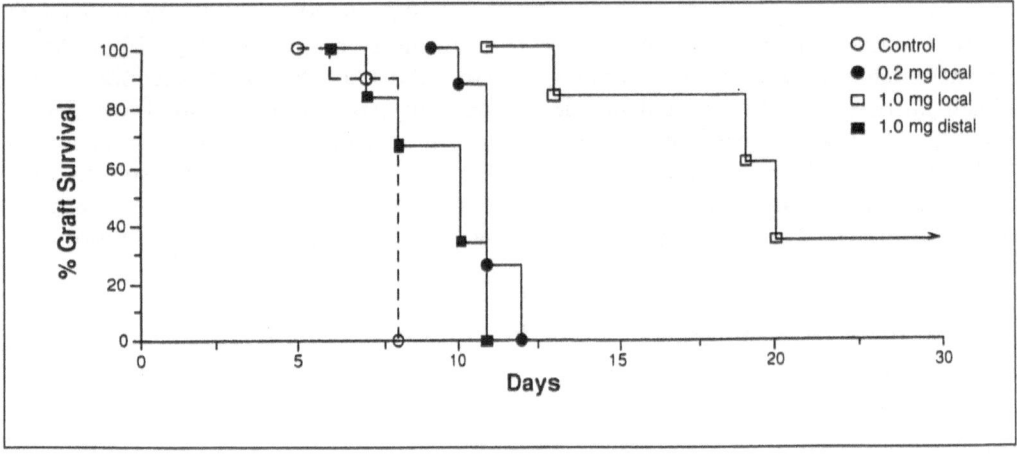

Fig. 16.2. *Cardiac allograft survival of Brown-Norway hearts transplanted into Lewis rats was significantly prolonged in both local release groups compared with that in untreated controls, while distal subdermal pouch implantation of the same release matrices did not result in prolongation of graft survival. Reproduced with permission from J Heart Lung Transplant 1991; 10:577-83.*

high cyclosporine levels in grafted heart tissue (> 9,000 ng/mg, Table 16.1). Importantly, neither cyclosporine (0.2 mg/kg/day) nor steroids (0.2%) released from a distal subcutaneous pouch prolonged allograft survival over that in untreated controls. Finally, on pathologic examination, all hearts harvested at the time of cessation of contractions had signs of typical rejection as demonstrated by lymphocytic infiltration and myocyte necrosis.

Interestingly, a cyclosporine (0.2 mg/kg/day) and dexamethasone (0.2%) combination controlled-release matrix was formed from polyanhydride and utilized in the same model. However, cyclosporine/dexamethasone combination matrices were not synergistic at the local level and did not increase efficacy beyond either drug alone. This may have been a local-release failure phenomenon of the matrix. In summary, local steroid controlled-release delayed

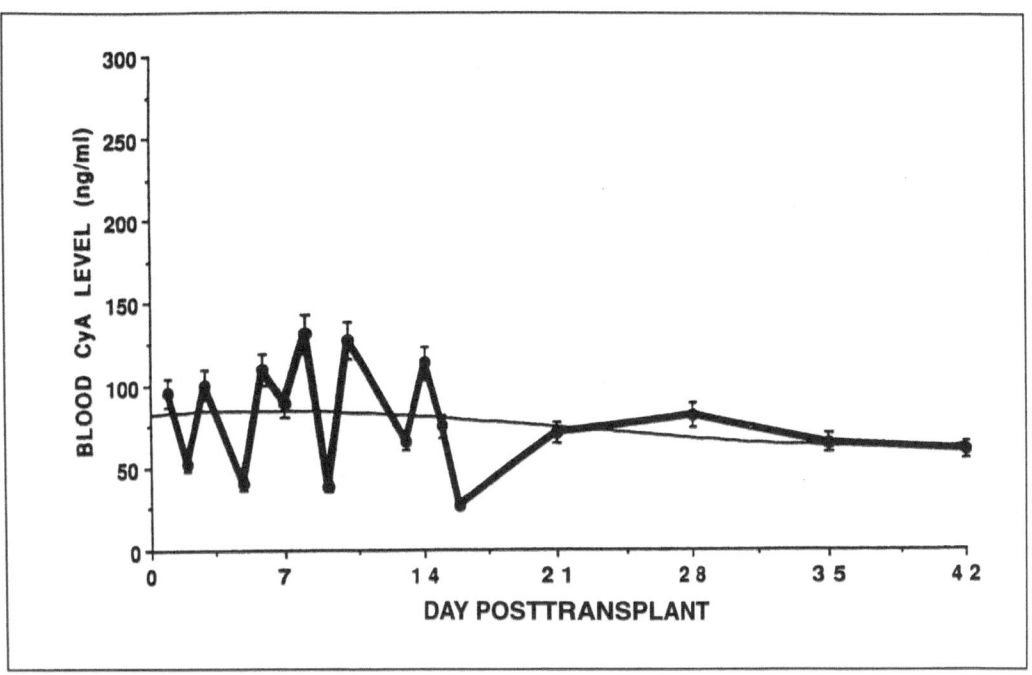

Fig. 16.3. Levels (mean ± SE) of whole-blood cyclosporine A obtained for 6 weeks following transplantation from animals with controlled-release cyclosporine matrices implanted around the rat heterotopic heart transplant. Reproduced from Polymers for Advanced Technology 1992; 3:45-50 by permission of John Wiley & Sons, Ltd.

transplant rejection and resulted in a significant survival advantage, without systemic immunosuppression. Distal steroid subdermal implantation did not prolong survival time, despite presumably equal plasma steroid levels when compared with the local-release groups. Local cyclosporine immunotherapy resulted in a significant survival advantage, was absorbed well into the myocardium and was effective with clinically negligible blood and kidney drug levels.

Others have also studied local-release immunosuppression. One study evaluated the effect of locally-delivered methylprednisolone on the systemic and local immune response in a sponge matrix allograft model.[17] Mice received two polypropylene sponge grafts seeded with either syngeneic or allogeneic spleen cells. Local immunosuppression was effected by placement on day 0 of cellulose/matrix pellets containing a preparation of increasing quantities of controlled-release methylprednisolone or by daily intrasponge injection of methylprednisolone. Absolute numbers of precursor cytolytic cells and mature cytolytic cells (determined by limiting dilution analysis) infiltrating the allografts were decreased in the sponges with local- release methylprednisolone. Local immunosuppression was achieved with decreased systemic steroid toxicity in the allogeneic sponge group. The presence of local methylprednisolone at the graft site prevented the animals from becoming specifically sensitized to the initial alloantigen, but did not keep the animal from developing a brisk rejection response to a third-party skin graft with first-set kinetics, demonstrating systemic immunocompetence with antigen-specific immuno-"tolerance". In this model, it appears that delivery of methylprednisolone locally at the site of antigenic challenge was an effective means of modulating alloreactivity.

Other immunosuppressive drugs have been studied for local effectiveness. Gruber et al[18] examined the efficacy of continuous local intraarterial versus systemic intravenous 6-mercaptopurine (6-MP) infusion in a mongrel canine renal allograft model and examined overall survival, incidence of systemic and renal toxicity and systemic drug exposure (chapter 9). A dose of 0.5 mg/kg/day 6-MP did not prolong survival over heparin-treated or untreated controls either locally or systemically. However, 0.75 mg/kg/day of 6-MP infused directly into the transplant renal artery significantly prolonged survival over both untreated and heparin-treated controls. In contrast, dogs receiving 2.0 mg/kg/day 6-MP intraarterially developed azotemia secondary to drug-induced nephrotoxicity. During 6-MP infusion, systemic exposure was significantly less in the locally-treated animals than in the systemically-treated dogs. In contrast to intravenous infusion, intraarterial 6-MP delivery dissociated immunosuppressive efficacy from the systemic toxicity of 6-MP.

Based on this work, our laboratory undertook the formulation of local 6-MP controlled-release matrices and studied their efficacy in the rat heterotopic cardiac allograft model. Ethylene vinyl acetate (EVA) matrices were loaded with 20% w/v 6-MP. One-hundred mg 6-MP and 400 mg purified EVA were dissolved in 10 ml methylene chloride and solvent casted in a teflon-coated petridish. Solvent was evaporated in a hood. The matrices formed were of 180-200 μ thickness and were characterized for in vivo release under physiologic conditions in phosphate buffer saline. About 4.2% of the incorporated drug was released over a period of 2 weeks (Fig. 16.4). Each animal received a 200 mg matrix. Local immunosuppression with 6-MP in a controlled-release matrix resulted in a significant survival advantage (mean survival time = 18.2 days; control = 6.9 days, P < 0.001), but unfortunately, survival was also quite good in a remote 6-MP matrix implanted group (mean sur-

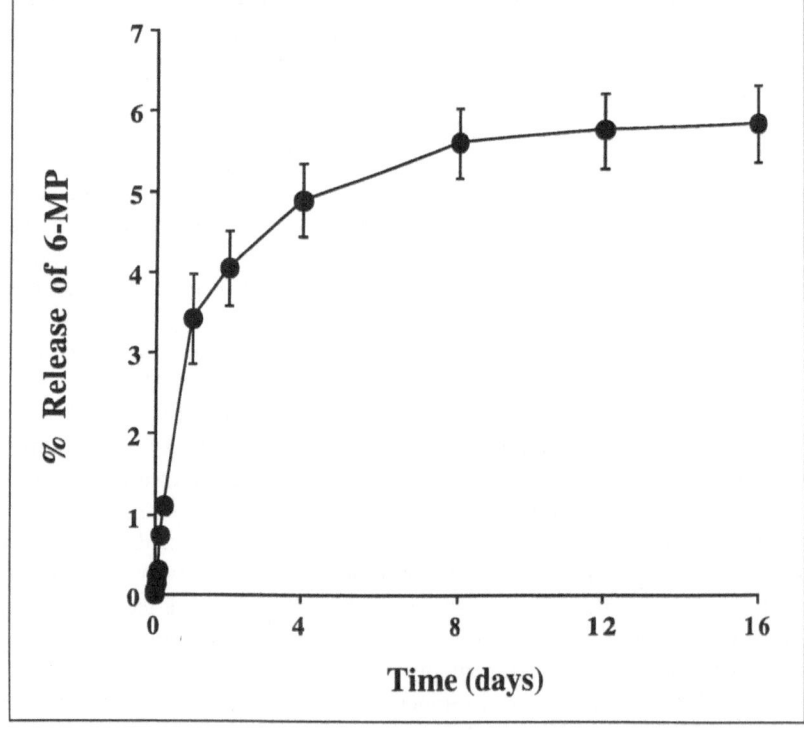

Fig. 16.4. In vitro release curve at pH 7.4 of 6-MP from EVA matrices indicating an initial burst release followed by an exponential declining rate.

vival time = 15.0 days). Thus, at the dose utilized, intragraft drug levels resulting from the distally implanted matrix were adequate to provide effective immunosuppression.

FUTURE PERSPECTIVES

It is conceivable that novel agents more ideally suited for local administration could be developed. For example, one might utilize immunosuppressive agents that would be highly toxic if administered systemically and could not be used except in a regional local-release configuration. Presently, we are undertaking this approach with many chemotherapeutic agents, such as BCNU and auranofin. For example, Gruber and colleagues[19] have recently demonstrated that mizoribine, administered by intraarterial infusion, could delay renal allograft rejection with limited systemic toxicity. A further example of this might include controlled-release systems containing monoclonal antibodies to cytokines, chemokines and adhesion molecules, which have been shown to effectively delay rejection alone[20] or in combination with cyclosporine,[21] but must be administered almost continuously to be effective. Sustained local delivery of monoclonal antibodies is feasible and may be appropriate for controlled-release strategies.

REFERENCES

1. Bolling SF, Putnam JB, Abrams GD et al. Hemodynamics vs. biopsy findings during cardiac transplantation rejection. Ann Thorac Surg 1991; 51:552.
2. Johnston TP, Bove EL, Bolling SF et al. Controlled release of 1-hydroxyethylidene diphosphonate: in vitro assessment and effects on bioprosthetic calcification in sheep tricuspid valve replacements. Int Journal of Pharmacology 1989; 52:139.
3. Sintov A, Scott W, Dick M et al. Cardiac controlled release for arrhythmia therapy: Lidocaine-Polyurethane studies. Journal of Cont Rel 1988; 8:157.
4. Radovsky AS, Van Vleet JF, Stokes KB et al. Paired comparison of steroid eluting and non-steroid endocardial pacemaking leads in

dogs: Electrical performance and morphologic changes. PACE 1988; 11:1085.
5. Olanoff LS, Anderson JM, Jones RD. Sustained release of gentamycin from prosthetic valves. Trans American Society of Art Int Organs 1979; 25:334.
6. Stepkowski SM, Duncan WR. The role of T_{DTH} and Tc populations in organ graft rejection. I: Functional analysis of graft infiltrating T cells. Transplantation 1986; 42:406.
7. Strom TB, Tilney NL, Pardysz JM et al. Cellular components of allograft rejection: Identity, specificity and cytotoxic function of cells infiltrating acutely rejecting allografts. J Immunol 1977; 118:2020.
8. Sprent J, Miller J. Fate of H-2 activated T lymphocytes in syngeneic hosts: II. Residence in recirculating lymphocytes pool and capacity to migrate to allografts. Cell Immunol 1976; 21:303.
9. Bunjes D, Hardt C, Rollinghoff et al. Cyclosporine A mediates immunosuppression of primary cytotoxic T cell responses by impairing the release of interleukin 1 and interleukin 2. European Journal of Immunology 1981; 11:657.
10. Garanelli-Piperno A, Keane M, Steinman RM. Evidence that cyclosporine inhibits cell-mediated immunity primarily at the level of the T lymphocyte rather than the accessory cell. Transplantation 1988; 46:53S.
11. Klebanoff S, Vadas MA, Harlan JM et al. Stimulation of neutrophils by tumor necrosis factor. J Immunol 1986; 136:4220.
12. Ruers TJM, Burman WA, Von Boxtel CJ et al. Immunohistological observations in rat kidney allografts after local steroid administration. Journal of Exp Medicine 1987; 166:1205.
13. Black K, Patel M, Patel A et al. Mechanisms of site specific immunosuppression. Handbook of the International Congress of Transplantation 1990; 54.
14. Bolling SF, Lin H, Ning X et al. Local release polymeric-controlled immunotherapy improves survival of cardiac transplants in rats. J Polymers Adv Tech 1992; 3(6):345.
15. Lin H, Iannettoni MD, Goldblum JR et al. Heterotopic heart transplantation without ischemia or reperfusion. Journal of Heart Transplantation 1990; 9:720.

16. Bolling SF, Lin H, Boyd JA et al. Local cyclosporine immunotherapy improves survival of cardiac transplants in rats. J Hrt Lung Transplant 1991; 10:577.

17. Freise CE, Clemmings S, Clemens LE et al. Demonstration of local immunosuppression with methylprednisolone in the sponge matrix allograft model. Transplantation 1991; 52(2):318.

18. Gruber SA, Hrushesky WJ, Cipolle RJ et al. Local immunosuppression with reduced systemic toxicity in a canine renal allograft model. Transplantation 1989; 48(6):936.

19. Gruber SA, Erdmann GR, Burke BA et al. Mizoribine pharmacokinetics and pharmacodynamics in a canine renal allograft model of local immunosuppression. Transplantation 1992; 53(1):12.

20. Lin H, Chensue SW, Streiter RM et al. Anti-tumor necrosis factor antibody prolongs heart allograft survival in the rat. J Hrt Lung Transplant 1992; 11:330.

21. Bolling SF, Kunkel SL, Lin H. Anti-TNF antibody and cyclosporine combination therapy prolongs cardiac allograft survival in the rat. Transplantation 1992; 53(2):283.

CHAPTER 17

GENE TRANSFER TO THE TRANSPLANTED ORGAN

Jonathan S. Bromberg and LiHui Qin

RATIONALE

Previous chapters detailed approaches in which physical methods are used to direct conventional immunosuppressive molecules to the local environment of the allograft. The advantages and limitations of these methods have been analyzed above. A consistent problem with these approaches is that there are some systemic effects of the immunosuppression, and biocompatible materials and devices are subject to mechanical failure and infection, especially in the immunocompromised host. We have pursued an alternative methodology of gene transfer and gene therapy of the allograft. In this approach, nucleic acids are delivered to the graft by viral vectors or by physical means. The nucleic acids are incorporated into the cells of the graft and direct the transcription of mRNA which is subsequently translated into a protein product. The local delivery of an appropriate vector will determine the local production of an immunosuppressive molecule. Translated protein products can be limited to the cytoplasm, the cell membrane, or secreted in concentrations low enough that physiologically significant systemic levels cannot be achieved. Furthermore, the half-life of most proteins, especially the ones considered relevant for immunosuppression, is very short so that secreted products will likely have negligible systemic effects. Gene transfer and gene therapy may therefore achieve the desired twin goals of local immunosuppression with decreased system i.e., side effects, while avoiding the mechanical and infectious complications of biocompatible materials (Table 17.1).

The elucidation of the structure of the genes and proteins of immunoglobulins, T cell receptors and major histocompatibility complex (MHC) molecules and of how these entities interact with intact or processed antigen demonstrates that there is an enormous amount of variation, heterogeneity and plasticity in the response to a single antigen or a single

MHC or haplotype difference. As a consequence, it currently seems unlikely that true antigen specific immunosuppression for transplantation using techniques such as peptide mimics or antibodies targeted to a single antigen or a particular alloantigenic difference, will be achieved in the near future. Therefore, less specific or nonspecific immunosuppression will still be required to target particular cells, receptors or pathways that are distributed in a nonclonal fashion. This approach can be imbued with a quasi-specificity by targeting only activated lymphocytes or lymphocytes that interact with relevant antigen. This quasi-specificity can be achieved in theory by a gene transfer approach because potent immunosuppressive molecules that would have global effects if administered systemically, will have relatively antigen-specific function when introduced only into the allograft at the site of antigen-specific lymphocyte activation.

Because the primary products of gene therapy are proteins, this technique will allow the delivery of molecules which are not ordinarily deliverable since most proteins tend to be unstable with short half lives, extremely expensive to manufacture and difficult to deliver. Further, the ability to administer protein products with genetic vectors increases the number and types of molecules available for immuno-suppression. Therapy will no longer be limited to small, stable, absorbable molecules that readily cross cell membranes. The proper development and use of vectors, promoters and gene products will permit the delivery of immunosuppressive molecules with exquisite specificity for particular cells, membranes, receptors or ligands.

GENERAL CONSIDERATIONS IN TRANSPLANTATION

The current major limitations of gene transfer and gene therapy (Table 17.2) are that most delivered genes can only be expressed transiently and expression is low or declines rapidly. While this is a major impediment for treating inborn errors of metabolism such as cystic fibrosis, it may be useful or even desirable for the transplant setting. Current notions of immune responsiveness and priming suggest that if costimulatory pathways for T cells and antigen presentation are disrupted at the time of initial antigen encounter, then the entire immune response can be shifted away from responsiveness toward nonresponsiveness, anergy, suppression and tolerance. Therefore the local, transient production of an immunosuppressive molecule may be desirable and extremely useful in this setting. For this reason, gene therapy may also be widely acceptable in therapeutic oncology: the transient expression of an immunostimulatory molecule may engage immunity and result in tumor destruction.

Another significant limitation of gene therapy is that introduced gene products may be immunogenic in the recipient. Using the example of cystic fibrosis, introducing the correct CFTR gene, which differs in a few amino acids from the patient's own defective CFTR, may result in an immune response against the new CFTR gene product. In this case the patient may require systemic immunosuppression to maintain gene expression. In the case of transplantation, inborn errors of metabolism are usually not being corrected and the transferred genes and gene products will be identical to those the individual already possesses. Therefore, there

---

Table 17.1. Rationale for gene therapy for transplantation

Local immunosuppression
Delivery of protein products
Decreased systemic side effects
Avoidance of mechanical and infectious complications
Quasi-antigen specificity

Table 17.2. Limitations of gene therapy

Low expression of gene products
Transient expression of gene products
Immunogenicity of gene transfer product

will be no immune response against the gene product.

EFFECTOR MOLECULES

It is important to consider which general and specific types of genes, and hence gene products, should be delivered to the allograft (Table 17.3). Two major categories of delivered sequences can be defined by the way transcribed and translated products are expressed. First, there are genes coding for products such as cytokines which are secreted from the target cell and therefore will have autocrine, paracrine and perhaps more distant effects, depending on the amount of protein produced. Second, there are genes coding for products which will be limited to the targeted cell. These proteins may be limited to intracellular membranes, extracellular membranes or the cytosol. Depending on the precise function and location of the product, only the targeted cell and other cells with which it directly comes in contact will be altered by the delivered sequences. This second category of genes could potentially encode proteins or anti-sense mRNA to inhibit cellular expression of a particular protein.

Considering the immunological effects of these different categories of transferred sequences, it is apparent that their functional activity will depend on the percentage of cells within the graft transfected by the vector and on the level of expression

Table 17.3. Effector molecules

Transcriptional Products
    Anti-sense RNA
    Sense RNA, translated to protein products

Translational Products
    Secreted, soluble proteins
    IL-10 (vIL-10)
      IL-13
      TGFβ

Target cell limited
    Extracellular membranes
    Intracellular membranes
    Cytosol

per cell. For example, if a gene encoding a soluble, immunosuppressive cytokine is transferred and expressed at a low level in only a small portion of the target cells, this might be adequate for preventing rejection and impeding lymphocyte activation since the entire graft may be "bathed" in the cytokine. In contrast, if a gene encoding anti-sense which disrupts costimulator or MHC expression, or encoding a sense strand which directs the production of an inhibitor of antigen processing or cytokine release, is transferred and expressed at a low level or in only a small portion of the target cells, it is unlikely that lymphocyte priming, activation and effector function can be inhibited. As mentioned above, the major problem with current vectors is the transient, low level expression of transferred genes. Therefore, with current technology genes directing the transcription and translation of secreted products are preferable over cell limited products for the treatment and prophylaxis of rejection. It is possible that future technological developments will change this view.

Soluble cytokines with immunosuppressive properties should therefore be considered the best current candidates for gene therapy of allografts. The current list of candidates includes interleukin-10 (IL-10), IL-13 and transforming growth factor-β (TGFβ). IL-10 was originally described as cytokine synthesis inhibitory factor. It is a T cell derived cytokine which inhibits T cell and antigen presenting cell functions such as cytokine synthesis, MHC class II expression, costimulator receptor expression, cell migration and effector function.[1-3] In addition, IL-10 is pleiotropic, as is true for most cytokines, and possesses costimulatory and proinflammatory activities for T and B cells in some assays.[4,5] These dual properties may limit the usefulness of IL-10. However, the Epstein-Barr virus BCRFI gene encodes a highly homologous protein, termed viral IL-10 (vIL-10), which possesses the inhibitory but not the costimulatory activities of human and murine IL-10.[4] Therefore, vIL-10 is felt to be an appropriate candidate for gene therapy trials. Our initial results (see below) support this notion.

IL-13 is a recently described cytokine produced by activated T cells. It can inhibit a range of monocyte cytokine responses and can suppress experimental autoimmune encephalomyelitis.[6,7] However, it also possesses some costimulatory activity for B cells[8] which may make its use in gene therapy problematic. To date there are no reports of its use in gene transfer experiments in transplantation.

TGFβ is another pleiotropic cytokine produced by many cell types. Many other cells also possess receptors for TGFβ, including leukocytes and organ parenchymal cells, so the immunologic plus nonimmunologic response to TGFβ may be quite complex. TGFβ is secreted as a procytokine, which must be activated by proteolysis in vivo, and is composed of a mixture of three distinct gene products: TGFβ1, β2 and β3. Well defined biological or physiological distinctions among the three variants are not currently known. TGFβ can decrease immunogenicity, inhibit T cell activation and effector function, and prolong allograft survival.[9-11] TGFβ may also protect against ischemic injury,[12] prevent atherosclerosis,[13] and improve tissue healing,[14] which are all important and desirable functions in allografting. Nonetheless TGFβ may also promote excessive fibrosis[14] or activate some T cell and macrophage functions.[15,16] Despite these potential drawbacks, TGFβ

did prolong allograft survival in conventional studies,[9] and our initial results (see below) support its use in gene therapy.

TRANSFER VECTORS

Once a candidate molecule has been selected for therapeutic use in a gene transfer protocol, it is then necessary to determine what vector to use and what other genetic elements to incorporate into the vector to promote expression (e.g., promoters, additional elements to promote genomic incorporation). Table 17.4 lists currently developed vectors and their characteristics.

Plasmid vectors consist of naked plasmid DNA, usually generated in bacteria, which are delivered by a variety of physical means to target cells. As Table 17.4 shows, the advantages of plasmid vectors over viral vectors are the inability to replicate in the host and the lack of immunogenicity since no viral capsid or core proteins are generated. The disadvantage of plasmids is that they are not as efficient as viral vectors in entering cells and directing expression. To date, the best expression of plasmid vectors has been in muscle cells[17] although other tissues have been successfully transfected in vivo.[18,19] Improvements in the expression of plasmid vectors will depend on an increased understanding of the molecular biology of the transfection process and development of improved physical means for plasmid delivery. Incorporation of plasmids into cat-

Table 17.4. Current gene transfer vectors

Vector	Cell Uptake and Expression	Replication Potential	Immunogenicity	Maintenance
Plasmid	±	−	−	Episomal, Genomic
Adenovirus	++	±	+	Episomal
Retrovirus	+	±	±	Genomic
HSV[1]	++	+	+	Episomal
AAV[2]	++	−	±	Genomic
Vaccinia	++	±	+	Episomal

[1] HSV- Herpes simplex virus
[2] AAV- Adeno-associated virus

ionic lipids has improved delivery to a variety of tissues,[20-23] presumably through cell-liposome fusion. Receptor mediated uptake by the asialoglycoprotein receptor of liver cells has been used to direct transfection of the liver.[24,25] This is accomplished by complexing the plasmid DNA with galactosylated poly(L-lysine) or asialo-orosomucoid-poly(L-lysine). This technique has been improved by combining it with the inclusion of replication defective adenovirus which carries adenospecific proteins that disrupt endosomal membranes, thereby increasing the transfer of DNA from the endosomal to the cytoplasmic compartment.[26] An alternative approach has been to complex the DNA with the nonhistone chromosome protein high mobility group 1 (HMG1), to act as a scaffold for DNA structure; liposomes; and Sendai virus, which possesses hemagglutinating activity that promotes liposome-cell fusion.[27-29] These techniques essentially create "artificial viruses" by incorporating ligand, fusion and endosomal escape mechanisms into a large macromolecular complex. An alternative approach is the development of particle bombardment or "gene guns" to physically introduce DNA into cells via accelerated gold particles.[30-33] Such guns are probably of limited value for organ transplants. Once plasmid DNA is successfully introduced into a cell, it is thought to remain episomal in the cytoplasm or nucleus and direct transcription. The molecular biology of episomal maintenance, structure and transcriptional control is currently unknown. However, it is considered likely that inclusion of genetic elements within the plasmid that promote incorporation into genomic DNA may improve its stability and expression.[34]

Viral vectors are derived from intact viruses and have the advantage over plasmid vectors of more readily entering cells and expressing delivered genes. The disadvantages of viral vectors are that they may replicate, carry a variety of immunogenic proteins, carry proteins which cause cytopathic effects unrelated to replication or immunogenicity and direct genomic incor-poration which could result in oncogenic transformation. Adenovirus (the cause of the common cold) is a DNA virus and the most frequently used current vector. It has a large genome which permits the delivery of large genes, and extremely high viral titers (> 10^{10}/ml) can be achieved.[35,36] Adenovectors can infect all cell types which further enhances their value. Problems with adenovectors include a low level of replication potential with currently used viral strains, episomal maintenance of DNA with only low level long term gene expression, viral induced cytopathic effects, and significant immunogenicity, particularly in light of the fact that most people have been exposed to and are serologically positive for adenovirus.

Retrovirus is a small RNA virus that is reverse transcribed upon cell entry and the DNA becomes incorporated into the cell genome. This may be an advantage for persistence of gene expression, but because genomic incorporation is a random event, it may result in oncogenic transformation of the cell. Retroviral vectors have a small potential for replication within the cell, and immunogenicity and cytopathicity are not major problems. However, retroviral vectors are only capable of infecting actively proliferating cells which significantly limits their range and utility.[37]

Herpes simplex virus type I (HSV) is a large DNA virus capable of infecting virtually all cell types and the vector DNA remains episomal.[38] Cytopathic effects and immunogenicity are potential problems. In these respects HSV vectors are similar to adenovectors, but they have not been as thoroughly investigated nor developed since current HSV vectors have significant replication potential and HSV titers are not nearly as high as adenoviral titers. A potential advantage of HSV vectors is that they can accommodate much more DNA than adenovectors and potentially deliver a large multigene complex.

Adeno-associated virus (AAV) is a small DNA virus that requires helper functions supplied by adenovirus or herpes virus. This means that AAV stocks can be generated from helper cells in vitro that supply helper function without contaminating infectious virus particles. AAV stably integrates into a single specific site on chromosome 19, therefore combining the expression advantage of genomic incorporation with markedly less potential for oncogenic transformation.[39] The small size of AAV, however, may limit the types of genes and regulatory sequences transferred. AAV can infect most cell types and cytopathic and immunogenic effects are not considered significant.

Vaccinia virus is a large virus that can infect most cells. Current strains have limited replication potential, and delivered DNA remains episomal.[40,41] A major disadvantage is that virtually all people are immune to vaccinia virus since it serologically cross-reacts with small pox virus. This will probably limit its usefulness in most gene therapy applications, except in oncology where augmented immune responses are desirable.

EXPRESSION

Expression of the transferred gene is the major problem with all current vectors (Table 17.5). It would be most desirable to have regulatable, long term tissue specific expression of the gene product. The current reality is that most expression is of a low level, transient in nature and not regulatable. The issue of genomic versus episomal maintenance was addressed above and it is likely that genomic incorporation will be a more reliable way to achieve long term expression. Use of tissue specific promoters will also likely enhance the level and maintenance of expression[42-45] and may also add a level of regulatory control.[42] However, because current expression levels are low, strong promiscuous (i.e., nonselective) viral promoters have been used in most systems.

The issue of immunogenicity of viral proteins as a result of prior infection or vaccination or as a result of viral replication was also mentioned above. Immune responses to vectors may lead to inflammation in the region of gene transfer. This is obviously an undesirable result in the setting of transplantation. Furthermore the anti-viral immune response may also lead to transfected cell death and place significant limitations on gene expression.[46-49] Improvements in gene expression may require not only improved genetic elements in the vector but also manipulation of anti-vector immune responses. A related issue is that if the transferred gene is not autologous to the recipient then immune responses directed to the gene product may limit its expression. For these reasons plasmid vectors encoding autologous genes are the best current candidates for gene therapy in this setting.

Additional safety issues in the evaluation of vectors concern toxicity of the vector or of the transferred gene product. Direct cytopathic effects of viral proteins or replicative virus or immune mediated damage directed toward a viral vector, may severely limit the usefulness of viral vectors. Similar analyses of plasmid vectors show no evidence for such negative effects.[50,51] This suggests that plasmid vectors will eventually supplant viral vectors unless major changes in the structure of viral vectors are achieved. The transferred gene products may also be immunogenic

---

Table 17.5. Determinants of expression of transferred genes

Maintenance
    Episomal
    Genomic
Promoters
    Tissue-specific
    Regulatable
    Promiscuous
Immunogenicity
    Vector coat proteins
    Recipient prior exposure
    Replicative virus
    Transferred gene product
Cytopathic effects
    Vector coat proteins
    Replicative virus
    Immune response
    Transferred gene product

or directly toxic. No firm evidence currently shows that the immunogenicity of the expressed gene limits expression or results in undesirable inflammatory responses. However, there is evidence that the immunosuppressive cytokine TGFβ, a good potential candidate for gene therapy in allografting, may induce arterial fibrocellular hyperplasia or glomerulosclerosis.[52,53] This suggests that studies of efficacy of gene therapy in any setting will have to include careful analyses of a variety of normal cell functions and structures to exclude the possibility of secondary toxic effects.

EXPERIMENTAL RESULTS

The general approach to gene therapy studies in transplantation requires the selection of a vector and therapeutic gene for transfer. Initial studies should include the use of reporter genes (such as β-galactosidase or luciferase) within the vector and syngeneic transplants to confirm that vector delivered nucleic acids can be transferred and expressed and that these will not be immediately toxic to a functioning, newly transplanted graft. Subsequent studies should then examine the ability of the therapeutic gene to influence allograft survival. If a therapeutic effect is evident, then follow-up studies should evaluate gene expression and the exact immunologic mechanisms of prolonged graft survival to determine ways to improve efficacy. In addition toxicity studies evaluating transformation, fibrosis, necrosis and inflammation are required and should include evaluation of vector effects in vitro on relevant cell types.

We have evaluated several different vectors in a heterotopic, nonvascularized cardiac transplant model. We first showed that both plasmid and viral vectors could express reporter β-galactosidase genes in a myocyte cell line in vitro and in syngeneic transplants in vivo. There were no toxic effects to cells in culture or on indefinite syngeneic graft survival in vivo (Table 17.6).

We next evaluated murine TGFβ1 incorporated into a plasmid vector under the control of the strong, promiscuous viral SV40 promoter (pSVTGFβ1) and viral IL-10 incorporated into a retroviral vector under the control of a retroviral promoter (MFG-vIL-10). The results show that both vectors were able to prolong graft survival[54,55] (Fig. 17.1) while control or inactivated vectors did not. Additional data revealed that the effect was specific and localized since remote injection of vector, or simultaneous transplantation of two grafts only one of which received vector, did not result in prolonged survival of grafts not receiving the vectors (Table 17.7). Serum levels of TGFβ1 or viral IL-10 were not measurable, further confirming the local effect, although local transcription of the transformed genes was demonstrated by polymerase chain reaction amplification and Southern blotting.[54,55] Preliminary studies now suggest that the direct intragraft expression of these cytokines results in decreased priming and/or recruitment of helper and cytotoxic T cells into the graft (not shown).

FUTURE DIRECTIONS

These encouraging initial results suggest that a gene transfer and gene therapy approach to transplantation rejection and tolerance will be feasible and useful. The major challenges involve the development of vectors which will allow long term, high to moderate level, regulatable expression of gene products while diminishing cytopathic, immune and replicative damage caused by vector components. Secondary issues are the determination of immune mechanisms at the cellular and molecular levels.

Table 17.6. Expression of reporter genes in myocytes

Vector	Myocyte In vitro	In vivo
Plasmid	+	+
Retroviral	+	+
Adenoviral	+	+
Herpesviral	+	+

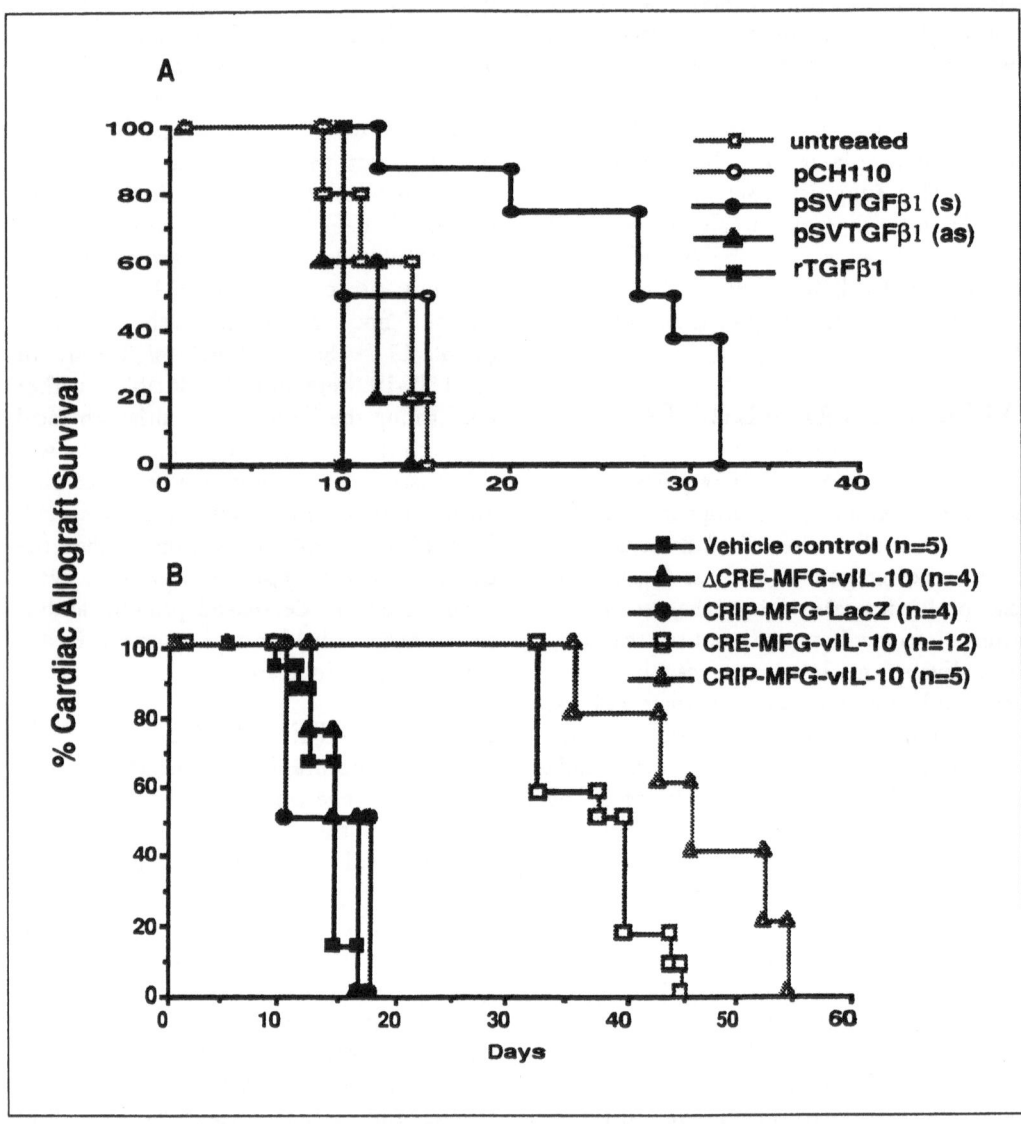

Fig. 17.1. (A) Gene transfection of TGFβ1 prolongs cardiac allograft survival. Donor neonatal C57BL/6 murine hearts were directly injected with 20 μg of the indicated plasmid DNA or 25 pmol of recombinant TGFβ1 protein and transplanted into CBA/J recipients. Survival of cardiac allografts was followed with EKG monitoring. rTGFβ1-recombinant protein; pCH110-control plasmid; pSVTGFβ1(s)-plasmid encoding TGFβ1; pSVTGFβ1(as)-plasmid encoding antisense TGFβ1. (B) Gene transfer of vIL-10 prolongs cardiac allograft survival. Donor C57BL/6 mice neonatal hearts were directly injected with 5000 pfu of the indicated retroviral vector and transplanted into CBA/J recipients. Survival of cardiac allografts was followed with EKG monitoring. Δ-heat inactivated virus; LacZ-virus encoding β-galactosidase; vIL-10-virus encoding viral IL-10; CRE and CRIP designate different packaging cell lines used to generate the retroviral vectors. They result in essentially equivalent vectors with slightly different tropisms for target cells.

Table 17.7. Graft survival in gene transfer

A. TGFβ1 gene transfer induces local immunosuppression

Treatment	Individual Survival Times (d)	MST ± (SE)	P
Untreated	9 ,11 ,14 ,14 ,15	12.6 ± 1.1	–
pSVTGFβ1	12, 20, 27, 27, 29, 32x3	26.3 ± 2.5	< 0.05
Remote injection			
pSVTGFβ1	11, 11, 11, 12, 21	13.2 ± 2.0	–
Double Transplant			
Left: untreated	11 x 5, 16	12.3 ± 0.7	–
Right: pSVTGFβ1	20 x 2, 22, 23 x 3, 29	23.0 ± 1.2	< 0.001

B. vIL-10 gene transfer induces local immunosuppression

Treatment	Individual Survival Times (d)	MST ± SE	P
Untreated	9, 11, 14, 14, 15	12.6 ± 1.1	–
MFG-vIL-10	32(x5), 37, 39(x4), 43, 44	36.7 ± 1.3	< 0.0001
Remote injection			
MFG-vIL-10	12, 12, 12, 14, 14	12.8 ± 0.5	–
Double Transplant			
Left: untreated	10(x2), 12, 13(x2), 15(x2), 17	13.1 ± 0.9	–
Right: MFG-vIL-10	27, 27, 29(x2), 31, 33, 36	30.3 ± 1.2	< 0.01

Remote injection: untreated C57BL/6 donor hearts were transplanted to CBA/J recipients, which were injected intramuscularly in the right thigh with plasmid or virus. Double transplant: two C57BL/6 donor hearts were transplanted into both ears of CBA/J recipients. Left side is the control untreated graft, and the right side is the graft injected with plasmid or virus. d-days. MST ± SE: mean survival time ± standard error. Comparison by Wilcoxon sign rank.

REFERENCES

1. Fiorentino DF, Zlotnik A, Vieira P et al. IL-10 acts on the antigen-presenting cell to inhibit cytokine production by TH1 cells. J Immunol 1991; 146:3444.

2. Jinquan T, Larsen CG, Gesser B et al. Human IL-10 is a chemoattractant for CD8⁺ T lymphocytes and inhibitor of IL-8-induced CD4⁺ T lymphocyte migration. J Immunol 1993; 151:4545.

3. Del Prete G, De Carli M, Almerigogna F et al. Human IL-10 is produced by both type 1 helper (TH1) and type 2 helper (TH2) T cell clones and inhibits their antigen-specific proliferation and cytokine production. J Immunol 1993; 150:353.

4. MacNeil IA, Suda T, Moore KW et al. IL-10, a novel growth cofactor for mature and immature T cells. J Immunol 1990; 145:4167.

5. Ishida H, Muchamuel T, Sakaguchi S et al. Continuous administration of anti-interleukin 10 antibodies delays onset of autoimmunity in NZB/W F¹ Mice. J Exp Med 1994; 179:305.

6. Minty A, Chalon P, Derocq JM et al. Interleukin-13 is a new human lymphokine regulating inflammatory and immune responses. Nature 1993; 362:248.

7. Cash E, Minty A, Ferrara P et al. Macrophage-inactivating IL-13 suppresses experimental autoimmune encephalomyelitis in rats. J Immunol 1994; 153:4258.

8. Zurawsi G, de Vries JE. Interleukin 13 elicits a subset of the activities of its close relative interleukin 4. Stem Cells 1994; 12:169.

9. Carel J, Schrieber RD, Falqui L et al. Transforming growth factor β decreases the immunogenecity of rat islet xenografts (rat

to mouse) and prevents rejection in association with treatment of the recipient with a monoclonal anitbody to interferon γ. Proc Natl Acad Sci (USA) 1990; 87:1591.

10. Wallick SC, Figari IS, Morris RE et al. Immunoregulatory role of transforming growth factor β (TGFβ) in development of killer cells: comparison of active and latent TGFβ1. J Exp Med 1990; 172:1777.

11. Ahuja SS, Paliogianni F, Yamada H et al. Effect of transforming growth factor-β on early and late activation events in human T cells. J Immunol 1993; 150, 3109.

12. Lefer AM, Tsao P, Aoki N et al. Mediation of cardioprotection by transforming growth factor-β. Science 1990; 249:61.

13. Grainger DJ, Kemp PR, Metcalfe JC et al. The serum concentration of active transforming growth factor-β is severely depressed in advanced atherosclerosis. Nature Medicine 1995; 1:74.

14. Border WA, Noble NA. Transforming growth factor β in tissue fibrosis. New Engl J Med 1994; 331:1286.

15. Lee HM, Rich S. Differential activation of CD8 T cells by transforming growth Factor-β1. J Immunol 1993; 151:668.

16. Noble PW, Henson PM, Lucas C et al. Transforming growth factor-β primes macrophages to express inflammatory gene products in response to particulate stimuli by an autocrine/paracrine mechanism. J Immunol 1993; 151:979.

17. Wolff JA, Malone RW, Williams P et al. Direct gene transfer into mouse muscle in vivo. Science 1990; 247:1465.

18. Sikes ML, O'Malley BW, Finegold MJ et al. In vivo gene transfer into rabbit thyroid follicular cells by direct DNA injection. Human Gene Therapy 1994; 5:837.

19. Hickman MA, Malone RW, Lehmann-Bruinsma K et al. Gene expression following direct injection of DNA into liver. Human Gene Therapy 1994; 5:1477.

20. Stribling R, Brunette E, Liggitt D et al. Aerosol gene delivery in vivo. Proc Natl Acad Sci (USA) 1992; 89:112771.

21. Zhu N, Liggit D, Liu Y et al. Systemic gene expression after intravenous DNA delivery into adult mice. Science, 1993; 261:209.

22. Alton EWFW, Middleton PG, Caplen NJ et al. Non-invasive liposome-mediated gene delivery can correct the ion transport defect in cystic fibrosis mutant mice. Nature Genetics, 1993; 5:135.

23. Nabel GJ, Nabel EG, Yang Z et al. Direct gene transger with DNA-liposome complexes in melanoma: Expression, biologic activity, and lack of toxicity in humans. Proc Natl Acad Sci (USA) 1993; 90:113071.

24. Perales JC, Ferkol T, Beegen H et al. Gene transfer in vivo: Sustained expression and regulation of genes introduced into the liver by receptor-targeted uptake. Proc Natl Acad Sci (USA) 1994; 91:4086.

25. Wu GY, Wilson JM, Shalaby F et al. Receptor-mediated gene delivery in vivo. J Biol Chem., 1991; 266:14338.

26. Cristiano RJ, Smith LC, Woo SLC. Hepatic gene therapy: Adenovirus enchancement of receptor-mediated gene delivery and expression in primary hepatocytes. Proc Natl Acad Sci (USA) 1993; 90:2122.

27. Kato K, Nakanishi M, Kaneda Y et al. Expression of hepatitis B virus surface antigen in adult rat liver. J Biol Chem 1991; 266:3361.

28. Tomita N, Higaki J, Morichita R et al. Direct in vivo gene introduction into rat kidney. Biochem Biophys Res Comm 1992; 186:129.

29. Morishita R, Gibbons GH, Ellison KE et al. Single intraluminal delivery of antisense cdc2 kinase and proliferating-cell nuclear antigen oligonucleotides results in chronic inhibition of neointimal hyperplasia. Proc Natl Acad Sci (USA) 1993; 90:8474.

30. Burkholder JK, Decker J, Yang N. Rapid transgene expression in lymphocyte and macrophage primary cultures after particle bombardment-mediated gene transfer. J Immunol Methods 1993; 165:149.

31. Fynan EF, Webster RG, Fuller DH et al. DNA vaccines: Protective immunizations by parenteral, mucosal, and gene-gun inoculations. Proc Natl Acad Sci (USA) 1993; 90:11478.

32. Woffendin C, Yang Z, Udaykumar et al. Nonviral and viral delivery of a human immunodeficiency virus protective gene into primary human T cells. Proc Natl Acad Sci (USA) 1994; 91:11581.

33. Andree C, Swain WF, Page CP et al. In vivo transfer and expression of a human epidermal growth factor gene accelerates wound repair. Proc Natl Acad Sci (USA) 1994; 91:12188.

34. Philip R, Brunette E, Kilinski l et al. Efficient and sustained gene expression in primary T lymphocytes and primary cultured tumor cells mediated by adeno-associated virus plasmid DNA complexed to catioinic liposomes. Molec Cell Biol 1994; 14:2411.

35. Herz J, Gerard RD. Adenovirus-mediated transfer of low density lipoprotein receptor gene acutely accelerates cholestrol clearance in normal mice. Proc Natl Acad Sci (USA) 1994; 90:2812.

36. Grubb BR, Pickles RJ, Ye H et al. Inefficient gene transfer by adenovirus vector to cystic fibrosis airway epithelia of mice and humans. Nature 1994; 371:802.

37. Ferry N, Duplessis O, Houssin D et al. Retroviral-mediated gene transfer into hepatocytes in vivo. Proc Natl Acad Sci (USA) 1991; 88:8377.

38. Kaplitt MG, Kwong AD, Kleopoulos SP et al. Preproenkephalin promoter yields region-specific and long term expression in adult brain after direct in vivo gene transfer via a defective herpes simplex viral vector. Proc Natl Acad Sci (USA) 1994; 91:8979.

39. Flotte TR, Afione SA, Conrad C et al. Stable in vivo expression of the cystic fibrosis transmembrane conductance regulator with an adeno-associated virus vector. Proc Natl Acad Sci (USA) 1993; 90:10613.

40. Ramsay AJ, Kohonen-Corish M. Interleukin-5 expressed by a recombinant virus vector enhances specific mucosal IgA responses in vivo. Eur J Immunol 1993; 23:3141.

41. Ramsay AJ, Husband AJ, Ramshaw IA et al. The role of interleukin-6 in mucosal IgA antibody responses in vivo. Science, 1994; 264:561.

42. Kitsis RN, Buttrick PM, McNally EM et al. Hormonal modulation of gene injected into rat heart in vivo. Proc Natl Acad Sci (USA) 1991; 88:4138.

43. von Harsdorf R, Schott RJ, Shen Y et al. Gene injection into canine myocardium as a useful model for studying gene expression in the heart of large mammals. Circ Res 1993; 72:688.

44. Hafenrichter DG, Ponder KP, Rettinger SD et al. Liver-directed gene therapy: Evaluation of liver specific promoter elements. J Surg Res, 1994; 56:510.

45. Rettinger SD, Kennedy SC, Wu X et al. Liver-directed gene therapy: Quantitative evaluation of promoter elements by using in vivo retroviral transduction. Proc Natl Acad Sci (USA) 1994; 91:1460.

46. Yang Y, Nunes FA, Berencsi K et al. Cellular immunity to viral antigens limits E1-deleted adenoviruses for gene therapy. Proc Natl Acad Sci (USA) 1994; 91:4407.

47. Engelhardt JF, Ye X, Doranz et al. Ablation of E2A in recombinant adenoviruses improves transgene persistence and decreases inflammatory response in mouse liver. Proc Natl Acad Sci (USA) 1994; 91:6196.

48. Yang Y, Nunes FA, Berencsi K et al. Inactivation of E2a in recombinant adenoviruses improves the prospect for gene therapy in cystic fibrosis. Nature Genetics, 1994; 7:362.

49. Yang Y, Ertl HCJ, Wilson JM. MHC class I-restricted cytotoxic T lymphocytes to viral antigens destroy hepatocytes in mice infected with E1-deleted recombinant adenoviruses. Immunity, 1994; 1:433.

50. Stewart MJ, Plautz GE, Del Buono L et al. Gene transfer in vivo with DNA liposome complexes: Safety and acute toxicity in mice. Human Gene Therapy, 1992; 3:267.

51. Nabel EG, Gordon D, Yang Z et al. Gene transfer in vivo with DNA liposome complexes: Lack of autoimmunity and gonadal localization. Human Gene Therapy, 1992; 3:649.

52. Nabel EG, Shum L, Pompili VJ et al. Direct transfer of transforming growth factor β1 gene into arteries stimulates fibrocellular hyperplasia. Proc Natl Acad Sci (USA) 1993; 90:10759.

53. Isaka Y, Fujiwara Y, Ueda N et al. Glomerulosclerosis induced by in vivo transfection of transforming growth factor β or platelet-derived growth factor gene into the rat kidney. J Clin Invest 1993; 92:2597.

54. Qin L, Chavin KD, Ding Y et al. Gene transfer for transplantation: Prolongation of allograft survival with transforming growth factor β1. Ann Surg 1994; 220:508.

55. Qin L, Chavin KD, Ding Y et al. Multiple vectors effectively achieve gene transfer in a murine cardiac transplantation model: Immunosuppression with TGFβ1 or vIL-10. Transplantation, 1995; 59:809.

CHAPTER 18

IMMUNOMODULATION OF ISLET ALLOGRAFTS WITH GENETICALLY MODIFIED MUSCLE CELLS

Ming Yu, A. Alfred Chahine,
Christian Stoeckert and Henry T. Lau

Localized perigraft delivery of immunosuppressive molecules can prolong islet allograft survival. This finding rests on three concepts: (1) immune recognition of an allograft can be modulated at the host-wwwwgraft interface; (2) immunosuppressive molecules can be delivered to the perigraft site by genetic engineering of carrier cells distinct from the islet allograft and (3) cotransplantation of genetically engineered myoblast carrier cells secreting immunosuppressive molecules with pancreatic islet cells can promote islet allograft survival.

IMMUNE RECOGNITION

Transplantation of tissue across strain or species barriers results in rejection of the graft. The basis of this process is immunological and is the result of the recognition by the host of the foreignness of the graft.[1] This foreignness is ascribed to the expression of polymorphic major histocompatibility complex (MHC) molecules by nearly all nucleated cells. The expression of these MHC molecules enables an organism to have an internal map of self and its polymorphism imparts an evolutionary survival advantage. In transplanting foreign tissue, we are disrupting the host internal map of self and in turn initiating the self defensive immunological rejection process. However, through the work of pioneer transplantation immunologists, we know that allogenicity does not always imply immunogenicity. Seminal work by Lafferty and others showed that antigen presenting cells (APCs) residing within the graft are in the main

Local Immunosuppression of Organ Transplants, edited by Scott A. Gruber.
© 1996 R.G. Landes Company.

responsible for the immunogenicity of allografts and that manipulations such as in vitro culture can render endocrine grafts hypoimmunogenic.[2] These investigators described the concept of graft immunogenicity as requiring not only the presentation of alloantigens by APCs, but also the delivery of a costimulatory signal which they believed was an inherent property of APCs residing within the graft. Although the molecular nature of these signals was not elucidated until recently, the concept that inactivation or deletion of APCs within an allograft can attenuate its immunogenicity was an important point of departure for many transplantation experiments.[3-5] Despite the ignorance of the nature of this costimulatory signal, we knew that these APCs were class II antigen positive and UV-radiation sensitive. Such treatment with anti-class II sera and UV irradiation was indeed effective in attenuating islet allograft immunogenicity and permitted prolonged graft survival without further immunosuppression.[6,7] This laid the groundwork for the concept that modulation of the graft alone can attenuate the allogeneic rejection process.

Despite the success in applying this concept of deletion and/or inactivation of APCs to prolong graft survival, it was an obvious over-simplification of in vivo immune activation. There is no question that intragraft APCs play a central, if not a pivotal, role in graft immunogenicity; however, their elimination does not equal rejection-free survival. Currently, we believe that an allograft can trigger host immune response by the direct interaction of graft APCs with host T cells. Additionally, graft antigens can be presented to host T cells indirectly by host APCs.[8] With increasing molecular understanding of T cell-APC interaction, it is now possible to set the stage for direct molecular manipulation of this interface.

APC - T CELL INTERACTIONS

Antigen-specific activation of T cells can be broadly divided into four stages. The first stage involves nonspecific T cell-APC adhesion, which occurs randomly to a lesser or greater degree depending on the activation state of the T cell and APC.[9,10] These interactions are mediated by a large family of adhesion molecules as shown in Figure 18.1. The adhesion receptor:ligand interaction join APC and T cell together permitting the second stage to occur, which is presentation of processed antigen by APC in the context of MHC molecules to the T cell receptor (TCR). At this juncture, it is believed that signals transduced by the TCR complex initiate low level transcription and expression of IL-2 and IL-2 receptor (IL-2R).[11,12] In stage 3, the B7 family of molecules (and other as yet unidentified molecules) on APC delivers the costimulatory signal to its counter receptors CD28 and CTLA4 on T cells.[13] This costimulatory signal significantly up-regulates IL-2 production and IL-2R expression.[14,15] In stage 4, specifically-activated T cell expansion occurs resulting in the expression of a wide variety of activation markers and receptors. Recent work suggests that expression of the B7 counter receptor CTLA4 on activated T cells may actually deliver negative regulatory signals.[16] At this stage, there are many levels of control which can lead to up- or down-regulation of the immune response in addition to elements controlling the divergence of T cells to the T helper 1 (Th1) or T helper 2 (Th2) phenotype.[17]

LEVELS OF INTERVENTION

Within this framework, intervention with antibodies or soluble receptors to each of the molecules involved with adhesion, TCR-antigen/MHC interaction and co-stimulatory signals is now possible.[13] Some of the possible outcomes are listed in Table 18.1. Blockade of APC-T cell adhesion with anti-ICAM-1, anti-LFA-1 and anti-CD2 results in complete abrogation of the T cell's ability to receive signals through its TCR. However, these T cells can respond to subsequent rechallenge after removal of the blocking reagent. In the vascularized heart transplant model in the mouse, prolonged graft survival was

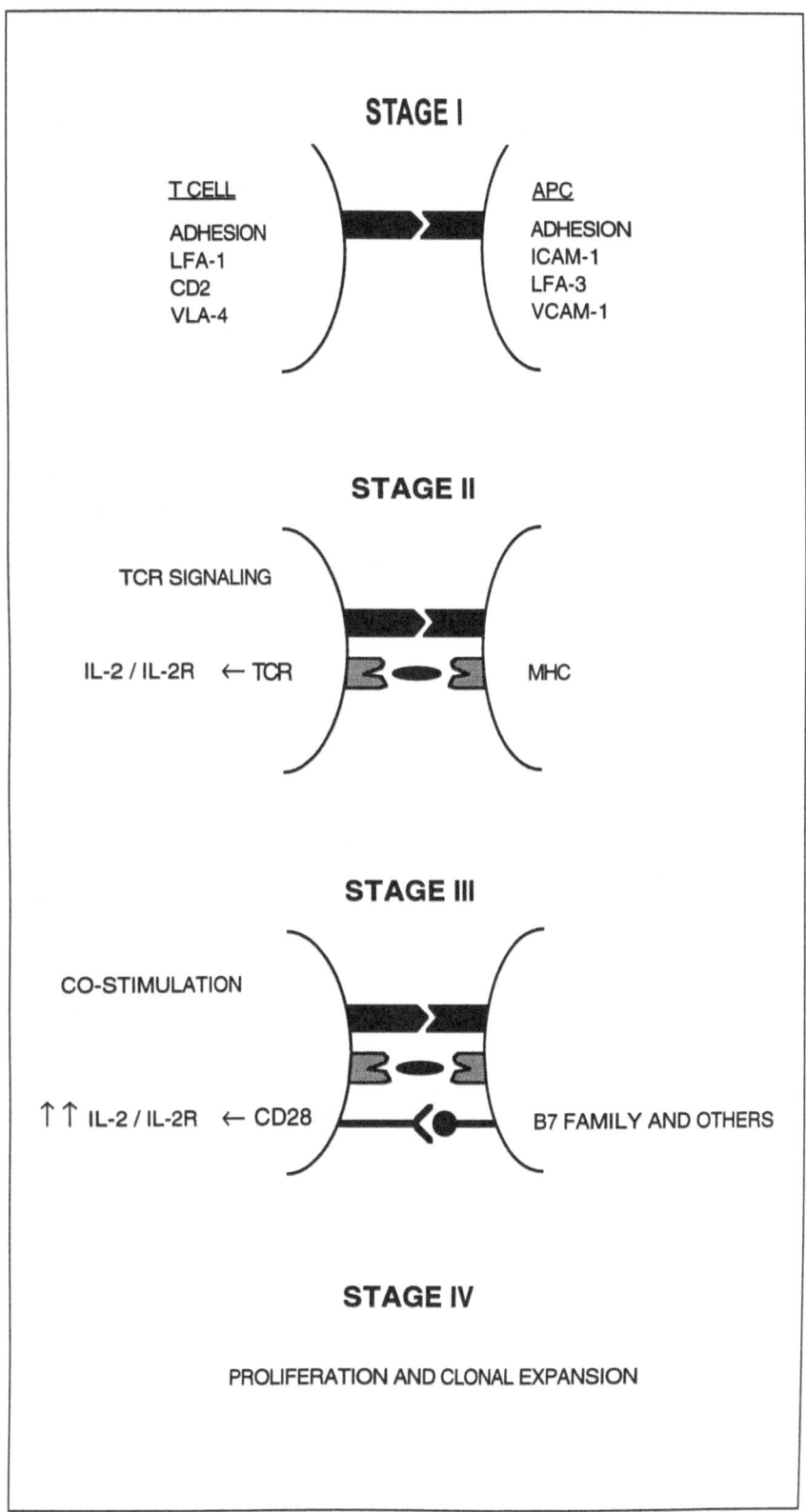

Fig. 18.1. The four stages of T-cell:APC interaction (after Guinan et al.[13])

Table 18.1. Possible outcomes of different blocking reagents on the T-cell activation cascade

Adhesion Blockade Reagents	Possible Outcome		
	Antigen Recognition	Proliferation	Proliferation on Rechallenge

Anti -   ICAM -1
            LFA-1
            LFA-3
            CD2
	-	-	+

TCR blocking reagents Anti- TCR MHC class I/II	-	-	+
Co-stimulatory blocking reagents Anti- B7 CD28 Soluble - CD28Ig/CTLA4Ig	+	-	-

achieved using a combination of antibodies directed at LFA-1 and its counter receptor ICAM-1.[18] Although this approach was very successful in the mouse, similar blockade did not result in such dramatic graft prolongation in the rat.[19] Blockade of T cell receptor signaling either with anti-TCR or anti-MHC antibodies results in abrogation of the T cell response but again does not prevent proliferation upon subsequent rechallenge.[20]

An important dichotomy occurs with the blockade of costimulatory signals. In vitro reagents capable of blocking the B7 family of molecules and its counter receptor CD28 can not only abrogate T cell response, but more importantly, can also result in a state of specific anergy.[21,22] That is, these T cells which have recognized antigen in the context of MHC will be anergic upon subsequent rechallenge with the same antigen. These in vitro findings were in part already demonstrated by success in transplantation of grafts with modulated APCs.[5,6,7] With present molecular understanding of these costimulatory events, it is now possible to directly manipulate the delivery of these costimulatory

signals. During the last 5 years, a large body of experimental evidence has accumulated supporting a major costimulatory role for the B7 family of molecules on APCs and its ligand CD28 on T cells.[13] CTLA4 was cloned from activated T cells with homology to CD28 although its function was not well understood. A fusion molecule incorporating the gamma portion of IgG with the extracytoplasmic portion of CTLA4 (CTLA4Ig) was found to bind all known members of the B7 family of costimulatory molecules.[23] In vitro, CTLA4Ig was able to block delivery of costimulatory signals and effect specific anergy of T cells.[24] When administered in vivo, CTLA4Ig was able to prolong human islet xenograft survival in mice and was moderately effective in prolonging rat heart allograft survival.[25,26]

In reviewing the coordinated cascade of events leading toward T cell activation, it is obvious that there are many control points that may be manipulated to promote allograft survival. With an eye toward local manipulation of this T cell activation cascade, there is evidence to suggest that acute allograft rejection requires a preponderance of T cells of the Th1 phenotype.[17] It has been suggested that if lymphokines attributed to the Th2 phenotype, namely, IL-4 and IL-10, are provided within the milieu of an allograft, then the T cell response may be shifted toward the more allograft-accommodating Th2 phenotype. One of the more powerful controlling elements within the immune activation cascade is transforming growth factor-β (TGFβ). As its name suggests, TGFβ is implicated in a wide variety of functions including embryogenesis, tumor growth, wound healing and control of inflammation and immune responses.[27,28] In vitro, TGFβ is an extremely potent inhibitor of T cell activation; however, in vivo it is also a powerful chemoattractant capable of recruiting monocytes and activating naive immune cells. Yet activated T cells also have increased expression of TGFβ receptor; therefore, TGFβ is not only able to initiate an immune response, but also can keep it in check.[29] Additionally, there is a suggestion that TGFβ given in a local fashion creates a gradient which promotes inflammation and that systemic administration promotes immunosuppression.[30] These attributes make TGFβ an intriguing molecule to use in a local fashion for the control of an allograft reaction.

LOCAL DELIVERY OF IMMUNOSUPPRESSIVE MOLECULES

With this background, we initially hypothesized that if we could deliver high levels of an immunosuppressive molecule, such as CTLA4Ig, in a paracrine fashion to the immediate vicinity of a graft, we might be able to prolong its survival without global immunosuppression. One method would be to directly engineer grafts with the use of viral constructs to secrete recombinant immunosuppressive molecules. There are limitations to this approach in that transfection of end stage cells such as pancreatic islets with retroviral constructs would be ineffective and adenoviral constructs have been shown to allow for only transient expression.[31] Concomitant with the inherent risk of using viruses, there is the problem of host response to viral products that may contribute to decreased efficacy.[32]

Another approach which would preclude genetic manipulation of the graft would be to engineer a carrier cell derived from the host to manufacture recombinant immunosuppressive molecules. In order for this concept to have any potential clinical application, these carrier cells should fulfill the following criteria:

1. Have the potential to be maintained in culture with high cloning efficiency.
2. Be readily transfected with expression vectors.
3. Contain the synthetic machinery necessary to manufacture secretable recombinant protein.
4. Remain nonmalignant.

Muscle cells would appear to fulfill all these criteria. Using the C3H mouse-derived muscle cell line C2C12, it was possible to obtain stable clones transfected with the cDNA for human growth hormone. When these cells were injected into syngeneic mice, they continued to produce detectable levels of human growth hormone for a protracted period of time.[33] More importantly, within the muscle bed injection site, these cells were able to integrate with the native myotubules. More recently, it was shown that primarily derived rat muscle cells can be genetically engineered to secrete dopamine within the brain.[34] It would appear that muscle cells have all the synthetic machinery necessary for the continued expression of recombinant protein in vivo. Of particular importance is the observation that it does not appear to be necessary for these genetically modified muscle cells to be within a muscle bed for their continued survival and synthesis of recombinant protein.

This foundation allowed us to investigate whether muscle cells genetically engineered to produce immunosuppressive molecules can be used as platforms for the delivery of local immunosuppression in a model of islet cell transplantation.

MUSCLE CELLS AS PLATFORMS FOR DELIVERY OF IMMUNOSUPPRESSION

The characteristics of the C3H mouse-derived muscle cell line C2C12 have been well described.[35] It can be grown continuously in culture and will differentiate into fused myotubules in low serum media. Using this prototypical muscle cell line, we initiated our initial transfection experiments with the πLN vector containing the cDNA for murine CTLA4Ig.[36] Additionally, these cells were cotransfected with the plasmid SV2neo containing the neomycin resistance gene which was used as a selectable marker for transfection. G418 resistant clones were initially screened by ELISA specific for the Ig segment of the fusion protein CTLA4Ig. One clone CC15 was selected for further study. In order to ascertain whether the secreted molecule was functional, FACS analysis was used to detect binding of the CTLA4 portion of the fusion molecule to Raji cell lines which are known to express B7 (Fig. 18.2). Additionally, supernatant from the CC15 clone was able to block T cell proliferation in a mixed lymphocyte culture (MLC) (Fig. 18.3). Having obtained the stable muscle cell clone CC15 which produces functional CTLA4Ig, we were now set to perform composite muscle-islet cell transplantation experiments using this clone as carrier cells in the delivery of CTLA4Ig in a paracrine fashion.

In initial experiments, we noted that when the transfected muscle cell clone CC15, which is of H-2^k background, is cotransplanted with syngeneic C3H islets into streptozotocin-induced diabetic allogeneic C57BL/6 mice, no prolongation of islet allograft survival was observed (Table 18.2). However, when the CTLA4Ig secreting muscle cell clone is syngeneic to the diabetic recipient, composite grafting with allogeneic C57BL/6 islets into diabetic C3H mice resulted in prolonged islet allograft survival. Histologically, intact

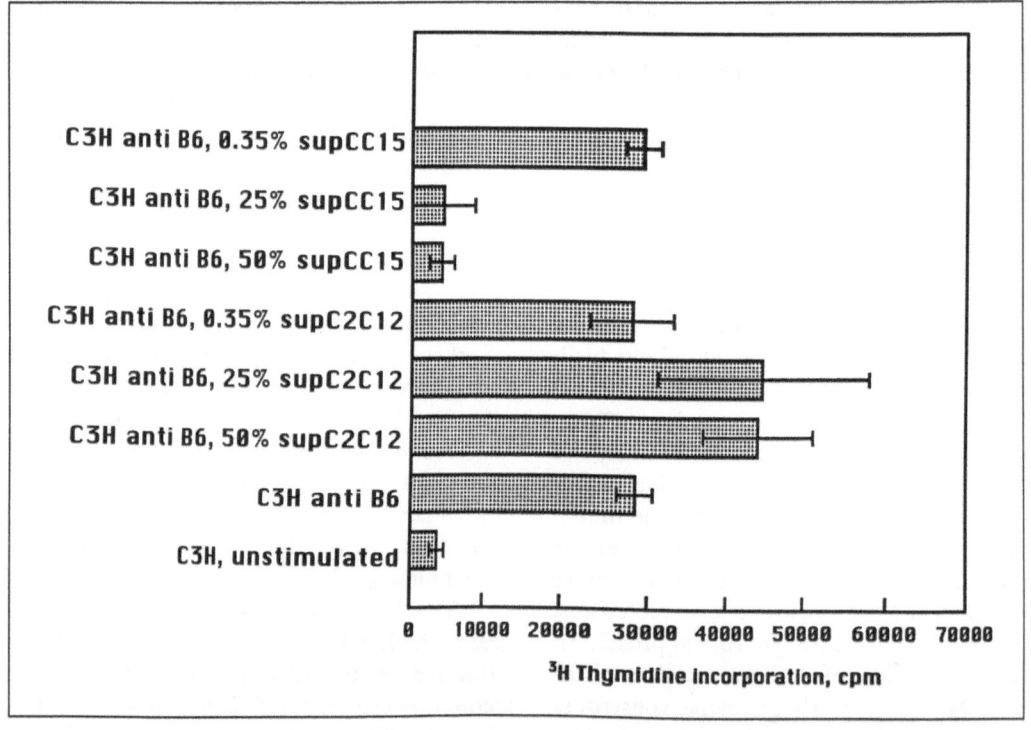

Fig. 18.2. FACS analysis of CTLA4Ig binding to Raji cell line which expresses B7. Panel A, control supernatant from C2C12 cell line. Panel B, supernatant from BAC1 (primary C57BL/6 muscle cell secreting CTLA4Ig). Panel C, supernatant from CC15 cell line.

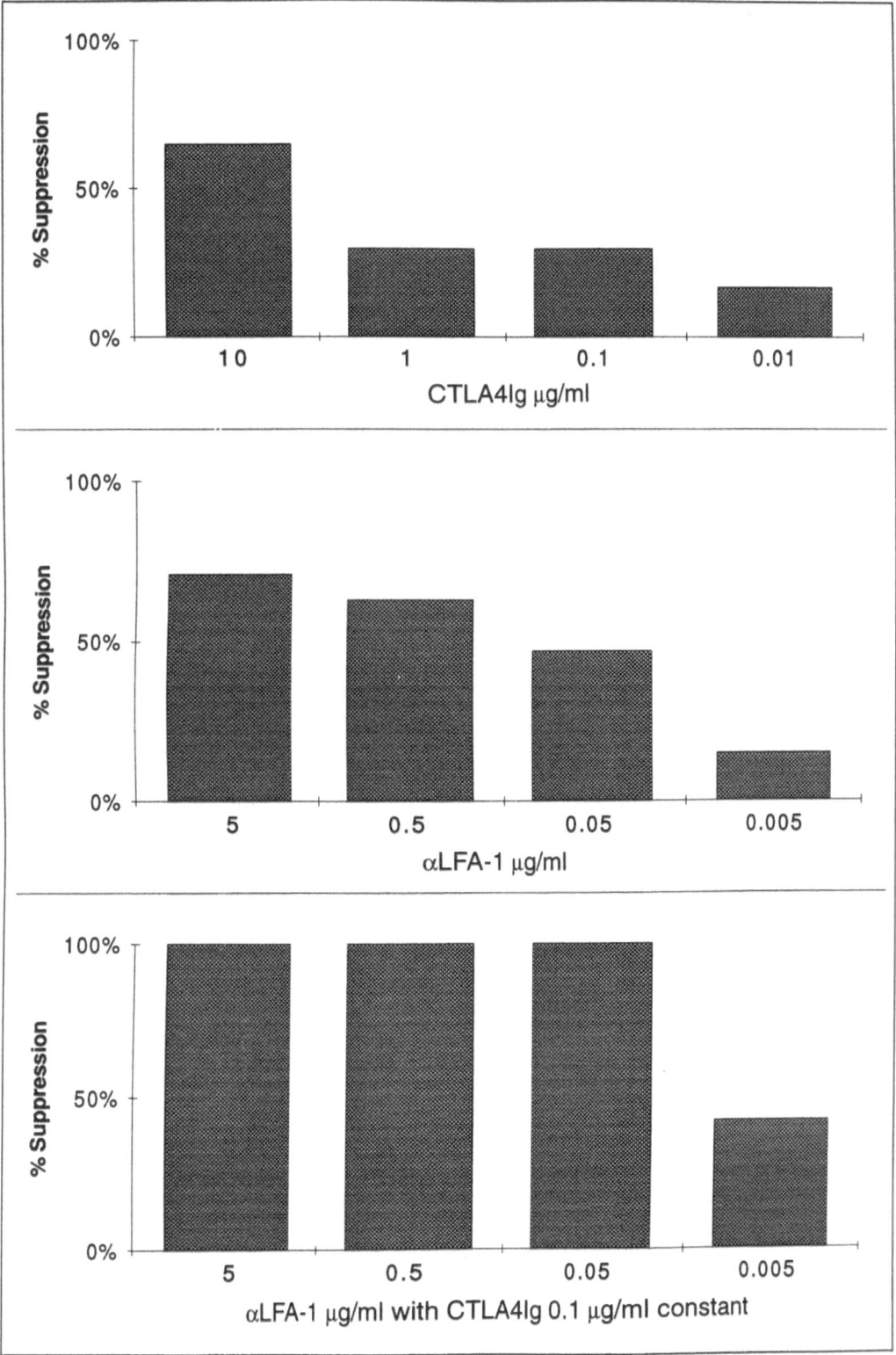

Fig. 18.3. Supernatant from CC15 abrogates an allogeneic MLC. Responder C3H lymphocytes were cultured in triplicate with irradiated C57BL/6 splenocyte stimulators for 4 days. Supernatant from C2C12 (nontransfected cell line) or CC15 (CTLA4Ig-secreting clone) was added as per cent of total culture volume (200 μl).

islets were found under the kidney capsule interspersed amongst muscle cells.

The limited degree of prolongation obtained from this initial series of experiments could be due to multiple factors: (1) inadequate production of CTLA4Ig by the muscle cells; (2) in vivo inactivation of the transfected gene and (3) redundancy of the in vivo alloresponse whereby multiple costimulatory signals are operative. In addressing the last of these possibilities, we ascertained whether blockade of adhesion molecules such as the LFA-1/ICAM-1 receptor/counter receptor pair, which may also act like costimulatory signals, may be synergistic with the use of CTLA4Ig in attenuating the alloimmune response. Using the mouse monoclonal antibody (mAb) M17.4 directed at the LFA-1 molecule, we found that there was synergism with CTLA4Ig in abrogating T cell proliferation in a MLC (Fig. 18.4).

With these results, we reasoned that brief systemic administration of an anti-LFA-1 antibody at the time of composite transplantation of islets with the CC15 clone may be synergistic in promoting islet allograft survival. Table 18.3 lists the results of experiments showing that indeed one dose of anti-LFA-1 in conjunction with cotransplantation of CC15 muscle cells and allogeneic islets can significantly prolong islet graft survival when compared with the singular use of CC15 cells or anti-LFA-1. Under these transplant conditions, the host response to antigenic challenge with KLH was comparable to normal animals, indicating that despite transient systemic administration of anti-LFA-1, it did not result in global immunosuppression. Yet, it was synergistic with local delivery of CTLA4Ig in promoting survival of cotransplanted islet allografts.

PRIMARY MUSCLE CELLS AS PLATFORMS FOR DELIVERY OF IMMUNOSUPPRESSION

In thinking about extending these findings to different strains of mice or animal models, we needed to be able to apply these concepts using primary muscle cells. Intramuscular injection of bupivacaine can result in a large population of myoblasts as a response to injury.[37] This makes adult animals suitable as myoblast donors. In conjunction with the use of basic fibroblast growth factor as a myoblast growth factor,[38] we were able to obtain

---

Table 18.2. Syngeneic CTLA4Ig-secreting muscle cells can prolong survival of islet cell allografts

Composite Graft Left KC	Recipient	Survival (MST) (days)
C3H	B6	8,8,10,11,14,15 (11.0)
C3H/C2C12	B6	8,10,11,11,12 (10.4)
C3H/CC15	B6	8,12,13,13,15x6 (13.6)
B6	C3H	9,10,11,11,12x5 (11.2)
B6/C2C12	C3H	9,11,12,13,14 (11.8)
B6/CC15	C3H	16,17,18,21,22,23,24,40,51,>75 exp. (31.7[a])

5x10⁴ to 5x10⁵ muscle cells (H-2ᵏ) were cotransplanted with fresh islets as a composite graft under the left kidney capsule of diabetic recipients. C57BL/6J (B6)(H-2ᵇ) and C3H/HeJ(C3H)(H-2ᵏ) mice were reciprocally used as donors and recipients. KC, Kidney capsule; MST, mean survival time; C2C12, nontransfected muscle cell line; CC15, CTLA4Ig-secreting clone; exp., expired. [a]P < 0.05 compared with controls.

Fig. 18.4 (opposite). Synergism of CTLA4Ig and anti-LFA-1 mAb M17.4 (αLFA-1) in suppressing an allogeneic MLC. Responder C57BL/6 lymphocytes were cultured with irradiated C3H splenocytes in triplicate for 4 days. CTLA4Ig and mAb M17.4 were added at the beginning of culture.

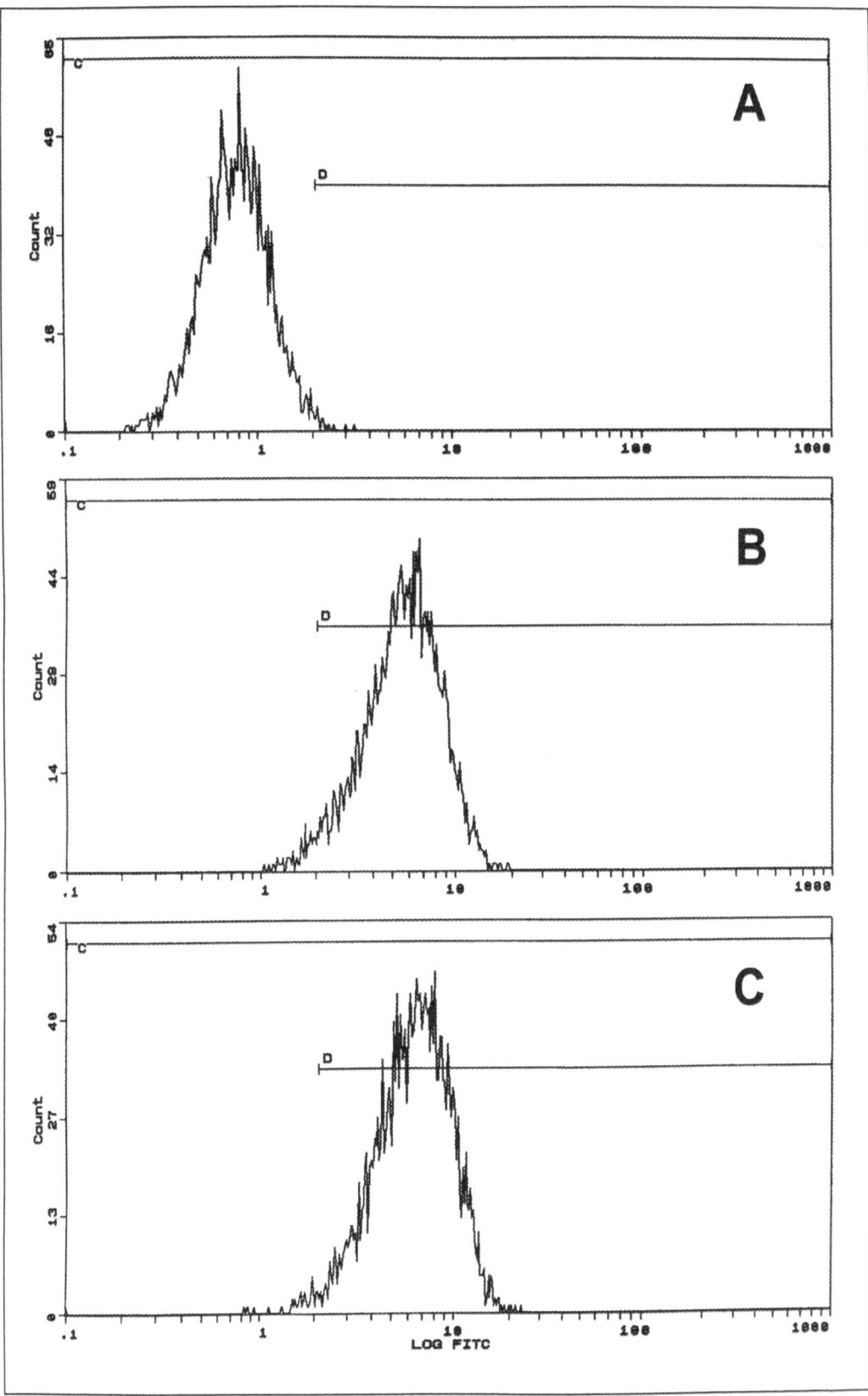

Table 18.3. Anti-LFA-1 is synergistic with local CTLA4Ig in achieving indefinite acceptance of composite islet allografts

Graft	Recipient	mAb	Survival (days)
C3H	B6	M17	10,11,13,13,14,26,43,77,>300
C3H-CC15	B6	M17	9,13,>51 exp,66,>90,>143,>200, >200,>183,>196,>205,>300
C3H	B6	SF1	9,9,12,13,14
C3H-CC15	B6	SF1	9,10,11,11,11,11,13
C3H-CC15	B6	ALS	11,12,12,14,15, 33

mAb SF1 (anti-H2-K^d) and rabbit anti-mouse anti-lymphocyte serum were used as controls.

C57BL/6 mouse myoblast cell lines from adult animals pretreated with bupivacaine. These myoblast cells express desmin and retain the ability to differentiate into myotubules in low serum media. Using this primary muscle cell line designated B6a, we obtained stable transfectants expressing CTLA4Ig designated BAC-1. These cells, like the previously-described CC15, produce biologically active CTLA4Ig (Fig. 18.2). In cotransplantation experiments using the BAC-1 cell line and C3H islets, we were able to promote islet allograft survival in diabetic C57BL/6 recipient mice. Again, the addition of peritransplant administration of anti-LFA-1 antibody was synergistic.

Having defined the optimal conditions for growth and transfection efficiency of primary mouse muscle cells, we are exploring whether other immunosuppressive molecules may be delivered in a similar manner. TGFβ, a pleiotrophic cytokine, is a powerful immunosuppressant in addition to its many other functions in modulating wound healing and inflammation. In the use of this immunosuppressive molecule, timing of administration may be a key factor in creating a local immunosuppressive environment. Using the pPK9a plasmid, which contains the cDNA of a mutant TGFβ under control of the zinc-sensitive metallothionein promoter, we have obtained stable muscle cell transfectants expressing biologically active TGFβ.[39] With the ability to control the promoter with zinc, it is possible to control the delivery of this recombinant immunosuppressive molecule in a temporal fashion. With TGFβ, a level of intervention can be pursued distinct from CTLA4Ig and anti-LFA-1. Combining these approaches may lead to the most effective local immunosuppression.

CONCLUSION

With the continued molecular description of immune activation, it is now possible to block selected and successive steps in the rejection cascade. We propose that it is possible to deliver recombinant immunosuppressive molecules by genetically engineering recipient type muscle cells such that they become carrier cells for the production of recombinant protein. The additional advantage would be that these cells would not be immunogenic since they are syngeneic to the host. Such genetically-engineered muscle cells, when cotransplanted with an islet allograft, can serve as platforms for the local delivery of immunosuppressive molecules. Besides the obvious goals of promoting allograft survival by the use of this technique, this concept allows us to manipulate an immunogenic environment locally as a means of further understanding immune activation.

References

1. Klein J. Immunology, The science of self-nonself discrimination. New York: Wiley, 1982.
2. Lafferty KJ, Prowse SJ, Simeonovie CJ. Immunology of tissue transplantation: a

return to the passenger leukocyte concept. Ann Rev Immunol 1983; 1:143.

3. LaRosa FG, Talmage DW. The abrogation of thyroid allograft rejection by culture in acid medium. Transplantation 1987; 44(4):592.

4. LaRosa FG, Talmage DW. The failure of a major histocompatibility antigen to stimulate a thyroid allograft reaction after culture in oxygen. J Exp Med 1983; 157:898.

5. Lechler RI, Batchelor JR. Restoration of immunogenicity to passenger cell-depleted kidney allografts by the addition of donor strain dendritic cells. J Exp Med 1982; 155:31.

6. Lau H, Reemtsma K, Hardy MA. Prolongation of rat islet allograft survival by direct ultraviolet irradiation of the graft. Science 1984; 223:607.

7. Faustman D, Hauptfeld V, Lacy P et al. Prolongation of murine islet allograft survival by pre-treatment of islets with antibody directed to Ia determinants. Proc Natl Acad Sci USA 1981; 78(8):5156.

8. Shoskes DA, Wood KJ. Indirect presentation of MHC antigens in transplantation. Immunol Today 1994; 15:32.

9. Van Seventer GA, Shimizu Y, Horgan KJ et al. The LFA-1 ligand ICAM-1 provides an important co-stimulatory signal for T cell receptor-mediated activation of resting T cells. J Immunol 1990; 144:4579.

10. Damle NK, Klussman K, Linsley PS et al. Differential co-stimulatory effects of adhesion molecules B7, ICAM-1, LFA-3, and VCAM-1 on resting and antigen-primed CD4+ T lymphocytes. J Immunol 1992; 148:1985.

11. Nishizuka Y. Intracellular signaling by hydrolysis of phospholipids and activation of protein kinase C. Science 1992; 258:607.

12. O'Keefe SJ, Tamura J, Kincaid RL et al. FK-506 and CsA-sensitive activation of the interleukin-2 promoter by calcineurin. Nature 1992; 357:692.

13. Guinan EC, Gribben JG, Boussiotis VA et al. Pivotal role of the B7:CD28 pathway in transplantation tolerance and tumor immunity. Blood 1994; 84(10):3261.

14. June CH, Ledbetter JA, Linsley PS et al. Role of the CD28 receptor in T cell activation. Immunol Today 1990; 11:211.

15. Gimmi CD, Freeman GJ, Bribben JG et al. B cell surface antigen B7 provides a co-stimulatory signal that induces T cells to proliferate and secrete interleukin 2. Proc Natl Acad Sci USA 1991; 88:6575.

16. Walunas TL, Lenschow DJ, Bakker CY et al. CTLA-4 can function as a negative regulator of T cell activation. Immunity 1994; 1:405.

17. Kelso A. Th1 and Th2 subsets: paradigms lost? Immunol Today 1995; 16(8):374.

18. Isobe M, Yagita H, Okumura K et al. Specific acceptance of cardiac allograft after treatment with antibodies to ICAM-1 and LFA-1. Science 1992; 225:1125.

19. Paul LC, Davidoff A, Benediktsson H et al. The efficacy of LFA-1 and VLA-4 antibody treatment in rat vascularized cardiac allograft rejection. Transplantation 1993; 55(5):1196.

20. Burlingham WJ. Prospects for anti-idiotype therapy in transplantation. In: Burlingham WJ, ed. Monoclonal antibody therapy in transplantation. Boca Raton: CRC, 1992: 101.

21. Schwartz RH. T cell anergy. Sci Am 1993; 269:62.

22. Schwartz RH. Co-stimulation of T lymphocytes: The role of CD28, CTLA-4, and B7/BB1 in interleukin-2 production and immunotherapy. Cell 1992; 71:1065.

23. Linsley PS, Brady W, Urnes M et al. CTLA-4 is a second receptor for the B cell activation antigen B7. J Exp Med 1991; 174:561.

24. Tan P, Anasetti C, Hansen JA et al. Induction of alloantigen-specific hyporesponsiveness in human T lymphocytes by blocking interaction of CD28 with its natural ligand B7/BB1. J Exp Med 1993; 177:165.

25. Lenschow DJ, Zeng Y, Thistlethwaite JR et al. Long-term survival of xenogeneic pancreatic islet grafts induced by CTLA4Ig. Science 1992; 257:789.

26. Turka LA, Linsley PS, Lin H et al. T cell activation by the CD28 ligand B7 is required for cardiac allograft rejection in vivo. Proc Natl Acad Sci USA 1992; 89:11102.

27. Wahl SM. Transforming growth factor beta (TGF-β) in inflammation: a cause and a cure. J Clin Immunol 1992; 12(2):61.

28. Roberts AB, Sporn MB. Physiological actions and clinical applications of transforming growth factor-β (TGF-β). Growth Factors 1993; 8:1.

29. Kehrl JH, Wakefield LM, Roberts AB et al. Production of transforming growth factor β by human T lymphocytes and its potential role in the regulation of T cell growth. J Exp Med 1986; 163:1037.

30. Wahl SM, Allen JB, Costa GL et al. Reversal of acute and chronic synovial inflammation by anti-transforming growth factor-β. J Exp Med 1993; 177:225.

31. Simon RH, Engelhardt JF, Yan Y et al. Adenovirus-mediated transfer of the CFTR gene to lung of nonhuman primates: toxicity study. Hum Gene Ther 1993; 4:771.

32. Yang Y, Nunes FA, Berencsi K et al. Inactivation of E2a in recombinant adenoviruses improves the prospect for gene therapy in cystic fibrosis. Nature Genet 1993; 7:362.

33. Barr E, Leiden JM. Systemic delivery of recombinant proteins by genetically modified myoblasts. Science 1991; 254:1507.

34. Jiao S, Gurevich V, Wolff JA. Long-term correction of rat model of Parkinson's disease by gene therapy. Nature 1993; 362:450.

35. Koh GY, Klug MG, Soonpaa MH et al. Differentiation and long-term survival of C2C12 myoblast grafts in heart. J Clin Invest 1993; 92:1548.

36. Chahine AA, Yu M, McKernan MM et al. Immunomodulation of pancreatic islet allografts in mice with CTLA4Ig-secreting muscle cells. Transplantation 1995; 59:1313.

37. Cantini M, Massimino ML, Catani C et al. Gene transfer into satellite cell from regenerating muscle: Bupivacaine allows β-gal transfection and expression in vitro and in vivo. In Vitro Cell Dev Biol 1994; 30A:131.

38. Rando TA, Blau HM. Primary mouse myoblast purification, characterization and transplantation for cell mediated gene therapy. J Cell Biol 1994; 125:1275.

39. Koh GY, Kim SJ, King MG et al. Targeted expression of transforming growth factor β1 in intracardiac grafts promotes vascular endothelial cell DNA synthesis. J Clin Invest 1995; 95:114.

CHAPTER 19

SERTOLI CELLS IN ISLET TRANSPLANTATION: TESTICULAR IMMUNE PRIVILEGE

Helena P. Selawry

The transplantation of pancreatic islets is the most physiologic and desirable form of therapy for establishment of normoglycemia and prevention of complications in the diabetic patient. In rodents, long-term survival of islet allo- and even xenografts can be achieved with a high degree of success.[1-6] The promising results reported in rodents were met with optimism and enthusiasm, and advances toward clinical application of islet transplantation were predicted at regular intervals. Unfortunately, successful islet transplantation in larger animals, and in particular, in humans, has been extremely difficult to accomplish. Some of the most disappointing results were in canine recipients, who initially showed signs of excellent isograft function with complete normalization of blood glucose levels, only to relapse after an interval of about 2 years.[7]

High failure rates of islet transplantation in higher animals have been attributed to various causes, including detrimental effects of immunosuppressive drugs such as cyclosporine (CsA) on islet revascularization,[8,9] grafting of unpurified islet cell preparations contaminated with exocrine tissue,[10] inability to rid islet cells of highly immunogenic passenger leukocytes resulting in a rejection response to alloantigens,[11] loss of function of grafted islets caused by agents such as lymphokines, free oxygen radicals and higher levels of immunosuppressive agents within the portal system[12] and grafting of insufficient quantities of islet cells.[13] It is generally accepted, though, that islet allogenicity is the single most important obstacle to successful clinical islet transplantation.[11]

Thus, a critical need exists for evaluation of novel methods of immunosuppression developed explicitly for prevention of rejection of islet cells. A potentially very promising method is the local delivery of immunosuppressive agents directly at the graft site.[14] Such agents can be relatively nontoxic to the host and selected not to interfere with beta cell function.

THE ABDOMINAL TESTIS AND ISLET ALLOGRAFT SURVIVAL

In our laboratory, we started exploring techniques which would avoid the use of toxic immunosuppressive drugs about ten years ago. The first series of experiments were designed to identify an ideal organ site for implantation of islet cells. It was felt that such an organ site should provide the graft with an abundance of blood supply and with all of its nutritional needs. If possible, the site should also "hide" the grafted cells from the immune response of the host.[15] Several different organ sites were considered, including immunologically privileged sites such as the brain, eye and testis. It was known since the early part of this century that the testis, in particular, is an immunologically privileged site. Greene[16] demonstrated in an elegant series of experiments that human breast tumor cells survived for extended periods in the testes of guinea pigs.

Our first study was designed to test comparative survival of islets of ACI donor rats in various organ sites in major histocompatibility complex (MHC)-incompatible Wistar-Lewis (W-L) hosts.[17] The islets were isolated from ACI rats and incubated for 4 days at 37°C. W-L rats were made diabetic by means of a single intravenous (i.v.) injection of streptozotocin. Islets were injected into three different organ sites: the testis, in its original scrotal position, the liver and the renal subcapsular space. The rats were not immunosuppressed. The results were disappointing: Average duration of normoglycemia in all three groups of rats did not exceed 3 days, suggesting very rapid immune destruction of the grafted cells.

In the next series of experiments, the grafted testes were surgically translocated into the abdominal cavity immediately following injection of islets. Our rationale was that in the mammal, the lower scrotal temperature of 33°C-34°C is essential for sperm cell differentiation but not necessarily optimal for beta cell function. The results were remarkable: Five of six rats treated in this manner became normoglycemic within 24 hours and remained so until the end of the study (300 days). Surgical removal of grafted testes even after a year of transplantation resulted in rapid reversal to hyperglycemia within 24 hours. Microscopic examination of islet allografts revealed the presence of viable and well granulated beta, alpha and delta cells.

The early success achieved in rats with chemically-induced diabetes prompted studies of the transplant technique in BB/Wor dp rats, an animal model with autoimmune diabetes. The critical question was whether islets grafted into the abdominal testis would also be protected from recurrence of the original disease process. It had been previously shown that islets grafted into conventional sites in the BB/Wor dp rat were extremely susceptible to immune destruction.[18]

The approach used was to isolate islets from several different strains of rats, including ACI, W-L, Fisher and Sprague-Dawley (S-D) and to incubate the cells for 4 days at 37°C.[19] No attempt was made to remove passenger leukocytes. Fifteen BB/Wor dp rats with duration of hyperglycemia varying between 13 and 145 days were grafted with mixtures of cultured islets into the abdominal testis. Postoperatively, they were given four injections of antilymphocyte serum (ALS) at weekly intervals. Insulin injections were stopped a day before transplantation. A control group of 14 rats was given intratesticular islet allografts with testes in their original scrotal position and four injections of ALS postoperatively.

The results showed that 13 of 15 rats in the experimental group with abdominal intratesticular islet allografts became normoglycemic within 48 hours and remained so in excess of 65 days. Only 1 of 14 control rats became normoglycemic for a total of 42 days when it reverted to hyperglycemia. Of particular interest was the finding that translocation of grafted testes from the scrotal location into the abdominal cavity on days 5 through 12 following implantation of islets led to prompt reversal to normoglycemia. Microscopic examination of grafted testes on days 130, 132 and 215 following transplantation revealed some interesting findings. The most consistent of these was the location of the grafts; a mass of viable endocrine cells was found always in close association with atrophic seminiferous tubules. The interstitial areas showed evidence of extensive new vascularization, large Leydig cells and no evidence of an inflammatory reaction.

Besides the histologic appearance, there were several other aspects of allograft survival in the BB/Wor dp rat which were unexpected and unusual. Intratesticular allograft survival was independent of the duration of diabetes at the time of transplantation. In contrast, rats with diabetes of prolonged duration were shown to be more amenable to grafting than acutely ill animals, the reason being that the autoimmune disease process apparently diminishes in intensity with time.[18] Furthermore, the source of islets appeared irrelevant to the outcome of the grafts. Thus, mixtures of islets from several donor strains were used to transplant the rats. Islet allograft acceptance was thus independent of the degree of histoincompatibility between different rat strains.

Despite excellent graft survival, we observed that the grafted rats, albeit normoglycemic, remained susceptible to upper respiratory infections. Susceptibility to bacterial and mycoplasmic infections in these rats was postulated to have been caused by defective T cell dependent immune responses characteristic of the BB/Wor dp rat,[20] including marked lymphopenia.[21] The altered T cell-mediated immunity was shown to precede the onset of hyperglycemia and was apparently not caused by metabolic derangements associated with diabetes. Our studies were in agreement with these theories, and clearly showed that long-term reversal of the diabetic process by means of islet transplantation did not restore to normal the abnormal immune effector cells.

In a follow-up study, we showed that islets obtained from MHC-compatible diabetes-resistant donors were likewise not destroyed when grafted into the abdominal testis of acutely diabetic BB/Wor dp rats.[22] Identical results were obtained whether freshly isolated or incubated islets were used as a source of transplantation material. Heavy contamination with passenger leukocytes thus had no effect on graft survival. The BB/Wor dp rats were not immunosuppressed. Grafted rats became insulin independent within 24 to 48 hours, suggesting excellent beta cell function within the testicular environment.

Taken together, the above two studies showed, for the first time, that it was feasible to protect both MHC-compatible and -incompatible islet grafts from autoimmune destruction in an experimental animal with typical insulin-dependent diabetes without maintenance immunosuppression.

ABDOMINAL INTRATESTICULAR ISLET XENOGRAFT SURVIVAL

The question asked next was whether the abdominal testis was also a suitable organ site for transplantation of xenogeneic islets. The plan was to examine survival of islets of hamster donors in the abdominal testes of three different strains of rats: BB/Wor dp rats with diabetes of spontaneous onset and two other strains of rats with streptozotocin-induced diabetes: ACI and W-L.[23] Islets were isolated from hamster donors and cultured briefly at 37°C. No attempt was made to remove passenger leukocytes. Some of the grafted rats were immunosuppressed with ALS, while others were treated with CsA for 30 days following transplantation. All therapy was then stopped.

The results showed that all rats treated with ALS remained diabetic, while 74% of those treated with CsA became normoglycemic within 24 to 48 hours following transplantation. With cessation of CsA, the ACI and W-L rats remained normoglycemic for a mean of more than 130 days. In contrast, BB/Wor dp rats reverted to diabetes within 2 days following withdrawal of CsA.

We postulated that extended survival of abdominal, intratesticular, islet xenografts in ACI and W-L rats following withdrawal of immunosuppression may have been due to development of unresponsiveness to the transplants. Graft survival in the presence of CsA was shown to lead to a state referred to as "CsA-induced tolerance".[24] This tolerance involves generation or programming of antigen-specific suppressor cells, which in turn was shown to require a normally functioning thymus.[25] ACI and W-L rats are immunocompetent, while BB/Wor rats are not.[20] Georgiou et al[26] provided evidence that T-lymphocyte dysfunctions in the BB/Wor dp rat are caused by a thymus-derived defect. Therefore, we concluded that the thymus-derived defect of the BB/Wor dp rats prevented production of suppressor cells that would maintain a state of tolerance. Overall, the data suggested that the abdominal testes also offered a highly physiologic environment for prolonged survival of concordant islet xenografts. Furthermore, extended survival of xenografts allowed development of a state of tolerance. Most impressively, this state of tolerance was sustained after withdrawal of immunosuppression in rats with normal thymic function.

While tolerance was an attractive explanation for extended survival of islets of hamster donors in ACI and W-L recipients following cessation of immunotherapy, it had to be demonstrated. A group of 15 rats with established intratesticular islet xenografts in excess of 200 days was therefore studied.[27] Normoglycemic rats were divided into three groups and challenged with a secondary islet xenograft of hamster donors injected either into the liver, renal subcapsular space, or into the contralateral testis. The controls consisted of three groups of diabetic rats who were similarly grafted with primary rather than with secondary islet xenografts. Controls became normoglycemic only briefly for periods not exceeding 12 days. In contrast, secondary islet xenografts survived much longer; in the contralateral testis for a mean ± SE of > 99 ± 26 days, in the liver for a mean of > 48 ± 11 days and in the renal subcapsular space for a mean of 22 ± 6 days. The observation that secondary islet xenografts survived in some instances for longer than 100 days in rats who did not require maintenance immunosuppression strongly supported the contention that they had developed systemic tolerance.

We then asked whether "systemic tolerance" could be adoptively transferred. In order to accomplish this goal, a total of 26 ACI rats were made diabetic and 22 of 26 were then treated with a monoclonal antibody (mAb) directed against all T-lymphocytes, OX-19, for 10 days. Treatment was then stopped. The rats were divided into five treatment groups as follows: Group 1 consisted of four control rats who received no therapy except for intratesticular transplantation of islets of hamster origin. Group 2 consisted of four rats who received only OX-19 and who were then grafted with islets of hamster origin. Group 3 consisted of five rats who were pretreated with OX-19, then given an i.v. injection of 50 million splenic lymphocytes obtained from normal, nondiabetic ACI rats and then transplanted similarly with hamster islets. Group 4 consisted of five rats who were pretreated with OX-19, then given an i.v. injection of lymphocytes isolated from ACI rats that had rejected their islet xenografts and then also grafted with hamster islets. Group 5 consisted of eight rats who were pretreated with OX-19, injected with lymphocytes obtained from ACI rats with established islet xenografts of longer than 200 days and then grafted with hamster donors. None of the rats received any other immunosuppression. Duration of normoglycemia was closely monitored in the five groups of rats. The results showed that of the five groups, only those rats pretreated with a combination of OX-19 mAb and lymphocytes harvested from rats with established islet xenografts became normoglycemic for a mean ± SE of 166 ± 31 days. The mean ± SE survival of grafts in groups 1, 2, 3 and 4 was: 8 ± 1, 31 ± 12 , 18 ± 2 and 13 ± 5 days, respectively. The data clearly showed that only lymphocyte populations obtained from rats with established islet xenografts were able to promote graft acceptance in naive hosts, a critical test for demonstration of "tolerance". Identification of the subset of T cells responsible for adoptive transfer of tolerance awaits further investigation (Selawry, H., unpublished observations).

MECHANISM OF TESTICULAR IMMUNE PRIVILEGE

The mechanism(s) of testicular immune privilege had not been previously elucidated. In contrast, much is known about testicular morphology and function.[28] The so-called blood-testis barrier consists of occluding junctions that join adjacent Sertoli cells. This barrier provides a unique environment within the lumen of seminiferous tubules for developing sperm cells. The intercellular junctions form an impermeable barrier to blood-borne agents which may be damaging to spermatogenesis. Mature sperm cells are ejected into the adluminal compartment of the seminiferous tubule, where they are prevented from eliciting an immune response by factors produced by Sertoli cells. The interstitial compartment, in contrast, is exposed to the extracellular fluid and is not protected from the immune response of the host. The Leydig cell is the major cell found in this compartment and is responsible for the synthesis of testosterone. An abundance of macrophages, plasma cells and T- and B-lymphocytes is also found within the interstitial compartment. Thus, the protection of testis autoantigens from the immune system can be explained by their isolation in the immunologically-safe side of the

blood-testis barrier. Protection from antigens that reside on the vascular side of the blood-testis barrier is not understood.

Taking the above into account, the location of intratesticular islet grafts was one of the most surprising findings. The grafts were not located within the adluminal compartment, where one would have expected them to be, but rather within the interstitial compartment. Some of the other characteristics of grafted islets located within the interstitium were: (1) Whereas the graft prior to injection consisted of a suspension of individual islets, the in vivo graft formed a single mass of islet cells in which all three cell types were preserved; (2) The beta cells were unusually well granulated within 14 days; (3) There was evidence of angiogenesis within the graft; (4) The mass of islets was always adjacent to, and very closely associated with, atrophic seminiferous tubules and (5) There was a near total absence of an inflammatory reaction or infiltrating lymphocytes within the graft or within the interstitium (Figs. 19.1, 19.2 and 19.3).

The absence of a lymphocytic reaction was difficult to explain in view of the fact that the testis has an excellent lymphatic drainage system.[29] Antigens grafted into the testis stimulate both humoral and cellular immune responses, indicating the presence of an intact afferent limb of the immune response.[30] Evidence for an intact efferent limb was provided by the demonstration that intratesticular islet allografts are susceptible to immunologic destruction in presensitized recipients.[31] These studies led to the hypothesis that local factors produced within the testis might be responsible for the inhibition of the immune response. Head and Billingham[32] investigated the effects of testosterone production on parathyroid allograft survival in the testis. In rats with intact Leydig cell function, graft survival was prolonged. On the other hand, functional survival of parathyroid glands was impaired in rats pretreated with estrogen, which lowered serum testosterone levels. The concentration of testicular tes-

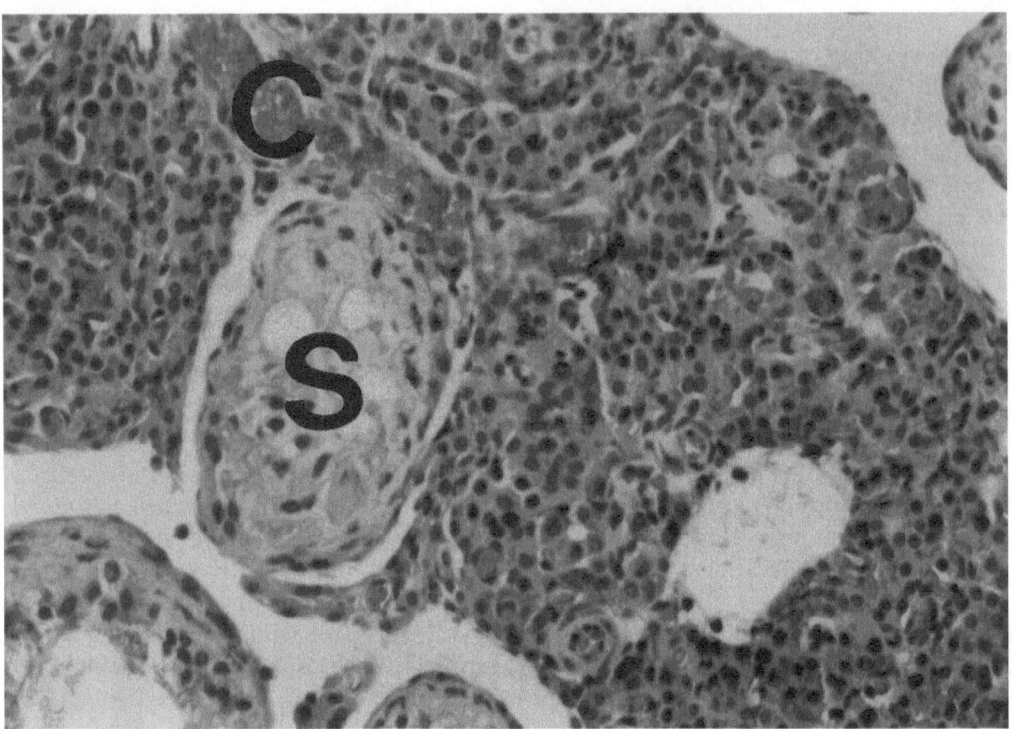

Fig. 19.1. Photomicrograph of an abdominal, intratesticular, islet graft in a BB/Wor dp rat 160 days following transplantation. A large mass of islet cells surround an atrophic seminiferous tubule (S). Note the capillary (C) within the islet tissue. There is no evidence of an inflammatory reaction or of fibrosis of the graft. Hematoxylin and eosin; x 250.

tosterone was not measured. They concluded, nonetheless, that the mechanism of testicular immune privilege involves an inhibition of the immune response by high local levels of testosterone.

Prolonged abdominal, intratesticular islet allograft survival made possible a study of the effects of local factors on immune responses in the testis. It was particularly helpful that these studies could be conducted in the absence of immunosuppressive drugs. Thus, we examined islet allograft survival in testes in which each of the cell components had been selectively destroyed. In the first group of rats, graft survival was assessed in testes in which Leydig cell function had been destroyed.[33] This was accomplished by means of administration of a GnRH agonist, leuprolide, known to cause severe depression of testosterone biosynthesis.

Male, diabetic S-D rats were pretreated with leuprolide and then transplanted with islets isolated from W-L rats. Grafted rats were not immunosuppressed. Continuous treatment of host rats with leuprolide assured prolonged inhibition of Leydig cell function. The fate of grafted islets was followed for 12 months postoperatively.

The results showed that leuprolide suppressed serum testosterone to below detectable levels and testicular testosterone concentrations to castrate levels. Despite extremely low levels of testosterone, intratesticular islet grafts remained viable without loss of function. In a follow-up study, similar experiments were done with a substantially more potent drug, ethanedimethylsulfonate, known to completely eliminate all Leydig cell function.[34] The outcome of these experiments was the same as described above and confirmed the ob-

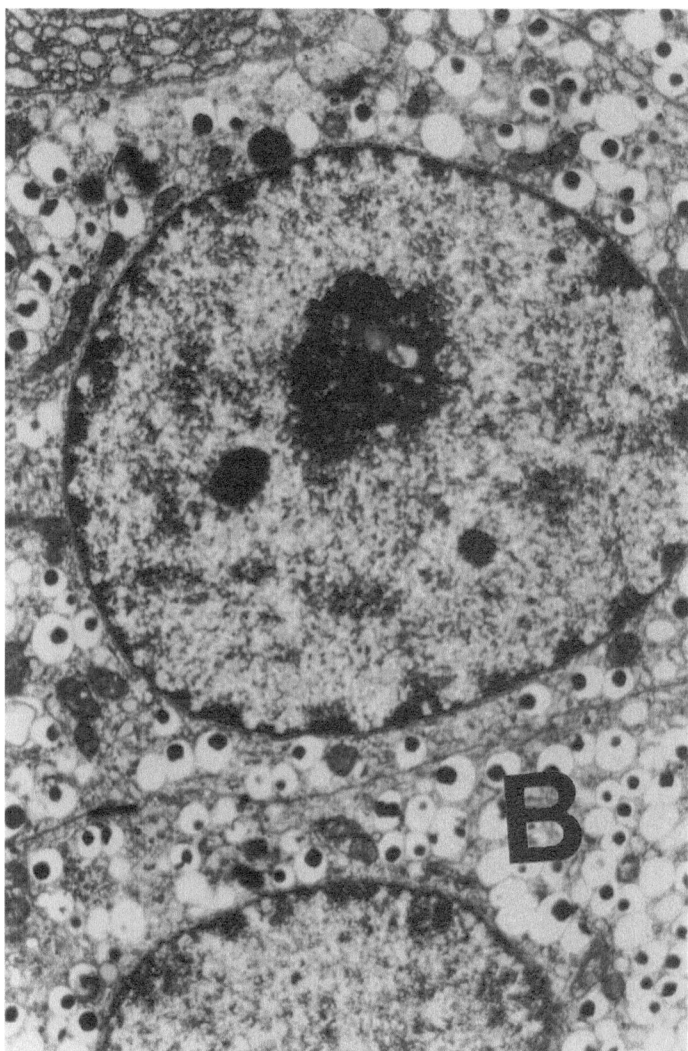

Fig. 19.2. This electron micrograph of a β-cell of an islet implanted into the abdominal testis of a BB/Wor dp rat contains many structurally normal insulin secretory granules (B) (x 30,400).

servation that abdominal testes provided immunoprotection of islet allografts by factors other than androgen hormone production.

The testis consists of three major cell components, germ, Leydig and Sertoli cells. Leydig cell function was felt not to be needed for protection of islet allografts against rejection.[33,34] It was not probable that germ cells were involved either because they are readily depleted in the abdominal testis and because allografts displayed prolonged survival within the testis subjected to experimental cryptorchidism.[23] By elimination of other cell types, the Sertoli cell became the most likely cell type involved in providing the testis with its unique immunological environment.

The Sertoli cell is the epithelial cell within the seminiferous tubule responsible for synthesis of factors required for differentiation of sperm cells. Unlike germ cells, Sertoli cells tolerate central body temperature quite well and can be cultured in vitro at 37°C without loss of their specialized secretory functions.[35] In order to evaluate the effect of Sertoli cell factors on T-lymphocyte proliferation, we initiated a series of experiments on cultured Sertoli cells.[36] The cells were isolated from testes of

Fig. 19.3. Electron micrograph of an alpha (A) [glucagon-producing] and delta (D) [somatostatin-producing] cell within islet shown in Figure 19.1. This electron micrograph shows that all three types of cells were preserved within the grafted intratesticular islet (x 2000).

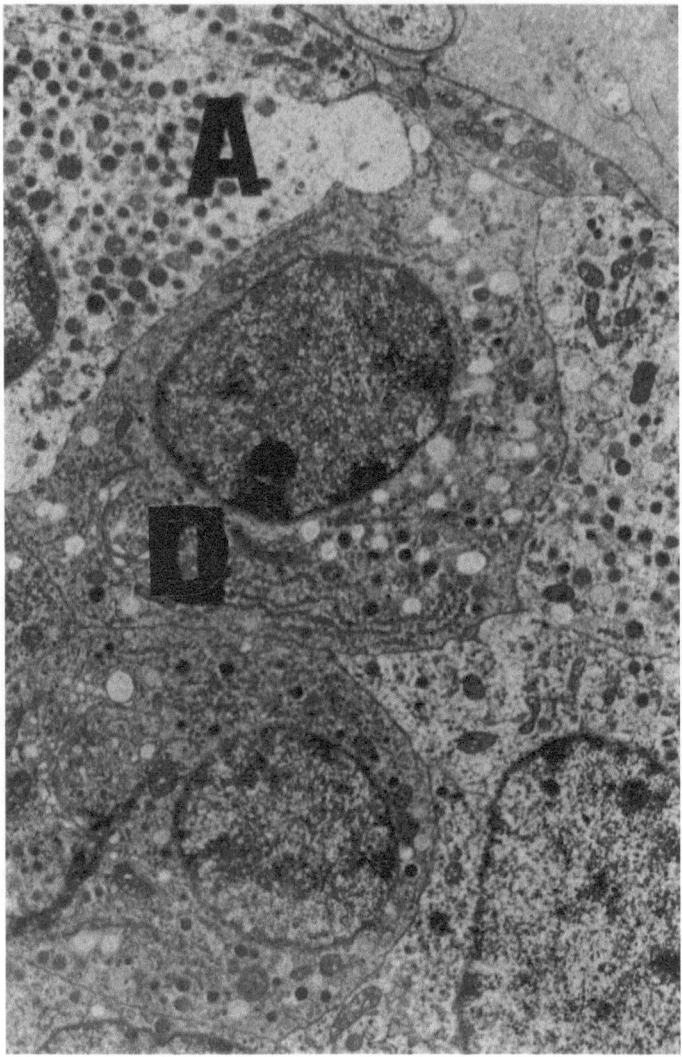

immature rats and cultured under a variety of conditions, including changes in temperature and exposure to hormones such as FSH and testosterone, known to influence their function. The effect of Sertoli-cell conditioned media on proliferation of activated T-lymphocytes was then determined.

The initial series of experiments demonstrated that Sertoli-cell enriched media inhibit lectin-induced proliferation in vitro in a dose-dependent manner. In addition, significant suppression of lymphocyte proliferation occurred only if the Sertoli-cell-enriched media was added within the

first 15 hours after initiation of culture (Fig. 19.4).

One of the most impressive findings was how temperature-dependent the phenomenon was. Thus, media collected from cells maintained at 37°C was significantly more suppressive than media collected from cells cultured at 32°C. The in vitro findings mimicked our in vivo observations exactly: Grafted islets were well preserved in the testis at 37°C while they were apparently not protected in the testis at a lower temperature. It was thus tempting to propose that inhibitory factor(s) produced by Sertoli cells may be responsible

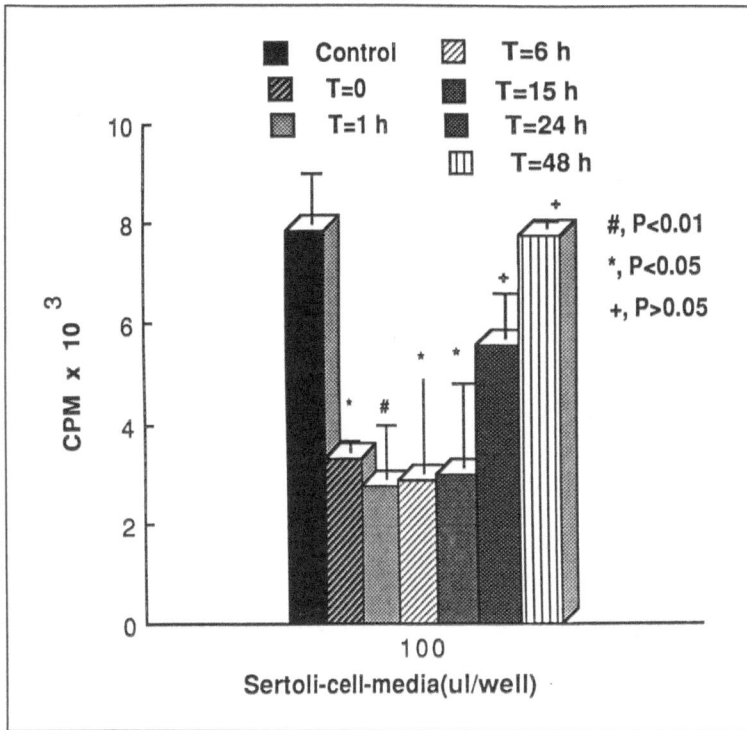

Fig. 19.4. Effects of timing of addition of Sertoli-cell-enriched media (SSC) on lymphocyte proliferation. The black bar to the left shows lymphocyte proliferation in the presence of media alone. The shaded bars from left to right show lymphocyte proliferation in the presence of 100 μl/well of SSC added at 0, 1, 6, 15, 24 and 48 h, respectively, after initiation of lymphocyte cultures. Significant suppression of lymphocyte proliferation occurred when SSC was added within 15 h of initiation of culture. SSC added between 24 and 48 h did not significantly suppress lymphocyte proliferation. Values are expressed as mean ± SE.

for protection of islet grafts from rejection at 37°C. We further observed that even presensitized lymphocytes, which are able to penetrate within the testis, are unable to initiate rejection of islet xenografts.[27]

The production of the inhibitor was also very hormone-dependent. Of various reagents tested, both testosterone and FSH enhanced production, although FSH was clearly the more potent of the two hormones (Fig. 19.5). FSH at low concentrations stimulated synthesis of the factor in serum-free medium in the absence of added testosterone. The lack of responsiveness to testosterone tended to confirm our earlier observations made in vivo that showed that neither induction nor maintenance of extended islet allograft survival required functioning Leydig cells.[33,34]

It is documented that FSH affects Sertoli cell function by binding to specific membrane receptors.[37] Interaction of FSH with Sertoli cells, moreover, is temperature-dependent, with optimal binding at 37°C and a sharp decline occurring at lower temperatures. FSH binding to Sertoli cell membranes results in activation of adenyl cyclase and rapid rise of intracellular cAMP levels. The synthesis of several factors such as inhibin is dependent on this cascade of reactions.[37]

The single most striking finding of the study was that inhibition of T lymphocyte proliferation by Sertoli cell media was caused by an inhibition of production of interleukin-2 (IL-2) (Fig. 19.6). The addition of exogenous IL-2 was not able to reverse this inhibition, suggesting that the inhibitory factor suppressed both IL-2 production and IL-2 responsiveness of T cells. This observation would explain near total absence of an inflammatory reaction in grafted testes. Allograft rejection is a T cell dependent response activated by donor histocompatibility molecules. T cell activation leads to production of the lymphokine IL-2. Release of IL-2 leads to further recruitment of macrophages and host lymphocytes that mediate graft destruction. mAbs directed against IL-2 receptor (IL-2R) were shown to be capable of delaying or preventing rejection of kidney

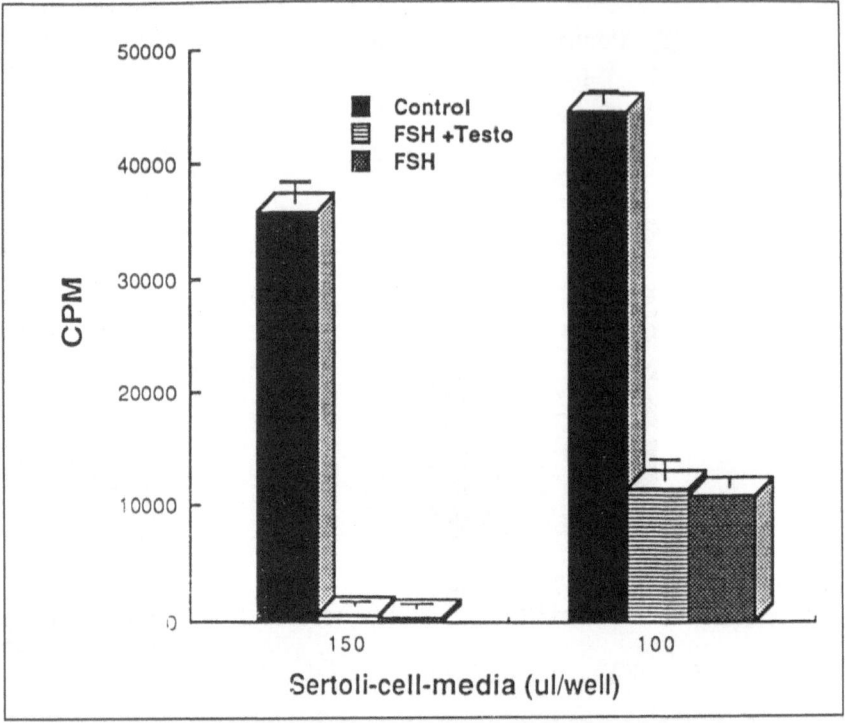

Fig. 19.5. Hormone dependence of production of the inhibitory factor(s) by Sertoli cells. Con-A-stimulated proliferation of splenocytes cultured in the presence of either 150 μl or 100 μl of SSC. The media were harvested from Sertoli cells cultured at 37°C in the presence of Ham-F_{12D}MEM, without additives (control, black bars) and in the presence of Ham-F_{12D}MEM supplemented with either testosterone (3 μg/dl) and FSH (10 μg/dl)[middle, hatched bar] or with only FSH(10 μg/dl)[right hatched bar]. The values are plotted as mean ± SE.

allografts in humans, monkeys and rodents.[38] In addition, following treatment with anti IL-2R antibody, immunologic tolerance was often noted.[38]

It was therefore postulated that extended islet allo- and xenograft survival could be attributed, in part, to production of an inhibitor by Sertoli cells which acted like a natural mAb to IL-2R. This conjecture is in accord with the findings of others who showed that Sertoli cells produced factors which were capable of suppressing phytolectin-stimulated proliferation of spleen lymphocytes. In a more recent report by an Italian group, it was noted that the inhibitory factor was specific for both B- and T cells but not for other lymphoid cells.[40] Furthermore, factors produced by immature rat Sertoli cells were shown to

suppress, in a dose-dependent manner, NK cell activity of mice, guinea pig and humans.[41]

INTRATESTICULAR ISLET ALLOGRAFT SURVIVAL IN PRIMATES

Past experience has demonstrated that successful grafting of islets is much easier to achieve in rats than in higher animals. Yet, application of a particular technique in higher animals is essential before clinical trials should be attempted. The objective of our next study was therefore to investigate the survival of islet allografts in the testis of the male Rhesus monkey, *Macaca mulatta*.[42] Six male monkeys were made diabetic by means of a 97% pancreatectomy and a single i.v. injection of

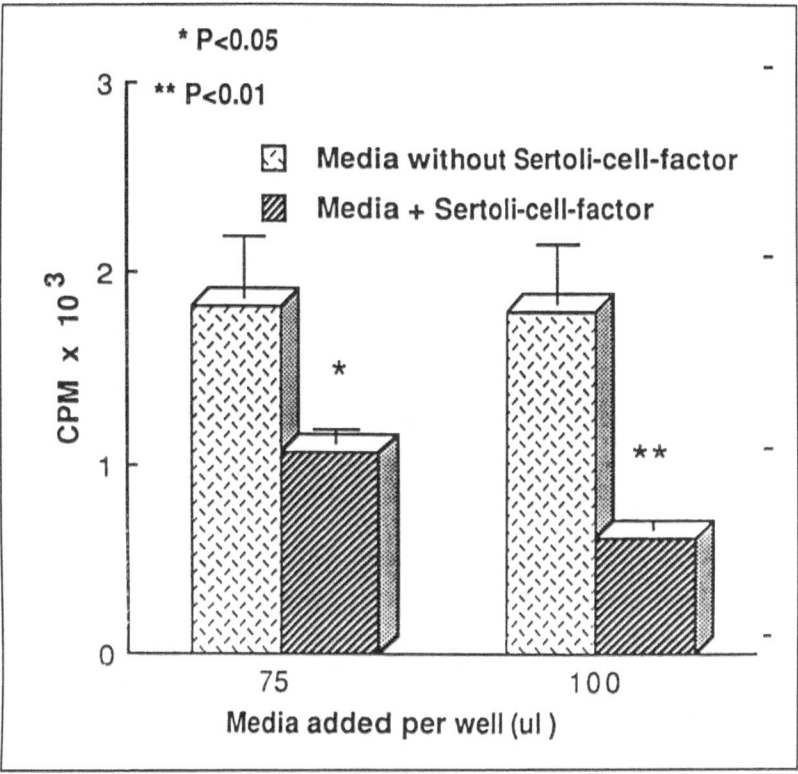

Fig. 19.6. Effect of Sertoli-cell-enriched media (SSC) on IL-2 production. Rat splenocytes were stimulated with 2 µg/ml of Con A in the presence and absence of SSC. At 24 hours, aliquots of culture supernatants were removed and assayed for IL-2 activity in a bioassay using CTLL. CTLL cells are known to proliferate in response to IL-2 but not to Con A. IL-2 activity is presented as cpm ^{3}H-thymidine uptake by CTLL cells exposed to media only (controls, shaded bars on left) and to variable concentrations of SSC (shaded bars on right). The values are expressed as mean ± SE.

30 mg/kg of streptozotocin administered immediately postoperatively. They became severely diabetic and ketoacidotic within 48 hours, and required insulin injections to survive. Islets were isolated from female donor monkeys and then incubated for 4 days at 37°C. No further purification of islets was attempted. Each of six diabetic male monkeys was given a total of approximately 10,000 islets per kg body weight injected slowly into both testes. The grafted organs were immediately anchored underneath the skin in the inguinal canal to expose them to a core body temperature of 37°C. Immunosuppression of the grafted primates consisted of a total of seven intramuscular (i.m.) injections of CsA, 20 mg/kg, on days -3 to +3 relative to the graft. Oral sustacal tolerance tests

were done prior to pancreatectomy, following pancreatectomy but before grafting, and at regular intervals posttransplantation.

Of the six grafted primates, three became normoglycemic within a week following transplantation. One of the grafted animals stayed normoglycemic for 8 months and then reverted to hyperglycemia. Two of the three monkeys have been normoglycemic now for periods exceeding 3 years. The mean ± SE fasting serum glucose level prior to pancreatectomy in the six animals was 45 ± 5 mg/dl. Following pancreatectomy, the level increased to a mean of 443 ± 30 mg/dl. In the successfully transplanted monkeys, the fasting serum glucose levels at 3 years posttransplantation have not changed and vary between 45 and 65 mg/dl. Prior to transplantation during their diabetic phase, serum C-peptide levels were less than 2.0 ng/ml. The C-peptide levels then increased to a mean of 5.5 ± 0.3 ng/ml for 3 years following transplantation.

The outcome of the primate studies was particularly important because it emphasized that the testicular environment is unusually conducive for extended survival of islet allografts, in contrast to other sites such as the liver.[7] While prevention of rejection is critical for an allograft to become established, preservation of the functional capacity of a highly specialized cell such as the insulin-producing beta cell is also extremely important. In this respect, the Sertoli cells may also play a primary role. These cells are responsible for the synthesis of potent growth-promoting factors and substances which may enhance angiogenesis.[43] The secretory products may play an important role in beta cell function. Furthermore, intratesticular concentration of immunosuppressive drugs such as CsA is much lower when compared with levels in the liver or kidney following administration of an identical i.v. dose.[44] CsA has been shown to impair beta cell function.[8,9] It has been suggested that release of insulin into the portal venous system is more physiologic than release of the hormone into the systemic circulation.[7] Prolonged secretion of insulin into the systemic circulation is believed to lead to a state of sustained hyperinsulinism, glucose intolerance and abnormal lipid metabolism. Remarkably, defective glucose and lipid metabolism have not become evident in the transplanted monkeys even with release of insulin for a period of 3 years into the systemic circulation.

DEVELOPMENT OF AN ECTOPIC IMMUNOLOGICALLY PRIVILEGED SITE WITH SERTOLI CELLS

Despite excellent results achieved with abdominal intratesticular islet allografts in both rodents and primates, there were some concerns expressed regarding this approach. Foremost, we had to consider the possibil-

ity that germ cells in the abdominal testis may undergo malignant transformation at 37°C.[45] Second, only males have Sertoli cells and our transplantation approach could not be used in half of the population which is female. These concerns prompted attempts at the development of a heterologous immunologically privileged site in vivo other than the testis. Our approach was based on the assumption that Sertoli cells would retain their function at an ectopic site, such as underneath the renal capsule, as they do in vitro.

Sertoli cells were isolated from two different strains of young male rats, PVG and S-D.[46] Islets were prepared from adult S-D rats. Islets and Sertoli cells were then grafted simultaneously into the renal subcapsular space of several groups of male and female diabetic PVG rats. Immunosuppression of the hosts was of short duration and consisted of a total of three injections of 25 mg/kg CsA on days 0, +1 and +2 relative to the graft. We demonstrated that 75% of either male or female recipients of a combination of islets and Sertoli cells grafted into the renal, subcapsular space became normoglycemic for periods exceeding 200 days. Moreover, normoglycemic female rats were able to conceive, carry pregnancies to full term and nurse their pups successfully. Control rats, on the other hand, who were grafted either with islets alone, or with Sertoli cells alone, remained hyperglycemic.

Examination of the grafts by light and electron microscopy revealed some interesting findings (Figs. 19.7, 19.8, 19.9). Large masses of well-granulated and viable beta cells were found directly underneath the kidney capsule. Most significantly, even though the kidney is not an immunologically-privileged site, there was no evidence of an inflammatory reaction within or surrounding the grafted islets. Instead, there was a high density of cells between and directly adjacent to the transplanted islets and kidney parenchyma. By light microscopy, they did not appear to be islet cells, kidney cells, nor cells of blood origin. When observed by electron microscopy, the

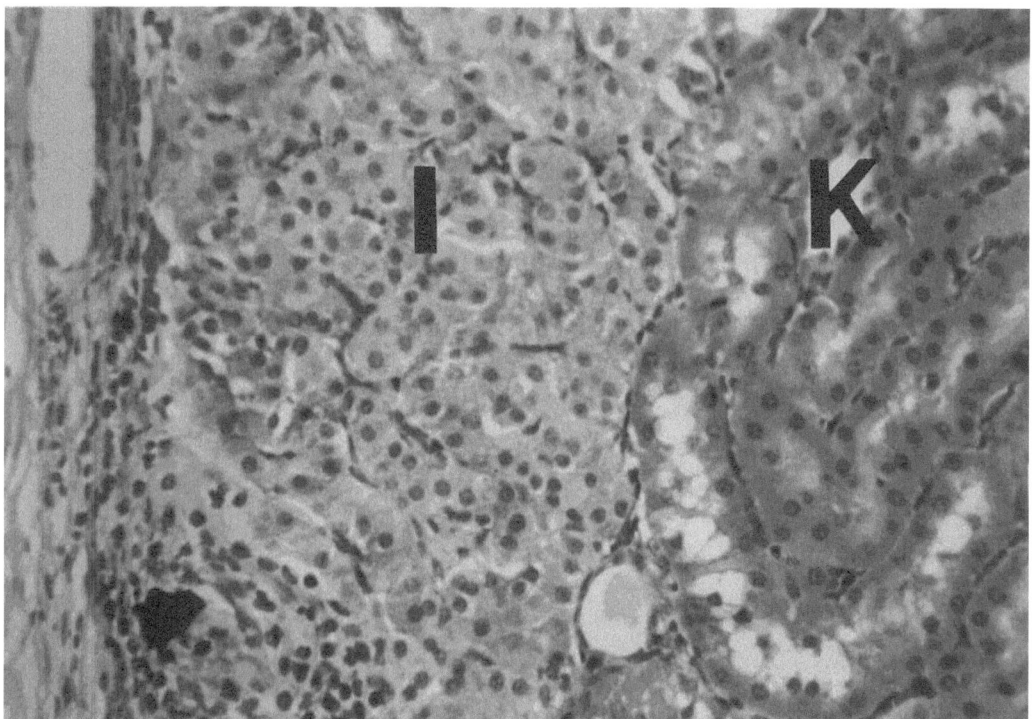

Fig. 19.7. Pancreatic islet allograft along with Sertoli cells was transplanted underneath the kidney capsule of a diabetic rat. As illustrated in this photomicrograph, the islet (I) appears structurally normal. The kidney parenchyma (K) also appears normal. Tissue was stained with toluidine blue (x 430).

cells were similar in ultrastructure to Sertoli cells in that their nuclei were irregular in profile and contained deep nuclear clefts, distinctive nucleoli were often present and mitochondrial structure was dense. Although these cells did not retain the typical polarity of Sertoli cells in vivo, they were, however, identical in appearance to Sertoli cells in vitro when the cells are not plated on a basement membrane. The cells were not associated with a basement membrane and appeared randomly organized. Cells showing ultrastructural features of either germ or Leydig cells were not observed.

Several conclusions were drawn from these results. First, Sertoli cells retained their specialized functions and apparently had the capacity to secrete immunosuppressive factor(s) in an organ other than the testis. Second, the renal subcapsular space in the rat provided an environment which allowed both islet and Sertoli cells to sur-

vive and to function for extended periods of time. Third, Sertoli cell secretions did not have an androgenic effect in female rats and did not affect ovulation adversely. Fourth, continuous functional survival of islet allografts long after immunosuppression was stopped suggested development of immunologic tolerance.

EFFECT OF TESTIS ENVIRONMENT ON GRAFTED ISLET FUNCTION

Successfully transplanted BB/Wor dp rats provided a unique opportunity to investigate several critical questions related to glucose metabolism and effects of long-term normoglycemia on development of diabetic complications. For the first time, to our knowledge, these questions could be addressed in grafted rats that were not on maintenance immunosuppression.

The goal of the first series of experiments was to examine the effect of known

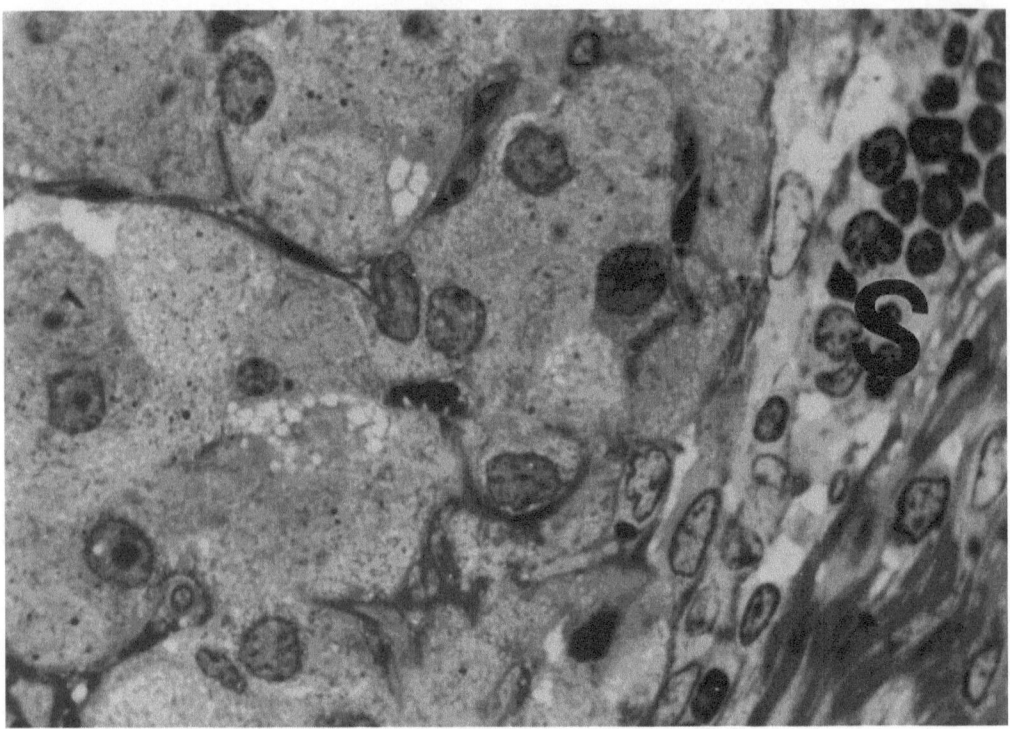

Fig. 19.8. This electron micrograph illustrates a high density of cells (S) between the renal and islet tissue shown in Figure 19.7. These cells do not appear to be of islet, renal or blood origin (x 2,000).

insulin secretagogues on insulin secretory patterns in BB/Wor dp rats with intratesticular islet allografts.[47] Oral glucose tolerance tests were done in control, BB/wor dr rats (resistant to development of diabetes) and in transplant-improved BB/wor dp rats who were normoglycemic for longer than 100 days. We found that the pattern of insulin release was identical to that in the control group, with a peak at 15 minutes and a rapid decline to basal levels at 30 minutes. Furthermore, liver enzymes associated with glycogenesis and glycogenolysis, glycogen synthase and glycogen phosphorylase, respectively, were restored to normal levels in rats with intratesticular islet grafts.[48] Microscopic and biochemical analyses of the grafted testes showed that the grafts contained not only beta cells, but also considerable amounts of glucagon and numbers of alpha cells.[49] Of three islet cell secretagogues tested, glucose by mouth was the most potent insulin-releasing agent.

Glipizide, given by mouth, had a minor effect on insulin secretion, but produced a significant suppression of glucagon. An i.v. infusion of arginine was the most potent glucagon releasing agent, while exerting only a minor effect on insulin secretion.

It was concluded from these studies that both beta and alpha cells were preserved in the abdominal testes following transplantation of islet preparations. Insulin secretory patterns were similar to those of control, never-grafted rats. Beta and alpha cells contained within the testis had the capacity to respond to insulin and glucagon secretagogues in a distinct and independent manner. Finally, there was no evidence of either graft failure or of development of glucose intolerance due to systemic delivery of insulin. The abdominal, intratesticular islet graft model also made possible an investigation of the impact of islet transplantation on secondary complications associated with diabetes. Our ob-

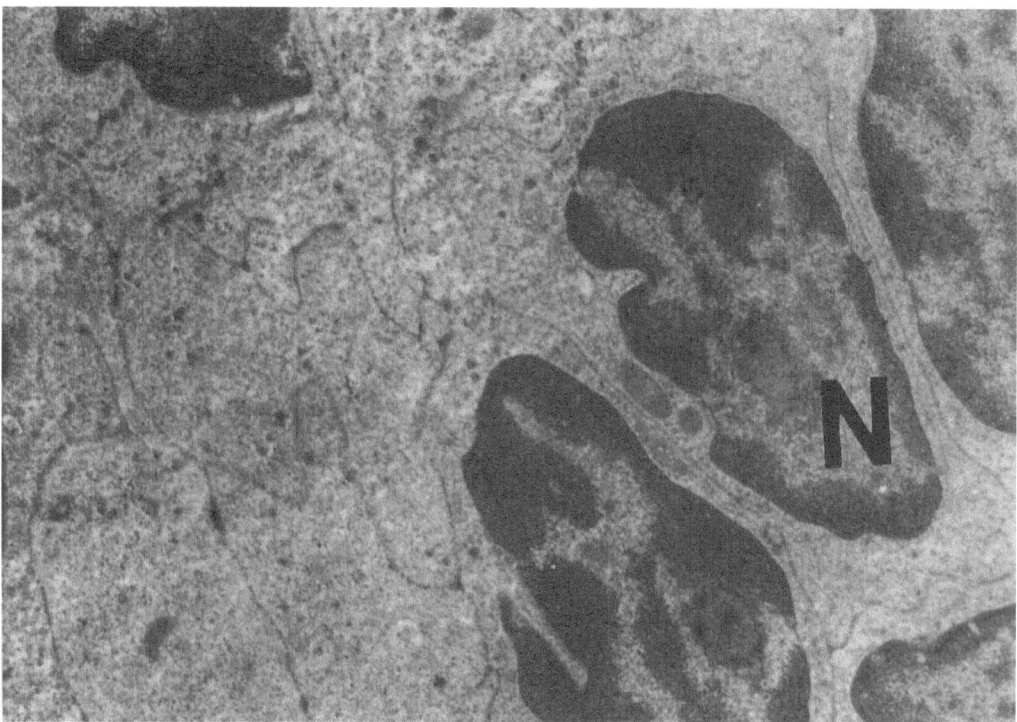

Fig. 19.9. This electron micrograph shows, at higher magnification, the fine structure of the extra-islet cells labeled "S" in Figure 19.8. Both the cell nucleus (N) and cytoplasm are similar in appearance to Sertoli cells in vivo, and are structurally identical to Sertoli cells in vitro (x 6,446).

jectives were to investigate the effects of abdominal, intratesticular allografts in BB/Wor dp rats on prevention of kidney disease and neuropathy.[50] BB/Wor dp rats were transplanted within a week following the onset of hyperglycemia without immunosuppression or any other therapy. At intervals following transplantation, urine total protein was quantitated and sural nerve morphometry and sexual function assessed. Nine of 16 rats were grafted successfully for a period of at least 6 months. Mean ± SE pretransplant glucose concentration was 394 ± 83 mg/dl and posttransplant glucose concentration was 115 ± 13 mg/dl. In the successfully grafted rats, glycosylated hemoglobin levels were not different from controls. Total urinary protein was significantly (P < 0.01) less than that in untreated diabetic rats (5.7 ± 2 versus 16.6 ± 3.7 mg/24 hours) and not different from controls. Penile reflexes and serum testosterone levels remained normal in islet-

transplanted rats. Sural nerve morphometry had 29.2% fewer abnormalities (paranodal swelling, paranodal demyelination, myelin wrinkling, Wallerian degeneration) than in untreated diabetic BB/Wor dp rats.

Previous studies in experimental diabetes have shown that proteinuria can be prevented or reversed by pancreatic islet transplantation.[51] To our knowledge, this was the first report that islet cell transplantation can prevent increased proteinuria in the BB/Wor dp rat. In addition, the improvement in metabolic control at 6 months was associated with normal total urinary protein, sural nerve morphometry and sexual function.

CONCLUSION

To date, the most promising immunologically-privileged site for islet transplantation for the cure of type I diabetes mellitus in experimental animals is the intraabdominal testis. Transplantation to the inguinal testis was performed in monkeys. Immunoprotection is provided by a substance or substances secreted by Sertoli cells. This substance is also operative when islet allografts are transplanted underneath the renal capsule of rats in the presence of Sertoli cells. This might well clear the way for initial clinical trials.

Much additional work needs to be done, including isolation and identification of immunosuppressive factor(s) secreted by Sertoli cells and identification of their physiologic and immunologic effects on transplants of islets and other tissues. Allotransplants of islets plus Sertoli cells under the renal capsule should be advanced to larger animals, preferably primates, and, if successful, could then be studied in clinical trials.

REFERENCES

1. Lacy PE, Davie JM, Finke EH. Prolongation of islet allograft survival following in vitro culture [24°C] and a single injection of ALS. Science 1979; 204:312.

2. Faustman D, Hauptfeld V, Lacy P et al. Demonstration of active tolerance in maintenance of established Islet of Langerhans allografts. Proc Natl Acad Sc USA 1982; 79:4153.

3. Selawry HP, Whittington K. Extended allograft survival of islets grafted into intra-abdominally placed testis. Diabetes 1984; 33:405.

4. Tze WJ, Tai J. Successful intracerebral allotransplantation of pancreatic endocrine cells in spontaneous diabetic BB rats without immunosuppression. Metabolism 1984; 33:785.

5. Sullivan FP, Ricordi C, Hauptfeld V et al. Effect of low-temperature culture and site of transplantation on hamster islet xenograft survival (hamster to mouse). Transplantation 1987;44:465.

6. Eloy R, Haffen K, Kedinger M. Chick embryo pancreatic transplants reverse experimental diabetes of rats. J Clin Invest 1979; 64:361.

7. Alejandro R, Cutfield RG, Shienvold FL et al. Natural history of intrahepatic canine islet cell autografts. J Clin Invest 1986; 78:1339.

8. Scharp D, Alderson D, Kneteman NM. The effects of immunosuppression on islet transplant function in dogs. Transplant Proc 1987; 19:952.

9. Rooth P, Dawidson I, Lafferty K et al. Prevention of detrimental effect of cyclosporine A on vascular ingrowth of transplanted pancreatic islets with verapamil. Diabetes 1989; 38(suppl 1):202.

10. Mehigan DG, Ball WR, Zudema GD et al. Disseminated intravascular coagulation and portal hypertension following pancreatic islet autotransplantation. Ann Surg 1980; 191:287.

11. Lafferty KJ, Prowse SJ, Simeonovic CJ et al. Immunobiology of tissue transplantation: a return to the passenger leukocyte concept. Ann Rev Immunol 1983; 1:143.

12. Hiller WF, Klempnauer J, Luck R et al. Progressive deterioration of endocrine function after intraportal but not kidney subcapsular rat islet transplanattion. Diabetes 1991; 40:134.

13. Cattral MS, Warnock GL, Evans MG et al. Transplantation of purified frozen/thawed canine pancreatic islet allografts with cyclosporine. Transplantation 1991; 52:457.

14. Gruber SA. The case for local immunosuppression. Transplantation 1992; 54:1.

15. Barker CF, Billingham RE. Immunologically privileged sites. Adv Immunol 1977; 25:1.

16. Greene HSN. Familial mammary tumors in the rabbit. IV. The evolution of autonomy in the course of tumor development as indicated by transplantation experiments. J Exp Med 1940; 71:305.

17. Selawry HP, Whittington K. Extended allograft survival of islets grafted into intra-abdominally placed testis. Diabetes 1984; 33:405.

18. Naji A, Silvers WK, Bellgrau D et al. Spontaneous diabetes in rats: destruction of islets prevented by immunological tolerance. Science 1981; 213:1390.

19. Selawry H, Fajaco R, Whittington K. Intratesticular islet allografts in the spontaneously diabetic BB/W rat. Diabetes 1985; 34:1019.

20. Bellgrau D, Naji A, Silvers WK et al. Spontaneous diabetes in BB rats: evidence for T-

cell-dependent immune response defect. Diabetologia 1982; 23:359.

21. Guttmann RD, Colle E, Michel F et al. Spontaneous diabetes mellitus syndrome in the rat. 11. T-lymphopenia and its association with clinical disease and pancreatic lymphocytic infiltration. J Immunol 1983; 130:1732.

22. Selawry H, Fajaco R, Whittington K. Extended survival of incubated MHC-compatible islet isografts in the spontaneously diabetc BB/W rat. Diabetes 1987; 36:1061.

23. Selawry HP, Whittington K, Bellgrau D. Abdominal, intratesticular islet-xenograft survival in rats. Diabetes 1989; 38(suppl 1):220.

24. Kupiec-Weglinski JW, Filho MA, Strom TB et al. Sparing of suppressor cells: a critical action of cyclosporine. Transplantation 1984; 38:97.

25. Beschorner WE, Namnoum JD, Hess AD. Immunopathology of rat thymus after cyclosporine A. Transplant Today 1986; 19:1230.

26. Georgiou HM, Lagarde AC, Bellgrau D. T cell dysfunction in the diabetes prone BB rat: a role for thymic migrants that are not T cell precursors. J Exp Med 1988; 167:132.

27. Bellgrau D, Selawry H. Cyclosporine-induced tolerance to intratesticular islet xenografts. Transplantation 1990; 50:654.

28. Pelletier RM, Byers SW. The blood-testis barrier and Sertoli cell junctions: Structural considerations. Micros Res Tech 1992; 20:3.

29. Head JR, Neaves WB, Billingham RE. Reconsideration of the lymphatic drainage of the rat testis. Transplantation 1983; 35:91.

30. Head JR, Neaves WB, Billingham RE. Immune privilege in the testis. I basic parameters of allograft survival. Transplantation 1983; 36:423.

31. Ferguson J, Scothorne RJ. Further studies on the transplantation of isolated pancreatic islets. J Anat 1977; 124:9.

32. Head JR, Billingham RE. Immune privilege in the testis. II. Evaluation of potential local factors. Transplantation 1985; 40:269.

33. Selawry H, Whittington K. Prolonged intratesticular allograft survival is not dependent on local steroidogenesis. Horm Metab Res 1988; 20:562.

34. Cameron DF, Whittington K, Schultz, RE et al. Successful islet/abdominal testis transplantation does not require Leydig cells. Transplantation 1990; 50:649.

35. Russell LD, Steinberger A. Sertoli cells in culture:Views from the perspectives of an in Vivoist and an in Vitroist. Biol Reprod 1989; 41:571.

36. Selawry HP, Kotb M, Herrod HG et al. Production of factor, or factors, suppressing IL-2 production and T cell proliferation by Sertoli cell-enriched preparations. Transplantation 1991; 52:846.

37. Means AR. Early effects of FSH upon testicular metabolism. Adv Exp Med Biol 1973; 36:431.

38. Bacha P, Williams DP, Waters C et al. Interleukin 2 receptor-targeted cytotoxicity. Interleukin 2 receptor-mediated action of diptheria toxin-related interleukin 2 fusion protein. J Exp Med 1988; 167:612.

39. Wyatt CR, Law L, Magnuson JA et al. Suppression of lymphocyte proliferation by proteins secreted by cultured Sertoli cells. J Reprod Immunol 1988; 14:27.

40. DeCesaris P, Filippini A, Cervelli C et al. Immunosuppressive molecules produced by Sertoli cells cultured in vitro: Biological effects on lymphocytes. Biochem Biophys Res Commun 1992; 186:1639.

41. Nikolova DB, Kancheva LS, Surneva MD et al. Species-specific effect of proteins secreted by cultured pre-pubertal rat Sertoli cells on natural killer cell activity. Immunopharm 1992; 23:15.

42. Selawry HP, Gaber O, Whittington K et al. Intratesticular islet allograft survival in the Rhesus monkey. Diabetes 1992; 41:155A.

43. Skalli M, Avallet O, Vigier M et al. Opposite vectorial secretion of Insulin-like Growth Factor I and its binding proteins by pig Sertoli cells cultured in the bicameral chamber system. Endocrinol 1992; 131:985.

44. Selawry HP, Whittington K, Forster H. Intratesticular islet xenograft survival in relation to tissue cyclosporine levels. Am J Med Sci 1988; 31:497.

45. Martin DC. Malignancy in the cryptorchid testis. Urol Clin N Am 1982; 9:371.

46. Selawry HP, Cameron DF. Sertoli cell-enriched fractions in successful islet transplantation. Cell Transplantation 1993; 2:123.

47. Selawry H, Whittington K, Forster H. Effects of islet grafts of MHC-compatible donors on glucose metabolism in the spontaneously diabetic BB/Wor rat. Diabetes Res Clin Pract 1988; 5:295.

48. Margolis RN, Holup JJ, Selawry HP. Effects of intratesticular islet transplantation on hepatic glycogen metabolism in the rat. Diab Res Clin Practice 1986; 2:291.

49. Whittington KP, Solomon SS, Selawry HP. Islet allografts in the cryptorchid testes of spontaneously diabetic BB/Wor dp rats: Response to glucose, glipizide, and arginine. Endocrinol 1991; 128:2671.

50. Murray FT, Beyer-Mears A, Johnson RD et al. Assessment of proteinuria and neuropathy in the nonimmunosuppressed BB diabetic rat after abdominal intratesticular islet transplantation. Transplantation 1993; 56:680.

51. Selawry HP, Pennel JP, Pardo V et al. The effects of culture-maintained pancreatic islets on metabolic parameters, renal function, and glomerular lesions in the diabetic rat. Metabolism 1980; 29:261.

Section E:
Conclusion

Scott A. Gruber

In light of the recent demonstration that intragraft mechanisms appear to be important in regulating virtually all phases of the rejection response, and that local immunosuppression achieves the goals of preventing rejection with reduced systemic drug exposure and toxicity in rodent and canine models, it is clear that the concept deserves continued exploration and eventual clinical application. Pharmaceutical companies must become interested in the development of immunosuppressant prodrugs that are selectively activated in and then rapidly eliminated by the transplanted organ of interest or the systemic circulation, and in the development of active agents that are pharmacokinetically tailored for pump-based local administration to a given target organ. New methods of local drug delivery, such as nanoparticle and magnetically-localized therapeutic carriers, should be applied to organ transplantation. Finally, research efforts must be continued towards the goal of utilizing gene transfer techniques to obtain stable, long-term local immunosuppression of immediately-vascularized solid-organ transplants in large animals and man.

INDEX

Page numbers in italics denote figures (f) or tables (t).